PERCUTANEOUS LOCAL ANAESTHESIA

ELLIS HORWOOD SERIES IN PHARMACEUTICAL TECHNOLOGY
incorporating Pharmacological Sciences
Series Editor: Michael H Rubinstein, Professor of Pharmaceutical Technology, School of Pharmacy, Liverpool John Moores University

Armstrong & James	UNDERSTANDING EXPERIMENTAL DESIGN AND INTERPRETATION IN PHARMACEUTICS (Available in Cloth and Paperback)
Bloomfield et al	MICROBIAL QUALITY ASSURANCE IN PHARMACEUTICALS, COSMETICS, TOILETRIES
Broadley	AUTONOMIC PHARMACOLOGY
Cartwright & Matthews	PHARMACEUTICAL PRODUCT LICENSING: Requirements for Europe
Cartwright & Matthews	INTERNATIONAL PHARMACEUTICAL PRODUCT REGISTRATION: Quality, Safety, Efficacy
Clark & Moos	DRUG DISCOVERY TECHNOLOGIES
Cole	PHARMACEUTICAL PRODUCTION FACILITIES: Design and Application
Cole, Hogan, Aulton	PHARMACEUTICAL TABLET COATING TECHNOLOGY
Cook	POTASSIUM CHANNELS: Structure, Classification, Function and Therapeutic Potential
Craig & Newton	DIELECTRIC ANALYSIS OF PHARMACEUTICAL SYSTEMS
D'Arcy & McElnay	PHARMACY AND PHARMACOTHERAPY OF ASTHMA
Denyer & Baird	GUIDE TO MICROBIOLOGICAL CONTROL IN PHARMACEUTICS
Doods & Van Meel	RECEPTOR DATA FOR BIOLOGICAL EXPERIMENTS: A Guide to Drug Selectivity
Evans et al	POTASSIUM CHANNEL MODULATOR DRUGS: From Synthesis to Clinical Experience
Field & Goldthorpe	DRUG RESISTANCE IN VIRUSES: Principles, Mechanisms and Clinical Perspectives
Ford & Timmins	PHARMACEUTICAL THERMAL ANALYSIS: Techniques and Applications
Glasby	DICTIONARY OF ANTIBIOTIC-PRODUCING ORGANISMS
Gould	PHYSICOCHEMICAL PROPERTIES OF DRUGS: A Handbook for Pharmaceutical Scientists
Hardy et al	DRUG DELIVERY TO THE GASTROINTESTINAL TRACT
Harvey	DRUGS FROM NATURAL PRODUCTS: Pharmaceuticals and Agrochemicals
Hider & Barlow	POLYPEPTIDE AND PROTEIN DRUGS: Production, Characterization, Formulation
Hutt	DRUG CHIRALITY: Chemistry, Biology, Regulation, Industrial Issues
Ioannides & Lewis	DRUGS, DIET AND DISEASE VOLUME 1 Mechanistic Approaches to Cancer
Izquierdo & Medina	NATURALLY OCCURING BENZODIAZEPINES: Structure, Distribution and Function
Junginger	DRUG TARGETING AND DELIVERY: Concepts in Dosage Form Design
Krogsgaard-Larsen & Hansen	EXCITATORY AMINO ACID RECEPTORS: Design of Agonists and Antagonists
Kourounakis & Rekka	ADVANCED DRUG DESIGN AND DEVELOPMENT
Kourounakis & Rekka	STEROIDS, DRUG RESPONSE AND METABOLISM: Pharmacochemical Approach to Defensive Steroids
Labaune	HANDBOOK OF PHARMACOKINETICS: The Toxicity Asssessment of Chemicals
Law	IMMUNOASSAY PROCEDURES: A Practical Guide
Macheras, Reppas & Dressman	BIOPHARMACEUTICS OF ORALLY-ADMINISTERED DRUGS
Martinez	PEPTIDE HORMONES AS PROHORMONES
Rainsford	ANTI-RHEUMATIC DRUGS: Actions and Side Effects
Ramabhadran	PHARMACEUTICAL DESIGN AND DEVELOPMENT: A Molecular Biological Approach
Ridgway Watt	TABLET MACHINE INSTRUMENTATION IN PHARMACEUTICS: Principles and Practice
Roth et al	PHARMACEUTICAL CHEMISTRY Volume 1 Drug Synthesis
Roth et al	PHARMACEUTICAL CHEMISTRY Volume 2 Drug Analysis
Rubinstein	PHARMACEUTICAL TECHNOLOGY Controlled Drug Release Volume 1
Rubinstein	PHARMACEUTICAL TECHNOLOGY Tableting Technology Volume 1
Rubinstein	PHARMACEUTICAL TECHNOLOGY Drug Stability
Russell & Chopra	UNDERSTANDING ANTIBACTERIAL ACTION AND RESISTANCE (Cloth & Paper)
Rutherford	PHARMACEUTICAL SPECIFICATIONS: Standards for Drugs
Taylor & Kennewell	MODERN MEDICINAL CHEMISTRY (Available in Cloth and Paperback)
Theobald	RADIOPHARMACEUTICALS: Using Radioactive Compounds in Pharmaceutics and Medicine
Thomas & Thurston	CHEMISTRY FOR PHARMACY, PHARMACOLOGY AND THE HEALTH SCIENCES (Available in Cloth and Paperback)
Tweed	CLINICAL TRIALS FOR THE PHARMACEUTICAL INDUSTRY
Van Meel, Hauel, Shelley	CARDIOTONIC AGENTS FOR THE TREATMENT OF HEART FAILURE
Vergnaud	CONTROLLED DRUG RELEASE OF ORAL DOSAGE FORMS
Washington	PARTICLE SIZE ANALYSIS IN PHARMACEUTICS AND OTHER INDUSTRIES
Washington et al	PHARMACOKINETIC MODELLING USING STELLA ON THE APPLE MACINTOSH (TM)
Wells	PHARMACEUTICAL PREFORMULATION
Wells & Rubinstein	PHARMACEUTICAL TECHNOLOGY Controlled Drug Release Volume 2
Wells & Rubinstein	PHARMACEUTICAL TECHNOLOGY Tableting Technology Volume 2
Wilson & Washington	PHYSIOLOGICAL PHARMACEUTICS: Biological Barriers to Drug Absorption

The above is a complete list of all Ellis Horwood titles in the pharmaceutical and pharmacological sciences, both published and in preparation. Further details can be obtained from Simon and Schuster International Group 0442 – 881900.

PERCUTANEOUS LOCAL ANAESTHESIA

DAVID WOOLFSON and DERMOT McCAFFERTY
both of the School of Pharmacy
The Queen's University of Belfast

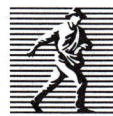

ELLIS HORWOOD
NEW YORK   LONDON   TORONTO   SYDNEY   TOKYO   SINGAPORE

First published in 1993 by
Ellis Horwood Limited
Market Cross House, Cooper Street,
Chichester, West Sussex, PO19 1EB, England
A division of
Simon & Schuster International Group

Printed and bound in Great Britain
by Bookcraft, Midsomer Norton

British Library Cataloguing in Publication Data

A catalogue record for this book is available from the British Library

ISBN 0–13–656372–4

Library of Congress Cataloging-in-Publication Data

Available from the publisher

Table of contents

Preface

Towards the end of 1980, we were approached by a consultant paediatric surgeon in Belfast, Victor Boston, who was concerned at the pain of frequent venepunctures experienced by young oncology patients during the course of their treatment. This 'needle pain' became, for many of these children, the most frightening aspect of their hospital experience. Clearly, a topical local anaesthetic preparation was required which would 'freeze' the skin, producing the kind of profound or stony anaesthesia familiar to any visitor to the dentist's chair. Unfortunately, formulation of a safe, effective and rapidly-acting preparation was not a simple task, since the skin provides an effective barrier to the percutaneous penetration of many topically applied drugs, including local anaesthetics. Indeed, the literature on the subject at that time was far from encouraging. Nevertheless, within a few months, we had produced a crude percutaneous anaesthetic cream containing a high drug content, lacking in pharmaceutical elegance and with poor chemical stability. This preparation did have one advantage, however. It worked! Thus encouraged, we have since spent much of our time on the development of safe, effective and convenient percutaneous anaesthetic preparations, which conform to accepted pharmaceutical and clinical standards. Often, the work has involved sticking needles in ourselves, so we can now claim to have genuine empathy with patients at the sharp end!

As our own work progressed, many other groups began to report effective skin anaesthesia achieved by topical application of local anaesthetics. In common with these groups, our experience of the clinical use of percutaneous local anaesthesia was that a short learning curve was necessary for most clinical staff, after which the technique was accepted with enthusiasm. Patients, of course, had no reservations about any method of pain prevention. In Belfast hospitals, the percutaneous anaesthetic rapidly became known as 'magic cream' by the children. Tubes of the preparation began to 'disappear' from the paediatric wards, miraculously turning up later on adult wards, sometimes in different hospitals. The popularity of this new method of pain prevention with both patients and staff has now been confirmed by the subsequent successful launch of the first commercially available percutaneous local anaesthetic preparation.

We are still some way, perhaps, from having the 'ideal' percutaneous local anaesthetic preparation, particularly one with a more rapid onset of action. In writing this book, we have attempted to draw together the current state of knowledge on all aspects of percutaneous local anaesthesia. We hope this will stimulate continued research on the topic and bring the clinical benefits of percutaneous local anaesthesia to the attention of a wider audience. This book, therefore, deals with many diverse scientific and clinical disciplines, all of which are directly relevant to percutaneous anaesthesia. Inevitably, in our attempt to cover the subject in a single, wide-ranging volume, we will have treated some areas in too much or too little detail for a particular, specialist reader. Nevertheless, we hope that all readers of this book concerned with the professional and scientific aspects of percutaneous local anaesthesia, including surgeons, anaesthetists, paediatricians, nursing staff, pharmacists and pharmaceutical scientists, will find it a useful source book on the subject.

During the course of our work on percutaneous local anaesthesia, we have been helped by many colleagues. In particular, we must acknowledge, once again, our debt to Mr Victor Boston of the Northern Ireland Paediatric Surgical Service, not only for bringing the subject to our attention, but also for all his advice and expertise in the clinical evaluation of candidate formulations. Similarly, Mr Roy Millar of the Burns Unit, Royal Victoria Hospital, Belfast and Mr James Small, of the Plastic Surgery Department at the Ulster Hospital, Belfast, did much to demonstrate the advantages of percutaneous local anaesthesia for the harvesting of split skin grafts. We must also acknowledge the enthusiastic support of the nursing staff at the Royal Belfast Hospital for Sick Children, particularly Sister Barbara Moneypenny, and the Belfast City Hospital, particularly Sister Leila Gibson. As academics, it was inevitable that our research and undergraduate students would be dragooned into playing their part. We gratefully acknowledge their collective contributions to the work and also the donation of their numerous arms for the inevitable needle challenge! In the latter part of the work, we also received much support and encouragement from colleagues at Smith and Nephew Pharmaceuticals Ltd, particularly Dr Michael Geraint, Group Medical Advisor.

In the production of this book, we are grateful to all those authors and publishers who kindly permitted us to reproduce their copyright material. We must give special thanks to Alan Robinson for carefully proof-reading the manuscript and computer typesetting the text. Finally, we would like to express our thanks to our families for their patience and understanding during the preparation of this book.

David Woolfson and Dermot McCafferty
School of Pharmacy
The Queen's University of Belfast

1

The need for effective percutaneous local anaesthesia

Any reader of this book who has ever had the experience of taking a young child to be immunised, or, worse still, for hospital treatment involving venepuncture or catheterisation, will need no convincing as to the need for effective percutaneous local anaesthesia. Although most adults will adopt a "grin and bear it" attitude to such procedures, children can be quite severely traumatised by unexpected pain. The trauma tends to be cumulative in that the painful episode is remembered, often in exaggerated form, and any attempt to repeat the procedure can then verge on the dramatic! Thus, the overall experience is distressing for the child, parents and, perhaps less obviously, for clinical staff who are required to perform the procedure and deal with its aftermath. Nursing staff, in particular, have been quick to recognise the benefits that painfree injection under percutaneous local anaesthesia has brought to their wards and clinics. Combined with a thoughtful and caring approach by staff, the use of effective percutaneous anaesthesia in children has reduced or eliminated needle trauma in most cases. Now the benefits of this pain prevention method are being applied to various surgical procedures, most notably in the area of split skin grafting. Increasingly, percutaneous local anaesthesia is now seen to have benefits not only in paediatric practice but also with adult patients.

Although some authors have used the term "skin analgesia" rather than anaesthesia, the method is, essentially, one of pain prevention rather than the relief of pain some time after its initial onset. This distinction suggests that the use of "percutaneous local anaesthesia" is preferable to "percutaneous local analgesia". A similar controversy might arise regarding the preferential use of "percutaneous" rather than the more usual "transdermal". Percutaneous ("through the skin") delivery is, in this case, intended to indicate drug absorption through the skin barrier layer, the stratum corneum, with the intention of producing a local effect on the skin. Transdermal ("across the skin") drug absorption is intended to allow the diffusing drug molecules to cross the skin barrier layer and the underlying epidermis before reaching the systemic circulation via absorption through the microcirculation in the dermis. Although the distinction in terminology is, perhaps, arbitrary, it is important to emphasise the distinction between percutaneous anaesthesia and transdermal drug delivery. Percutaneous anaesthetic systems must be designed to achieve a rapid biological response, minutes rather than hours or days, with a minimum systemic drug absorption. These differences impose additional constraints on the type of formulation which can be developed for the percutaneous delivery of local anaesthetics.

1.1 HISTORICAL DEVELOPMENT OF PERCUTANEOUS LOCAL ANAESTHESIA

Topical local anaesthetic preparations have been widely available for many years. Such products, which are usually available as over-the-counter remedies, are intended for anaesthesia of mucosal epithelia and of broken or abraded skin. They are quite without effect on healthy skin where the barrier function of the stratum corneum remains intact.

The first meaningful attempt at producing a topically applied preparation that would allow penetration of a local anaesthetic agent through the intact skin barrier, the stratum corneum, can be ascribed to Monash (1957). Monash had previously been interested in prolonging the activity of injectable local anaesthetic solutions by administering the drugs as their free bases rather than the more usual, water-soluble salts. By applying this approach to topical anaesthesia he was able to demonstrate that anaesthesia of unbroken skin could be produced within 45 minutes by using a 2% alcoholic solution of a local anaesthetic free base applied under occlusion. This compared to only partial anaesthesia achieved with a five hour application of the corresponding anaesthetic salt. Interestingly, the use of a local anaesthetic base at a higher concentration of 5% w/w in a hydrophilic ointment vehicle required twice as long to produce topical anaesthesia as the corresponding alcoholic solution. This fundamental observation, which really pointed the way to the successful formulation of percutaneous local anaesthetics, was, unfortunately, largely overlooked for some time thereafter. This was, perhaps, because much of the early experimental work on percutaneous anaesthesia was performed by dermatologists and anaesthetists who, by reason of their own particular clinical expertise and interests, did not fully appreciate the role of the drug delivery system with respect to the percutaneous absorption of local anaesthetic drugs.

Shortly after the publication of the paper by Monash, Campbell and Adriani (1958) investigated the penetration of local anaesthetics through various barrier membranes. The study was carried out in dogs, with the drugs being applied to subcutaneous tissues, abraded and burnt skin, mucous membranes or, alternatively, administered by intravenous injection. Absorption from the mucous membranes of the pharynx and trachea gave similar blood concentrations of local anaesthetics to those attained by intravenous injection, demonstrating the ease with which local anaesthetics can be absorbed via mucosal epithelia. However, no systemic absorption occurred when aqueous solutions of local anaesthetics, as their water-soluble salts, were applied to intact skin. This study concentrated on the toxicological properties of topical local anaesthetics rather than their percutaneous delivery. Nevertheless, it confirmed Monash's work in emphasising the importance, with respect to topical drug absorption, of the use of local anaesthetics in their free base, lipophilic form. Adriani, a distinguished American anesthesiologist, concluded from the study at the time that "local anaesthetics are without effect when applied to unbroken skin because of their inability to penetrate horny areas". This led to investigations into the use of solvents that were known to diminish the barrier function of the horny layer. Thus, Brechner *et al.* (1967) reported that tetracaine (amethocaine) base dissolved in dimethylsulphoxide was an effective percutaneous anaesthetic agent. However, the deliberate use of a skin barrier disrupting agent, dimethylsulphoxide, for what was, in essence, a prophylactic drug application, was never a realistic possibility, either clinically or commercially.

A significant advance in the formulation of local anaesthetics for percutaneous delivery was made by Lubens and Sanker (1964), who reported on the use of a 30% lignocaine cream applied in the form of a crude gauze patch impregnated with an undefined amount of the cream. This preparation was investigated for its ability to prevent the pain associated with intradermal allergy testing. Although not stated by the authors, it was clear that lignocaine was formulated in the cream base as its hydrochloride. A 30 minute application was claimed to produce adequate topical anaesthesia without "allergenic reactions, skin irritation or undesirable effects". The approach of using a high drug concentration to achieve an adequate concentration gradient for the drug at the barrier membrane interface was one which was subsequently adopted in a number of other studies.

Lubens and Sanker made a further contribution at this time to the development of percutaneous local anaesthesia by defining those properties which would be desirable in a local anaesthetic for topical administration to intact skin, although some of their suggested requirements were related specifically to the use of these preparations in an allergy-testing regimen. The desirable local anaesthetic properties were:

(1)   effectiveness on topical application to the skin
(2)   potency for abolition of pain sensation
(3)   adequate duration of anaesthesia
(4)   inability to cause allergic sensitisation
(5)   inability to diminish the dermal response of allergens
(6)   freedom from skin irritation
(7)   freedom from side effects.

A further contribution to the debate on how to achieve penetration of the skin barrier by local anaesthetics was made by John Adriani in 1971. In this new study, Adriani and Dalili (1971) studied the effects on over 150 volunteers of topically applied saturated solutions of local anaesthetic bases and salts. The base solutions were found to block the response to itch and burning induced by an applied electrical stimulus. By comparison, the salt solutions were ineffective in the same test. The study was extended to include some 30 local anaesthetic preparations then commercially available on the North American market. Only one such preparation, containing 20%w/w benzocaine, was found to be effective in the test. The lack of effect of most local anaesthetic preparations in the test was considered to be due to one or more of the following factors:

(1)   the preparation contained an insufficient amount of the active agent
(2)   instability of the anaesthetic base resulting in chemical change
(3)   adjuncts of the formulation modified the action of the local anaesthetics
(4)   the anaesthetics may have been retained by the vehicle, so reducing the drug available for penetration
(5)   ingredients in the preparation may have enhanced the barrier properties of the stratum corneum
(6)   the experimentally induced sunburn due to electrical stimulation of the skin may have altered the epithelial barrier, with a subsequent decrease in permeability.

With the benefit of hindsight, the importance of factors (1) and (4), in particular, can now be recognised. It is, of course, necessary to minimise the affinity of the vehicle for the drug and to maximise the concentration gradient achieved across the aqueous diffusion layer at the barrier membrane interface. The use of a readily saturable system, which can rapidly replenish drug lost from the diffusion layer as a consequence of penetration into and through the stratum corneum, is of prime importance in the formulation of percutaneous local anaesthetic preparations. These formulation factors are discussed in detail in Chapter 5.

Lubens and co-workers, since their development of the lignocaine cream saturated pad, had continued to use this system in their clinical practice. Some eleven years after their initial report on the topic, they produced an update on its use over the intervening period (Lubens *et al.*, 1974). By this stage the formulation had been shown to be effective for minor operations such as the excision of skin papilloma and the drainage of cervical abscesses. Longer application times of the pad were found to result in longer durations of skin anaesthesia. There were still no adverse reactions to the preparation. However, the unrealistically high drug concentration and the rather inconvenient method of application made the system commercially unattractive and no further development of the work appears to have occurred.

Much of the early work in the successful commercial development of local anaesthetic drugs, notably lignocaine, was due to a Swedish multinational pharmaceutical company, Astra Lakemedel Aktiebolag. It was, perhaps, inevitable, that this company should turn its attention to percutaneous anaesthesia, no doubt as a consequence of the early work of Monash, Lubens and Adriani in the USA. In the late 1970's Astra patented a percutaneous anaesthetic system based on the ether local anaesthetic, ketocaine, a proprietary drug of Recordati SpA in Milan, Italy. The formulation was to be marketed as "Ane-Pad" but was withdrawn before this stage was reached due, apparently, to unacceptable levels of skin irritation. Nevertheless, this formulation, discussed in Chapter 5, produced effective percutaneous anaesthesia in various clinical applications (Ponten and Ohlsen, 1977; Pettersson, 1978; Pettersson and Strombeck, 1978).

It was, perhaps, fortunate, that, about the time of the demise of "Ane-Pad", formulation scientists at Astra noticed by chance that, when two local anaesthetic bases were mixed together in the solid form, an oily liquid was produced at room temperature. It was quickly realised that local anaesthetic bases, which were amorphous rather than well-defined crystalline materials, readily formed these lower melting eutectic mixtures both with each other and similar amorphous solids. The direct emulsification of the eutectic mixture of lignocaine and prilocaine to form an oil-in-water percutaneous anaesthetic cream enabled Astra to eventually launch the first commercially available percutaneous local anaesthetic preparation, EMLA® (Eutectic Mixture of Local Anaesthetics) cream (Juhlin *et al.*, 1980; Broberg and Evers, 1981). The present licensed applications for EMLA® in the UK are listed in Table 1.1.

Table 1.1 — Dosage and administration of EMLA® in children and adults: Summary of recommendations contained in the ABPI Data Sheet Compendium 1992

procedure	dosage
Minor dermatological procedures, e.g. needle insertion and surgical treatment of localised lesions.	Approximately 2 g applied for a minimum of 60 minutes, maximum 5 hours.
Split skin grafting and other large area applications	Approximately 1.5 - 3 g per 10 cm^2 applied for a minimum of 2 hours, maximum 5 hours.
Surgical treatment of localised lesions on the genital mucosa	Approximately 10 g for 5 -10 minutes, followed immediately by the procedure

Since the basic parameters for the successful formulation of local anaesthetics for percutaneous delivery were established, a number of other systems capable of producing effective anaesthesia of the skin have been reported. These have included liposomal and iontophoretic drug delivery systems. During the past decade the authors have worked on the development of a percutaneous anaesthetic system based on the observation that amethocaine base undergoes a phase change from solid to liquid in an aqueous environment (McCafferty and Woolfson, 1988). Fortuitously, this phase change occurs just below normal skin surface temperature. This has allowed the development of effective percutaneous anaesthetic preparations, based on this amethocaine phase-change system, which are notable for producing profound skin anaesthesia lasting for several hours (Woolfson *et al.*, 1990).

1.2 PERCUTANEOUS LOCAL ANAESTHESIA: THE WAY FORWARD

The substantial body of published research now available allows the properties of the ideal percutaneous local anaesthetic preparation to be defined. Essentially, such preparations should be formulated to contain the minimum concentration of local anaesthetic agent consistent with producing the desired clinical benefit. Thus, they should provide rapid, deep and relatively long-acting anaesthesia of both the skin and underlying tissues, with no systemic effects or significant adverse local skin reactions. Of course, these ideals may never be fully reached, but substantial progress has already been made in that clinical efficacy and safety have now been reported with the use of several percutaneous anaesthetic systems.

The way forward lies largely in the direction of improved convenience of use with these preparations. In particular, a reduction in the onset time of anaesthesia would be highly desirable. At present, EMLA® has a recommended application period of one hour for venepuncture, with a minimum of 2 hours being required for applications involving the harvesting of split skin grafts. The amethocaine phase-change system effectively halves this period, requiring a 30 minute application period for pain prevention in paediatric venepuncture applications. Iontophoresis may produce a more rapid anaesthetic effect, perhaps within 10 minutes, but it is, at present, of short duration and further work is required to produce a realistic iontophoretic system for percutaneous anaesthesia. Iontophoretic delivery of local anaesthetics is considered fully in Chapter 5.

Systems that rely on passive drug diffusion along a concentration gradient may be rate-limiting in respect of achieving faster onset times with percutaneously delivered local anaesthetics. Perhaps a more realistic approach is to improve the design of the delivery system itself such that it can be, in most cases, self-applied by the patient before visiting the clinic. Alternatively, it can conveniently be applied to the patient by nursing staff well in advance of any intended clinical procedure or ward round. A pre-requisite for this approach, which is intended to minimise the inconvenience of the patient still waiting for the onset of skin anaesthesia when the clinical procedure is imminent, is that the anaesthetic effect, when it occurs, is prolonged. This is necessary to allow a sufficient "window" of anaesthesia, for example to take into account travelling time from home to clinic or delays at the clinic or ward level. The amethocaine phase-change system, which can be tailored to produce anaesthesia of the skin for several hours, is particularly suitable for this approach. Thus, the authors have further developed this system to produce a self-adhesive, film-like, local anaesthetic patch, which, unlike cream-based formulations, is easily self-administered and delivers a defined local anaesthetic dosage to the site. The patch system, which, at the time of writing, is completing final clinical trials, has been well-received by both nursing staff and patients. It is intended that this system will be commercially available in the future.

Although the availability of percutaneous local anaesthesia might be regarded as very much a first world luxury by a minority of practitioners, there is no reason to suppose that pain prevention in this form should not, eventually, be available on a worldwide basis. Thus, Hellgren et al. (1990) have commented on the usefulness of EMLA® in field studies on Tanzanian children where repeated, potentially painful blood sampling was frequently required. Wider availability of the technique will be a matter of economics. Certainly, in first world countries, where there is an increasing trend towards day-stay or office surgery for minor procedures, it is economic, as well as humane, considerations that are prompting the rapidly increasing use of percutaneous local anaesthesia (Dave, 1990).

REFERENCES

Adriani, J. and Dalili, H. (1971) Penetration of local anaesthetics through epithelial barriers. *Anesth. Analg.* **50** 834-841.

Brechner, V.L., Cohen, D.D. and Pretsky, I. (1967) Dermal anesthesia by the topical application of tetracaine base dissolved in dimethylsulfoxide. *Ann. N.Y. Acad. Sci.* **141** 524-531.

Broberg, B.F.J. and Evers, H.C.A. (1981) European patent 0 002 425.

Campbell, A.H. and Adriani, J. (1958) Absorption of local anesthetics. *J. Amer. Med. Ass.* **168** 873-877.

Dave, A.L. (1990) EMLA as a topical anaesthetic in the office. *Clin. Pediatrics* **29** 353-354.

Hellgren, U., Kihamia, C.M. and Rombo, L. (1990) Painless venepuncture in the field. *Trans. Roy. Soc. Trop. Med. Hyg.* **84** 352.

Juhlin, L., Evers, H. and Broberg, F. (1980) A lidocaine-prilocaine cream for superficial skin surgery and painful lesions. *Acta Dermatovener (Stockholm)* **60** 544-546.

Lubens, H.M. and Sanker, J.F. (1964) Anesthetic skin patch. *Ann. Allergy* **22** 37-41.

Lubens, H.M., Ausdenmoore, R.W., Shafer, A.D. and Reece, R.M. (1974) Anesthetic patch for painful procedures such as minor operations. *Am. J. Dis. Child* **128** 192-195.

McCafferty, D.F. and Woolfson, A.D. (1988) Percutaneous local anaesthetic composition for topical application and associated method. U.K. Patent 2163956.

Monash, S. (1957) Topical anesthesia of the unbroken skin. *Arch. Dermatol.* **76** 752-756.

Pettersson, L. (1978) Percutaneous anaesthesia for some minor surgical procedures. *Scand. J. Plastic Reconstruct. Surg.* **12** 283-286.

Pettersson, L. and Strombeck, J.O. (1978) Percutaneous anaesthesia for dermabrasion. *Scand. J. Plast. Reconstr. Surg.* **12** 287-290.

Ponten, B. and Ohlsen, L. (1977) Skin surface application of ketocaine to provide local anaesthesia for cutting split skin grafts. *Brit. J. Plastic Surgery* **30** 251-254.

Woolfson, A.D., McCafferty, D.F. and Boston, V. (1990) Clinical experiences with a novel percutaneous amethocaine preparation: prevention of pain due to venepuncture in children. *Br. J. Clin. Pharmac.* **30** 273-279.

2

Pain

Pain can be defined as an unpleasant sensory and emotional phenomenon which is associated with actual or potential tissue damage. The physiological function of pain is to prevent or limit injury to the individual by eliciting a variety of protective behaviours such as reflex withdrawal and future avoidance of noxious stimuli. The importance of this protective effect is dramatically illustrated by individuals who lack the neural apparatus for detection of noxious stimuli. This congenital insensitivity to pain can cause severe injuries, for example, loss of digits, pressure sores and damage to load-bearing joints. Sensory aspects of pain can be classified by both character and site of origin (Fig. 2.1). In this chapter discussion will centre around somatic superficial pain such as that caused by injury to the skin. The shaded area in Fig. 2.1 illustrates this particular area of interest.

Application of a noxious stimulus to the skin surface results in a series of complex chemical and electrical events before pain is experienced. These processes can be divided into four main areas: transduction, transmission, modulation and perception. Transduction can be defined as the process by which a noxious stimulus provokes electrical activity in appropriate sensory nerve endings. Transmission, as the term implies, involves relaying impulses from the site of transduction to their terminals in the spinal cord. From here transmission continues via a network of relay neurones to the brain stem, thalamus and cortex. Modulation concerns the neural activity providing control of the pain transmission neurones. An inhibitory pathway has been discovered in the central nervous system that selectively controls pain transmission cells in the spinal cord. When this system is activated, by stress, for example, noxious stimuli produce less activity in the pain transmission pathway. Perception, the final process, is much more difficult to define in physiological terms. Neural activity of the pain transmission neurones is interpreted, in some unknown way, by brain structures to provide the actual perception of pain.

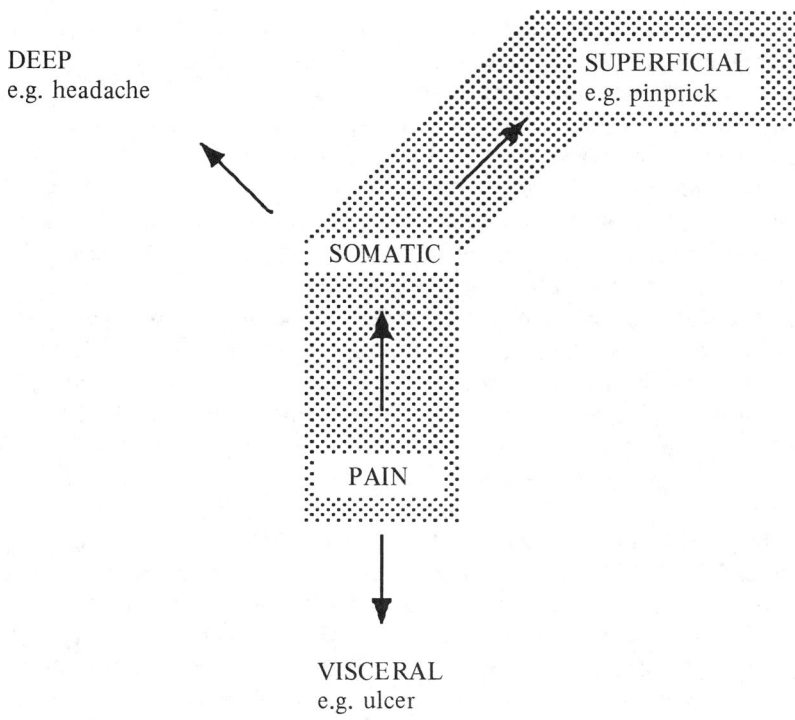

Fig. 2.1 — Pain quality

Due to the substantial increase in knowledge about pain physiology over the last 20 years, it is no longer possible to accept previous concepts of a simple, dedicated spinothalamic pain system. It would appear that, as well as the spinoreticular tract being an important afferent pathway for pain, complex neural connections involving diverse areas of the nervous system are also involved in pain perception. The response to a painful stimulus can be modified at the spinal cord in the periaqueductal gray matter and brain stem raphe nuclei before reaching relays and gating mechanisms in the thalamus.

2.1 CUTANEOUS SENSORY NETWORK

The cutaneous sensory network is a complex system which comprises a number of different afferents both from a functional and morphological viewpoint. This network includes large and small myelinated fibres (Aβ and Aδ respectively) as well as unmyelinated C fibres (Erlanger and Grasser, 1937; Iggo, 1982; Duthie, 1989). Classification of these fibres is shown in Table 3.7 (Chapter 3). There are two anatomically distinct groups of receptors; the "organised" receptors, where the nerve terminates in a group of sensory cells such as Pacinian or Meissner's corpuscles and the "free" unencapsulated nerve terminals (Sinclair, 1981). The latter arise from C fibres, which have been traced by careful electron microscopy and end primarily in the dermo-epidermal junction where they are exposed to the fluid-filled interstitial spaces. The C fibres comprise about 80% of all cutaneous afferents and most of them respond to varying intensities of mechanical stimulation (Keele and Armstrong, 1964). Three groups of mechanoreceptors have been identified within the skin structures and have been classified as low, medium and high sensitivity (Iggo, 1957a; 1957b). It has been shown that 20% of these C fibres required strong mechanical stimulation for activation, the threshold ranging from moderate to overtly damaging pressures. They showed little or no sensitivity to thermal stimuli including noxious heat.

Electrophysiological evidence indicates that there are several subgroups of nociceptors (Iggo, 1974). The two main subgroups of relevance include mechanical nociceptors, responding to pin-pricking, squeezing or crushing of the skin and mechanothermal, which respond to severe mechanical and high/low temperature stimuli (Iggo, 1982). Sinclair (1981) has suggested that nociception is primarily relayed via the free nerve terminal receptors. All cutaneous sensory afferents synapse in the dorsal horn of the spinal cord (Fig. 2.2), within which are both excitatory and inhibitory synapses (Schmidt, 1981). Some of the Aβ mechanoreceptor afferents send off collaterals, which enter the ascending dorsal columns on the same side (ipsilateral) as the dorsal root afferents. The other cutaneous sensory afferents cross the spinal cord and ascend in the anterolateral funiculus (contralateral). The anterolateral funiculus enters the reticular formation of the brain and the thalamus (Iggo, 1982). The axons of the dorsal column cross the spinal cord after synapsing on the neurones of the dorsal column nuclei in the medulla oblongata and then enter the thalamus.

The diversity of stimuli that can initiate pain has indicated that a chemical intermediary may be involved in the reception of the stimuli. It has been suggested that the essential mechanism is the release of substances from damaged cells. These released substances then stimulate the receptor (Sinclair, 1981). Intense mechanical stimulation of the skin causes the familiar triple response. This consists of white discolouration surrounded by a red flare, followed shortly by the appearance of a weal. The mediators of this inflammatory response, which are implicated in the stimulation of receptors, include bradykinin, hydrogen and potassium ions, histamine, leukotrienes, serotonin and prostaglandin E from damaged tissues, substance P and other neuropeptides from the sensory nerve endings themselves. The effects of bradykinin are potentiated in muscle in the presence of serotonin and prostaglandin E_2 (Wall, 1974; Sinclair, 1981). These chemicals stimulate nociceptors directly and sensitise them to further stimuli. A reduction in nociception threshold occurs, which results in an increased response to painful stimuli. It is possible that these mechanisms may explain the hyperalgesia induced by inflammation (Duthie, 1989).

Mechanoreceptors have high sensitivities to the indentation of skin or to the movement of hairs. They can be divided into the rapidly adapting and slowly adapting types. The former include Pacinian corpuscles. These are found in both hairy and glabrous skin and appear as small grey pearl-shaped structures in the deeper skin layers. They are 0.5 - 2 mm long, possess an onion-like lamellar structure formed of non-nervous tissue and contain an elongated nerve terminal at the core which is not derived from the dermal plexus. The most significant feature of the Pacinian corpuscle is that it is capable of detecting mechanical vibrations at high frequencies. It can, therefore, relay the sensations of pressure and vibration when the frequencies are greater than 100 cycles

per second. These can frequently be sensed in traumatised or anaesthetised skin because
their fibres are not derived from the dermal plexus (Brodal, 1981; Sinclair, 1981).

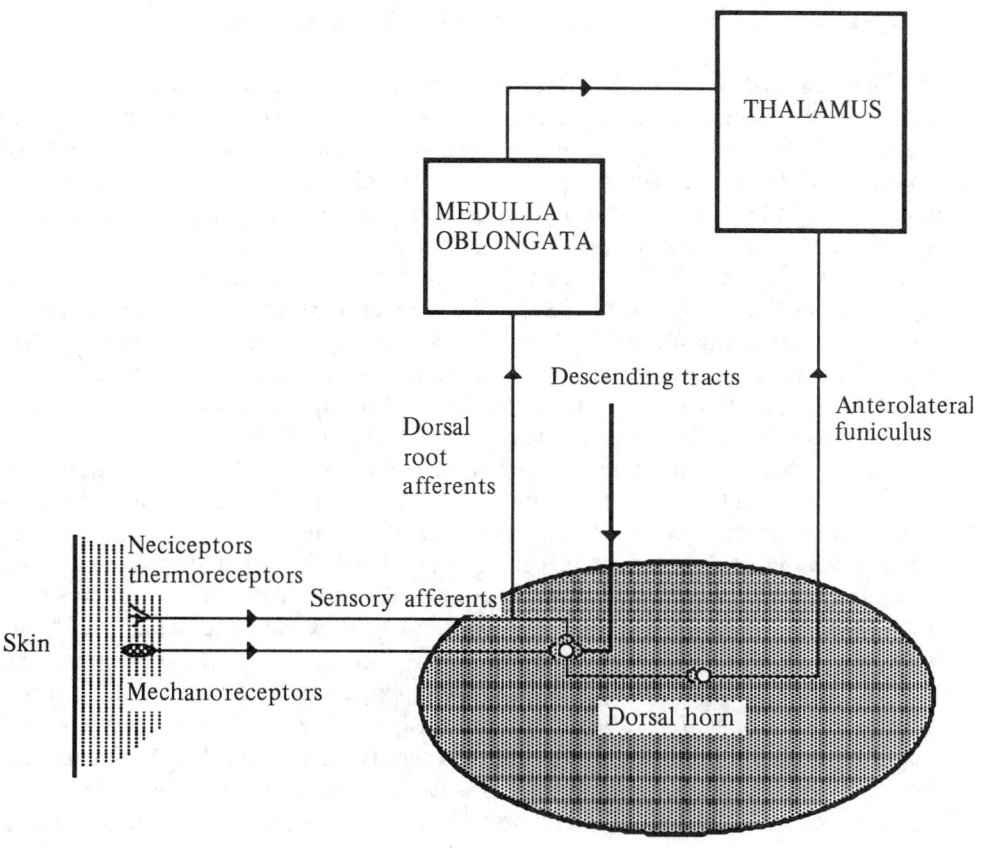

Fig. 2.2 — Diagrammatic representation of pathways for cutaneous sensory afferents

The Meissner corpuscle is an encapsulated receptor with a myelinated afferent fibre
which lies in the dermis of human glabrous skin, within the dermal papillae that fill the
grooves formed by epidermal ridges. These corpuscles are lobulated and tapered so that
the apical lobule is smaller than the basal one. The entire corpuscle is surrounded by a
connective tissue capsule, continuous with the perineurium which, in turn, is attached to
the basal projections of the epidermal cells by elastin fibrils. As a result, Meissner
corpuscles are capable of discriminating highly localised touch sensations, especially in
the palmar regions where they are most numerous.

Hair follicle receptors, which innervate hair follicles, are myelinated afferent fibres
that end in a circumferentially arranged complex of endings around the hair-route sheath,
just below the sebaceous glands. Large hair follicles can be supplied by up to 28 fibres.
Since each individual hair is positioned within its follicle, it is ideally placed to

stimulate its nerve collar and is primarily associated with tactile sensations. However, pain induced by, for example, pulling hair suggests that part of the mesh is sensitive to pain. It is probable that the free nerve terminals detect this type of sensory stimulation (Elliot, 1969). Although some hairy areas, such as the ears, contain only the follicle network and free nerve terminals, they can still discriminate sensations of warmth, pain and touch.

The slowly adapting mechanoreceptors respond during actual displacement of the skin and can also maintain a discharge of impulses whilst the skin is held static in the new position (Iggo, 1982). The slowly adapting mechanoreceptors include the Ruffini endings and the C mechanoreceptors. The Ruffini endings, which are encapsulated receptors found in the dermis of both hairy and glabrous skin, are usually more deeply placed than the Meissner corpuscle. They can provide a continuous indication of the intensity of the steady pressure or tension within the skin and are well situated to sense stretching of the skin (Brodal, 1981). The C mechanoreceptors have small receptive fields, approximately 6 mm^2, in hairy skin and can give a slowly adapting discharge when the skin is indented or the hairs moved. If they are continuously stimulated, there is a rapid reduction in excitability. After 20 to 30 seconds the receptors fail to respond since the receptor terminals are no longer excitable (Iggo, 1982).

Thermoreceptors are characterised by a continuous discharge of impulses at a particular constant skin temperature. As the temperature fluctuates there is a concomitant increase or decrease in the discharge of the impulses. However, these receptors are insensitive to both mechanical stimuli and pain-producing chemicals. The receptive fields of the thermoreceptors are spot-like and usually involve an area of less than 1 mm^2. There are two types of thermoreceptor, classified as "cold" and "warm" receptors. It has been suggested that the "cold" receptors are positioned more superficially in the skin structure at a depth of approximately 150 μm below the surface of the skin (Bazett *et al.*, 1930). In contrast, the "warm" receptors have been reported as being approximately 600 μm beneath the skin surface (Zotterman, 1959). The discharge frequency accelerates in "cold" receptors when the temperature decreases, whereas the opposite occurs for the "warm" receptors. The temperature range of maximum discharge for "warm" receptors is between 38 and 43°C, whereas the range for "cold" receptors is between 16 and 27°C (Hensel *et al.*, 1960). "Warm" receptors are inactive at normal skin temperature (approximately 33°C) and "cold" receptors are only slightly active (Iggo, 1977). A change in skin temperature of about 0.2°C is sufficient to cause a substantial increase in the discharge of "warm" or "cold" receptors. This corresponds with the thresholds of temperature which are sensed in man. Since the dynamic sensitivity of these receptors is high, this allows detection of both slow, less than 1°C in 30 seconds, as well as slight, changes in skin temperature (Iggo, 1982). Single fibres in the superficial branch of the radial nerve in man have been identified as "cold" fibres (Hensel and Boman, 1960).

When damaging, or potentially damaging, intensities of natural stimulation are applied to the skin, the mechano- and thermoreceptors can be substantially excited. However, it has been shown that they reach maximal activation by less intense stimulation. Therefore, these receptors cannot mediate pain, although they do contribute to the sensory quality of perceived pain.

2.2 PAIN PERCEPTION

When skin is pierced the pain produced is initially sensed as a sharp, rapidly localised flash which quickly fades. This initial or first pain occurs when the skin is penetrated to a depth of about 250 μm (Ranson and Clarke, 1959). If deeper penetration occurs (about 1000 μm) this initial pain is followed by delayed or second pain, especially at high stimulus intensities. This has a dull or burning character, is more diffuse spatially and fades gradually (Schmidt, 1981). If, for example, a contact injury to the foot takes place, the contact impulse travels via rapidly conducting Aβ myelinated fibres from the mechanoreceptors and arrives at the spinal cord within 10 ms. Impulses from the fastest pain receptors are 30 ms slower and the delayed pain is not sensed for a further 1500 ms. Perception of pain requires transmission to the conscious region of the brain. Therefore, by the time the first pain is perceived, the reflex withdrawal from touch brought about by skeletal muscle has already taken place (Ranson and Clarke, 1959). Sharp pain travels on A fibres whereas dull pain (which also has nauseating properties) is transmitted on C fibres (Iggo, 1974; Bowsher, 1979).

The localising effect of lateral or surround inhibition on the spatial distribution of excitation in the central nervous system (CNS) is shown in Fig. 2.3. Without lateral inhibition, the CNS perception of a point stimulus would become more and more diffuse at each successive relay station (top section of Fig. 2.3). This can happen in cases of strychnine poisoning since this chemical blocks the inhibitory synapses in the CNS. However, lateral inhibition (lower section of Fig. 2.3), which is mediated via interneurones, reduces this cascade effect and improves the sharpness of stimulus localisation (Zimmermann, 1981). Localisation of pain is the least accurate of all cutaneous sensations, partly because of the radiating quality of delayed pain (Iggo, 1982). Nociceptors have very small receptive fields. However, the neurones of the sensory pathway supply extensive receptor areas since the cutaneous afferents converge onto the spinothalamic tract neurones. Some of these can be excited by noxious stimuli at any part of a limb. Concurrent excitation of the lower threshold mechano- and thermoreceptors may aid localisation and contribute to the sensory quality of perceived pain.

Pain in the skin in the absence of any evident stimulus to the skin is termed referred pain. Angina pectoris, for example, which originates in the ischaemic tissues of the heart, is perceived on the anterior aspect of the thorax and may extend down the inner aspect of the forearm. Referred pain is usually aching or sharp and has a definite location on the skin surface. Various sites of referred pain are shown in Fig. 2.4.

2.2.1 Gate control theory

Although many theories of pain perception have been proposed, the Melzack and Wall (1965) gate control theory has now gained general acceptance (Beecher, 1957; Iggo, 1974; Wall, 1978; Sinclair, 1981; Schmidt, 1981). This theory suggests that information about the presence of injury is transmitted to the CNS by peripheral nerves. Various small diameter fibres (Aδ and C) respond only to injury while others with lower thresholds increase their discharge frequency if the stimulus reaches noxious levels. Cells in the spinal cord or fifth nerve nucleus, which are excited by these injury signals, are also facilitated or inhibited by other peripheral nerve fibres which carry information

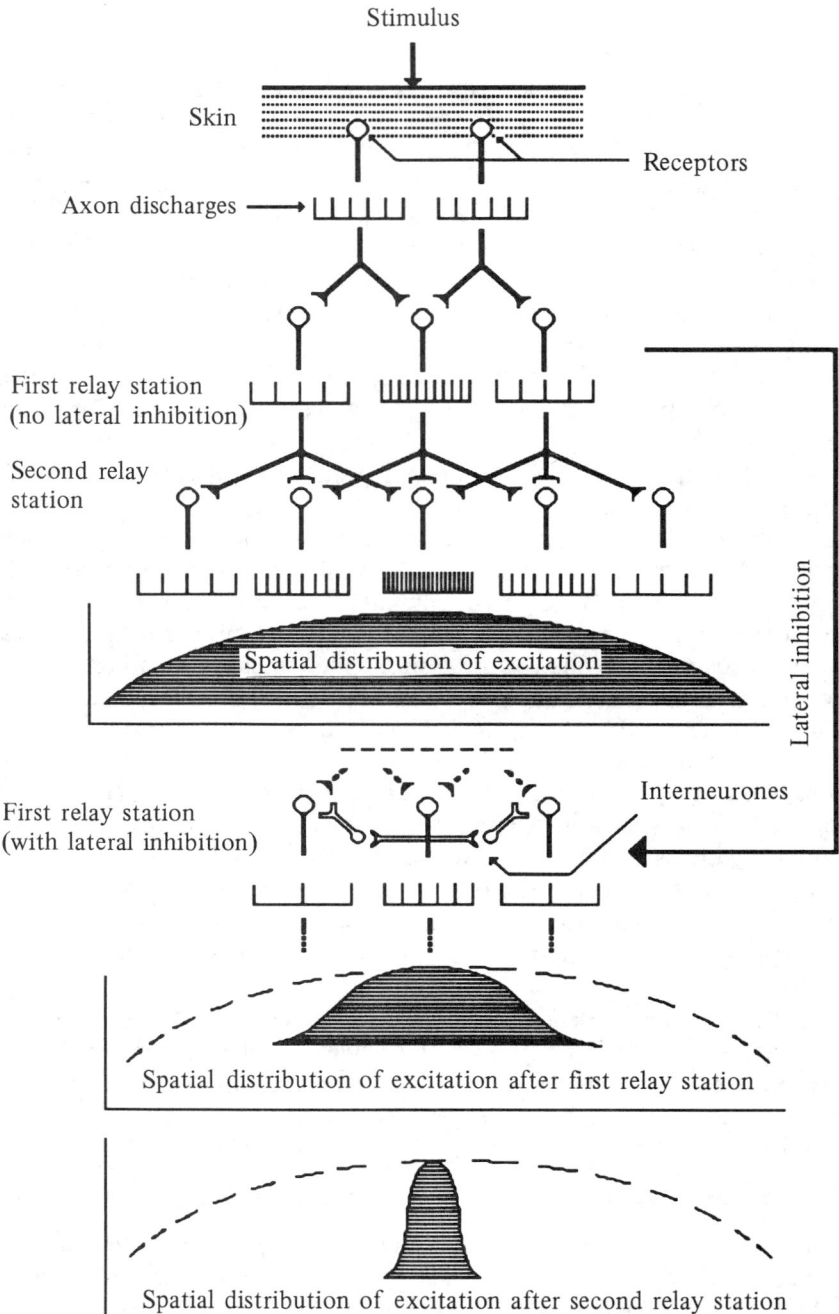

Fig. 2.3 — Spatial spread of excitation in a hypothetical CNS with, and without,
lateral inhibition (modified from Zimmermann, 1981)

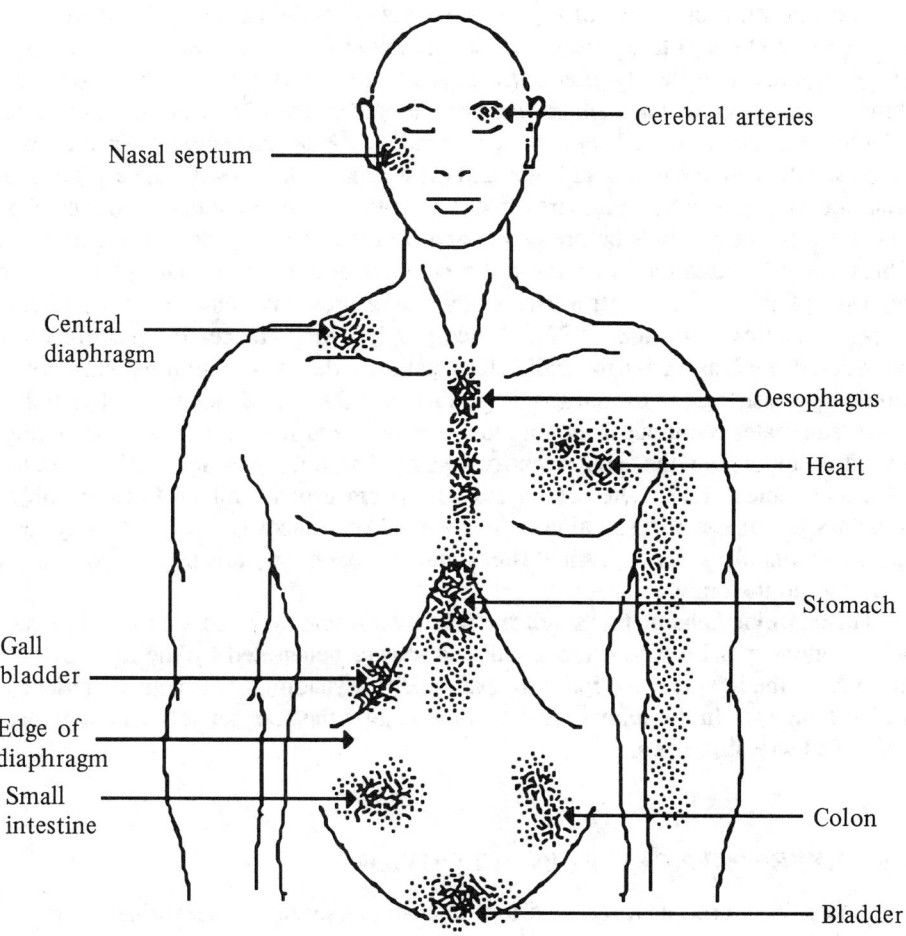

Fig. 2.4 — Sites of referred pain (modified from Ransom and Clarke, 1959)

about innocuous events. Descending control systems originating in the brain modulate the excitability of the cells that transmit information about injury. Therefore, the brain receives messages about injury via a gate controlled system, which is variously influenced by injury signals, other types of afferent impulses and descending control. It follows that pain could be relieved by stimulation of large fibres from the periphery or impulses from the brain through the editing mechanism (Sinclair, 1981). Brain stimulation anaesthesia, thought to involve the enkephalin-endorphin system, is possible under this theory (Iggo, 1982). Similarly, counter irritants and heat treatments can block nociception by segmental inhibition of the small fibres. Although the phenomenon of pain is, most usually, regarded as unpleasant, the theory also permits pain to be viewed in terms of excitation of the nociceptors. This excitation can sometimes be felt as a pleasant sensation and, hence, may not be recognised as pain by the subject.

The gate control theory of pain is particularly useful in the understanding of the responses of children to injections. Since it is now agreed that nerve tracts in children are able to function shortly after birth, although myelinisation is not complete, afferent impulses are processed in a similar manner for both children and adults. Pain caused by injection can be classified into two components. A needle penetrating the skin will mechanically activate the small fibres and the injected solution will also elicit a response from the small fibres by a pressure effect. A central control system is informed about an injury via the large fibres before processing occurs in the substantia gelatinosa. These fibres carry information concerning the position of the injury and activate selective sections of the central control system including previous memory of the injury and response tactics (Melzack, 1972). Since previous experiences of injections will be considered unpleasant by the child, it is unlikely that any inhibitory pain messages would be transmitted to the substantia gelatinosa at the specific spinal cord section. The T cell summates the input from both the excitatory and inhibitory fibres, including any inhibitory input from the central control system. Large fibres near injection sites tend to be inaccessible. Hence, the central control system usually fails to transmit inhibitory impulses to the specific spinal cord segment. Consequently, the T cell only receives excitatory impulses from the small fibres, the gate opens and this permits pain messages to be sent to the brain.

The neospinothalamic tracts indicate when and where the injection took place, as well as the intensity with which the small fibres were penetrated by the needle and then irritated by the injected solution. The paramedial ascending fibres activate reticular and limbic structures in the brain which, in turn, trigger the fear, anxiety and apprehension associated with injections.

2.3   EXPERIMENTAL PAIN INDUCTION

Induced pain is used as a research tool in both physiology, to examine reception and transmission of pain, and pharmacology, during testing of the efficacy of analgesics and anaesthetics. Consequently, many methods of pain induction have been reported (Beecher, 1957; Lindahl, 1961; Keele and Armstrong, 1964; Iggo, 1974; Sinclair, 1981; McCafferty *et al.*, 1988). The method of pain induction should be such that it can be measured to provide a comparison between different tests. The sensation of pain should be easily perceived without concomitant substantial tissue damage (Procacci *et al.*, 1974). The ideal experimental pain stimulus should have the following characteristics (Beecher, 1957; Gracely, 1989):

- cause minimum tissue damage
- have a rapid onset of action
- terminate rapidly
- be as natural as possible in origin
- provide a relationship between stimulus and pain intensity
- be repeatable with minimal temporal effects
- be easily applied
- produce distinct pain sensation
- allow quantifiable determination of pain quality

- be sensitive
- produce similar sensitivities in different individuals
- affect Aδ and C fibres only
- show dose-analgesic response relationship.

2.3.1 Pain threshold

Sensory thresholds for pain vary little between individuals but the tolerance level varies considerably between cultures, individuals and even in the same individual at different times (Bowsher, 1979). This occurs because the subjective intensity of pain depends not only on the stimulus intensity but also on the extent to which it preoccupies the subject. Redirection of attention can weaken the sensation and in extreme situations such as the stress of an accident, wounding in battle or hypnosis, can abolish it (Wall, 1974).

Most quantitative studies concerning pain sensation have utilised a radiant heat method since this involves no mechanical skin contact and activation of mechanoreceptors is, therefore, avoided. However, it is unavoidable that some non-nociceptive thermoreceptors are stimulated. The human thermal pain threshold is surprisingly reproducible. For example, a temperature pulse of 45°C lasting for 3 seconds will cause pain in about 50 percent of volunteers. Gybels *et al.* (1979) measured C fibre activity and subjective pain scores simultaneously in human volunteers. Using controlled thermal stimuli they found a direct relationship between C fibre discharge and the perceived pain intensity (Fig. 2.5). It is likely that C fibres detect the occurrence of thermal stimuli near the pain threshold and probably contribute to the perceived intensity of the heat stimulus. The Aδ mechanothermal nociceptors also probably contribute to this process. Evidence implicating both Aδ and C fibres in human pain perception originates from the observation that brief, intense stimuli applied to the skin provoke two distinct sensations. An initial sharp, and comparatively short, pricking sensation (first pain) occurs and this is followed by a more prolonged dull pain sensation (second pain). When brief thermal stimuli are used the second pain often has a burning quality (Price *et al.*, 1977). However, first pain is abolished when myelinated fibres are selectively blocked by pressure. In contrast, second pain can be prevented by selectively blocking unmyelinated fibres by using low concentrations of local anaesthetics. It has been suggested that first pain occurs by activation of Aδ fibres since it has been established that a minimum conduction velocity of 6 metres per second is required for the peripheral axons which mediate first pain. This conduction velocity is in the same range as that of Aδ fibres (Campbell and LaMotte, 1983). First pain is detectable using thermal stimuli to areas of skin not previously stimulated. Since high-threshold mechanoreceptors do not respond to thermal stimuli unless first sensitised, the mechanothermal rather than the high-threshold mechanical nociceptor must be the primary afferent class whose activity underlies first pain evoked by thermal stimuli. These observations suggest that both Aδ and C nociceptors contribute to pain sensation, as well as indicating that the activity of each receptor contributes in a specific manner to the quality of the pain sensation. However, it would be expected that any naturally occurring stimulus to the skin will activate a variety of receptors. For example, a mechanical stimulus will activate Aα mechanoreceptors in addition to nociceptors. Similarly, noxious heat will activate thermoreceptors and noxious chemicals may activate both mechanical and thermal receptors (Fields, 1987).

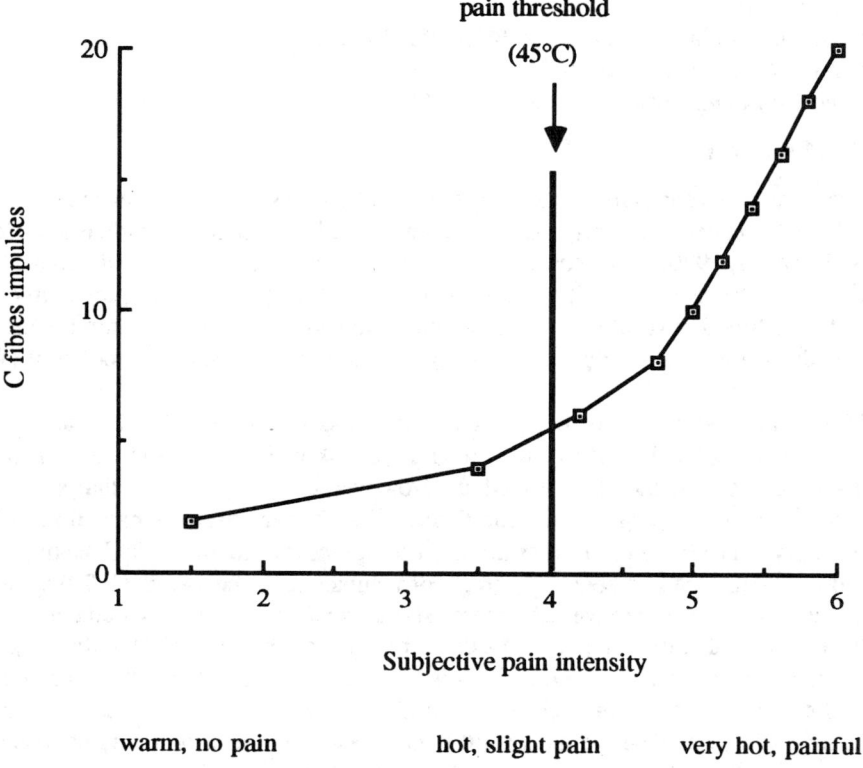

Fig. 2.5 — Effect of increasing C fibre discharge and perceived pain intensity
(modified from Gybels *et al.*, 1979)

It can be difficult to measure pain intensity if the pain threshold is high, for example pain associated with thermal radiation. Under these circumstances increasing the stimulus, in order to overcome the pain threshold, can cause tissue damage, as well as evoking significant emotional reactions to pain. These, in turn, can affect the actual perception of the painful stimulus. Ideally, although pain thresholds should be determined from the mean of the ascending and descending series of stimuli, in practice, often only the ascending series is used (Beecher, 1957). It is widely accepted that human volunteers provide more reliable results than animal models since pain intensities from human volunteers can be illustrated numerically or graphically (Keele, 1966; McCafferty and Woolfson, 1990). In contrast, pain assessment in animals requires the use of indirect methods such as reflex withdrawal or autonomic reactions (Schmidt, 1981). More recently, a study has described the determination of pain thresholds using a mechanical pain stimulation device (Kohlloffel *et al.*, 1991). Pain thresholds were calculated, using ten volunteers of both sexes (age range twenty-five - fifty years), from the linear regression of the stimulus response function or measured directly as the lowest velocity required to attain the pain threshold (Fig. 2.6). Both techniques produced similar values (average values of 12.5 ms^{-1} for the direct method and 11.6 ms^{-1} by extrapolation of linear regression curves) and distributions of the pain thresholds. There was little variation in the values obtained for the average pain threshold during subsequent testing.

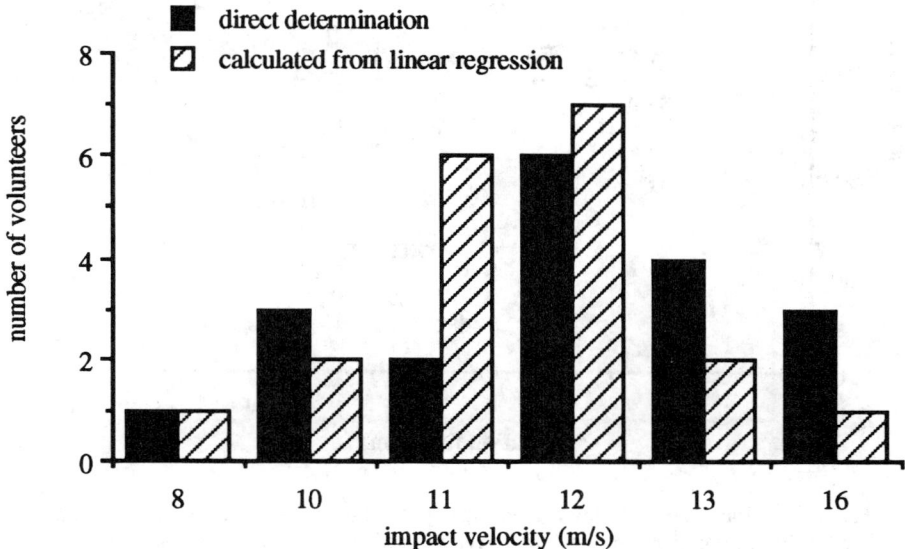

Fig. 2.6 — Determination of pain thresholds in human volunteers (modified from Kohlloffel *et al.*, 1991)

2.3.2 Methods of pain induction

Stimuli used to induce pain can be categorised as physical, chemical and electrical. One of the simplest methods for inducing pain is the pin-prick. This involves pricking the skin with a needle and many variations of this basic test procedure have been documented (Lubens and Sanker, 1964; Petterson, 1978; Juhlin *et al.*, 1980; Russo *et al.*, 1980; McCafferty *et al.*, 1988). This technique has been widely used to test for local anaesthesia of the skin. In one such study the effect of percutaneous local anaesthetic formulations on the reduction of pain caused by pin-pricking was examined using the cusum technique (McCafferty and Woolfson, 1990). An amethocaine gel formulation containing either 2 or 4% w/w active ingredient was applied for a randomly chosen time of between 10 and 25 minutes on trained adult volunteers. On removal of the gel the site was pricked six times in a random fashion using a sterile needle. Each volunteer was then asked to grade the pain on a 10 cm visual analogue scale (VAS) where 0 represented no pain and 10 represented the predetermined pain of injection. As can be seen from Figs 2.7 and 2.8, there was a considerable amount of scatter in the data thus obtained. For this reason conventional plotting and regression analysis were ineffective for determination of the minimum application time necessary for the anaesthetic formulations, in comparison to placebo, to reduce the pain response. However, when the cusum technique was used it was easy to interpret the effects of the local anaesthetic

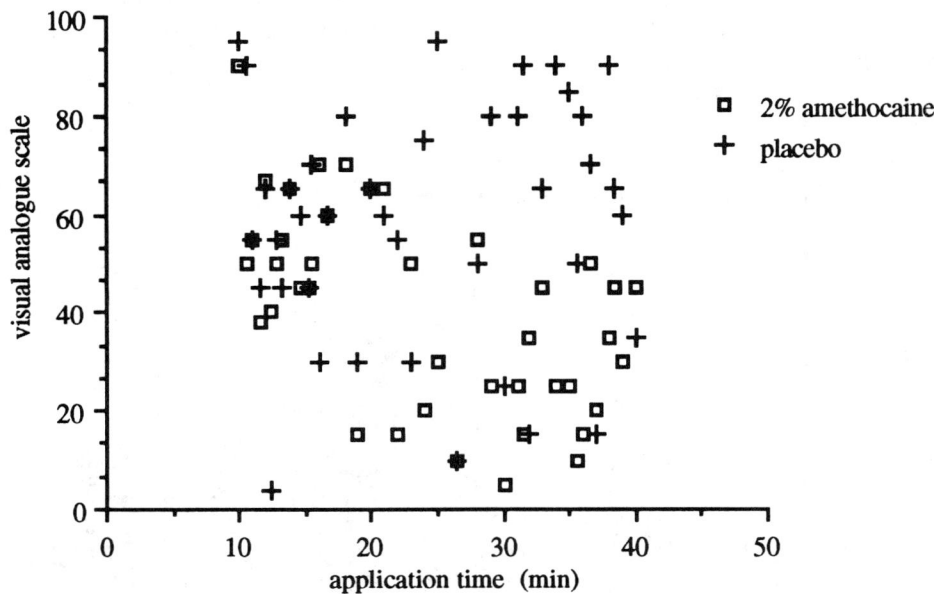

Fig. 2.7 — Pain scores following various application times of a 2% amethocaine formulation in comparison to placebo (reproduced from McCafferty and Woolfson, 1990, with permission of copyright owner, IBC Technical Services)

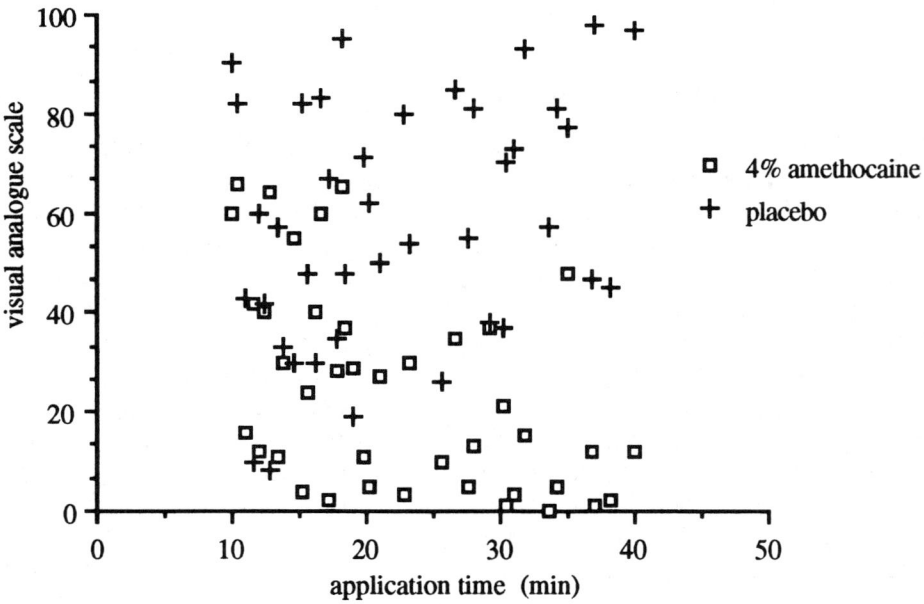

Fig. 2.8 — Pain scores following various application times of a 4% amethocaine formulation in comparison to placebo (reproduced from McCafferty and Woolfson, 1990, with permission of copyright owner, IBC Technical Services)

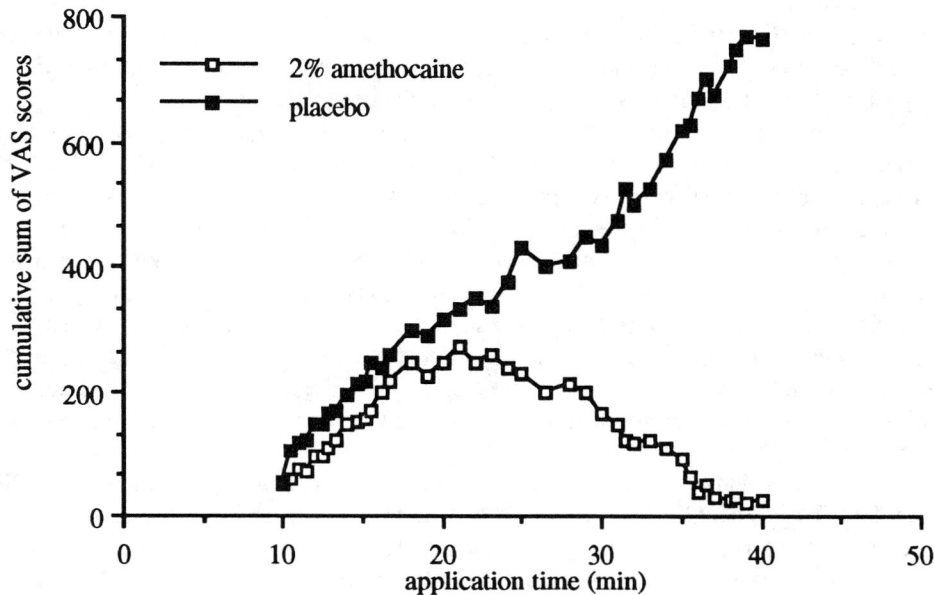

Fig. 2.9 — Cusum plot of pain scores following various application times of a 2% amethocaine formulation in comparison to placebo (reproduced from McCafferty and Woolfson, 1990, with permission of copyright owner, IBC Technical Services)

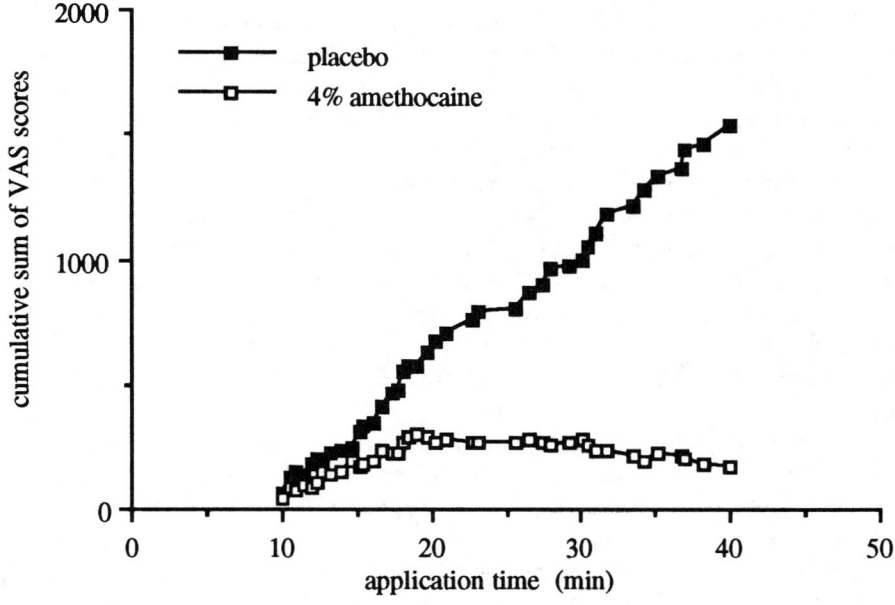

Fig. 2.10 — Cusum plot of pain scores following various application times of a 4% amethocaine formulation in comparison to placebo (reproduced from McCafferty and Woolfson, 1990, with permission of copyright owner, IBC Technical Services)

formulations on the overall pain scores (Figs 2.9 and 2.10). For example, it can be observed that both formulations caused a clear shift in the regression line, in comparison to placebo, after about 20 minutes. This can be interpreted as meaning that a minimum application time of 20 minutes was necessary to reduce the pain caused by pin-pricking.

Local anaesthesia of the skin is most frequently carried out prior to venepuncture. Hence, the experimental methods employed to mimic the pain responses in these situations should correspond to the actual procedure, i.e. penetration of the skin surface. Although, in an earlier study, the skin was fully penetrated with a needle (McCafferty *et al.*, 1988), this was probably not essential to evaluate the pain response since the nociceptors lie close to the surface of the skin. The degree of pin-pricking can be controlled more quantitatively by using a standard force of application such as a spring loaded system (Mongar, 1955). The pain threshold can also be determined using a technique based on pin-pricking. In these circumstances, a force generated gradually by weights or hydraulic pressure can be increased until a pain response has been evoked (Procacci *et al.*, 1974).

An apparatus that can be used to induce pain by mechanical stimulation has recently been described by Kohlloffel *et al.* (1991). The device resembles an air gun and it can accelerate an internal aluminium cylinder from its launch position to a predetermined final velocity. The barrel can be positioned perpendicularly to the skin surface and is connected to a pressure chamber via flexible tubing. As shown in Fig. 2.11 (a), the apparatus is operated by drawing the cylinder (C) to the top of the barrel by negative air pressure. This results from air escaping via the exhaust valves of the pressure chamber while, at the same time, air is drawn in by the barrel inlet valves. The cylinder is held in position by a magnetic rubber ring and can then be fired at the skin surface by closing the chamber exhaust valves. This is achieved by opening valve (V), which causes the piston to close the chamber pressure exhaust valves, after which the pressure increases and the cylinder is fired towards the surface of the skin as illustrated by Fig. 2.11 (b). The piston is then returned to its original position by means of a spring. The air, once again, can escape via the pressure chamber exhaust valve and the cylinder is returned to its launch position. The impact velocity of the aluminium cylinder, weighing 330 mg, can be accurately controlled to within a margin of 1% using this method. The apparatus was used in the evaluation of mechanical pain and hyperalgesia, where impact velocities ranging from approximately 8 - 23 m s^{-1} were employed. Although this device appears to be an excellent tool for the evaluation of mechanical pain and hyperalgesia, its use may be less suitable for the quantifying of pain reduction caused by the topical application of local anaesthetics. This is due to the fact that the area of stimulation is approximately 0.28 cm^2 and hence small areas of patchy anaesthesia might be difficult to detect.

Heat can also be used for pain induction and, in certain circumstances, can be controlled quantitatively. For example, an infrared source, where the subject directly controlled the stimulus, has been used. The noxious stimulus could be maintained at a threshold level where tissue damage did not occur (Schmidt, 1981). Infrared radiation warmed a blackened area of skin on the forehead of the subject who controlled the intensity of the radiation. Skin temperature was monitored via a chart recorder as shown in Fig. 2.12. However, the disadvantage of the apparatus was that it was unwieldy and subjects required prior training in order to discriminate among sensations (Sinclair, 1981). Ultraviolet radiation has also been employed to produce small areas of first

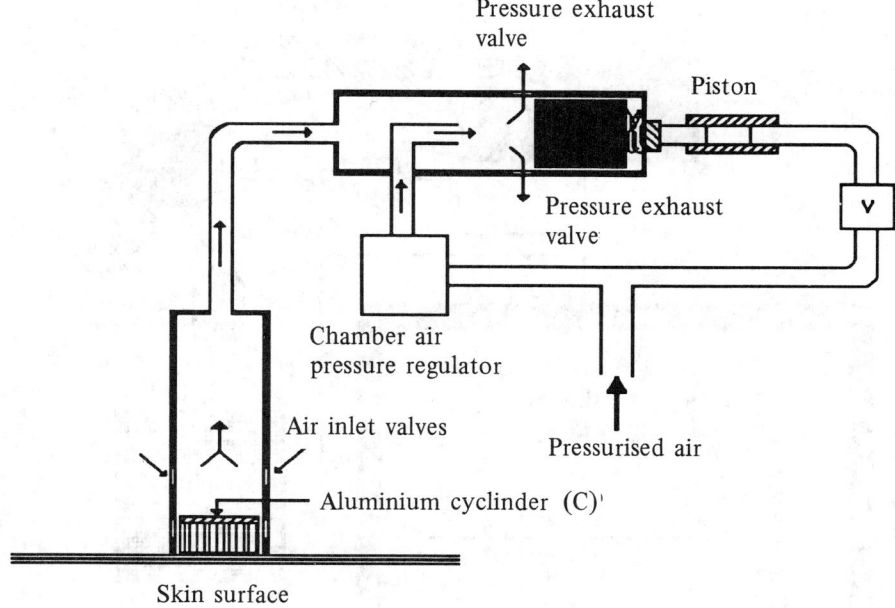

(a)

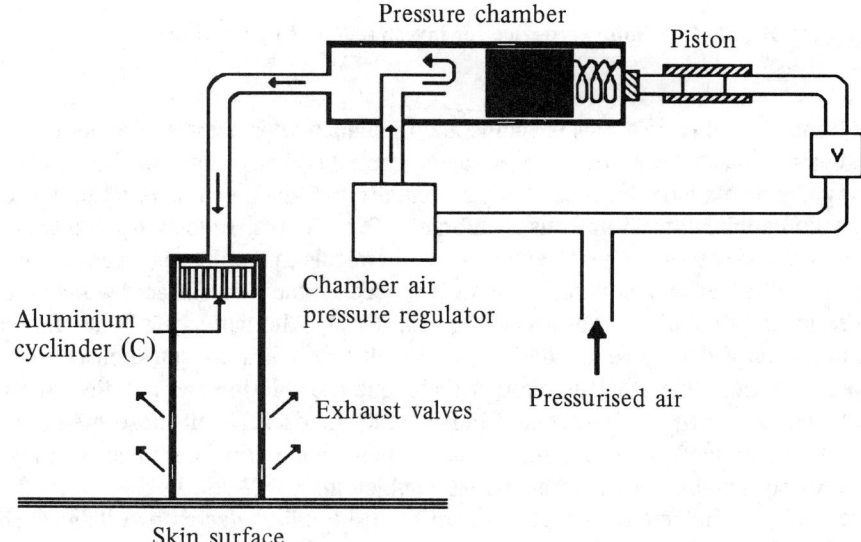

(b)

Fig. 2.11 — Apparatus for inducing pain by mechanical stimulation (modified from
Kohlloffel *et al.*, 1991)

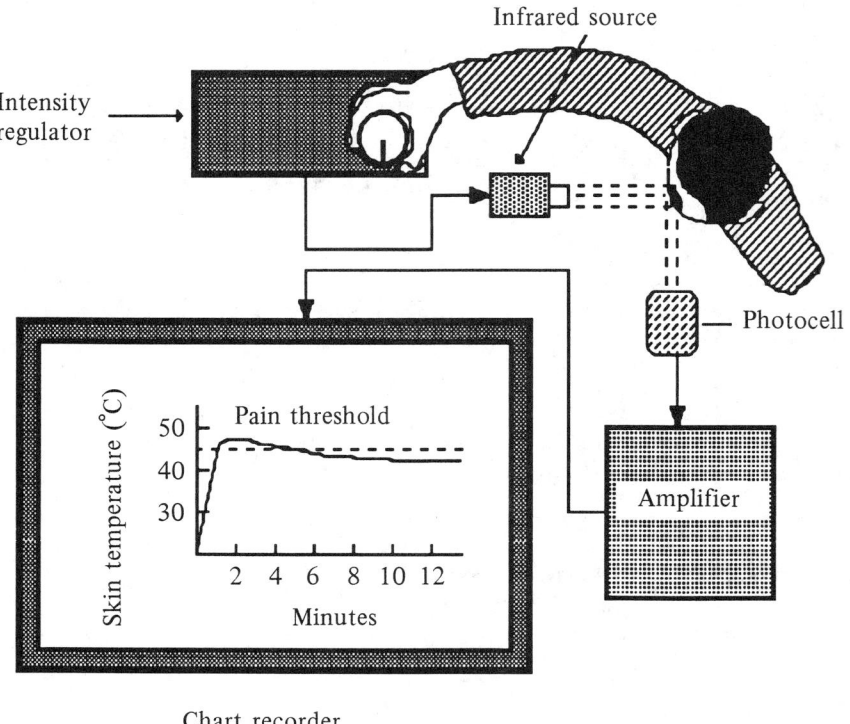

Fig. 2.12 — Infrared device for investigation of pain thresholds

degree burns but, of course, this is against the fundamental principles of experimentally induced pain in that substantial tissue damage is caused (Adriani and Dalili, 1971).

Many chemicals have been used experimentally to induce pain and, although some are active on application to mucous membranes, few can penetrate skin. A number of methods have been used to promote access of chemicals to the dermis. The substance, after being dissolved in a suitable solvent, is placed on the skin surface, which is then scratched until the solution is absorbed (Lindahl, 1961). Alternatively, a blister has been raised and removed to bare the dermis, to which test solutions can then be applied (Armstrong *et al.*, 1957). Using another technique the solution can be injected either intracutaneously or by jet injection (Lindahl, 1961). Clearly, all these methods are invasive by nature and can cause significant tissue damage. For these reasons they are not particularly suitable for experimental pain induction.

Electrical pain induction has been undertaken using microelectrode systems such as that employed by Hallin (1974) when investigating the effect of ketocaine on the C fibre afferent system. Notermans (1966), who also used electrical pain induction in the determination of pain thresholds by means of square wave current impulses, found that data generated in this way were reproducible. The technique was used to examine the pain sensed by neurological and neurosurgical patients (Notermans, 1967). By comparing affected and unaffected dermatomes, areas of altered sensation could be mapped with greater accuracy than could be achieved using the pin-pricking method.

Disadvantages associated with this technique are that it is time consuming to place the microelectrodes into the nerves and, further, electrical induction evokes responses that are not really representative of the natural situation where several nerve fibres will be triggered.

More recently, Kushla and Zatz (1990) reported the use of a Vitality Scanner to investigate the onset of skin anaesthesia following treatment by both infiltration anaesthesia (using both 1 and 2% lignocaine solutions) and topically applied local anaesthetics (using 5% lignocaine in either a cream base or as a solution in 40% propylene glycol). The instrument delivered a current of 0.1 mA through a 2 mm diameter flat metal probe. The former was automatically activated when electrical contact was made with skin. Voltage increased slowly (the rate of increase could be preset) from 15 to a maximum of 300 V. The electrical stimulation was delivered in a pulsed manner until a maximum digital reading of 80 was achieved. The scanner was removed from the skin once a mild "buzz" was felt. The results of the study are summarised in Figs 2.13 and 2.14. Clearly, the device was capable of demonstrating the different anaesthetic effects of infiltration and topical anaesthesia. For example, intradermal infiltration of lignocaine provided rapid onset of anaesthesia, in contrast to topically applied formulations which were left in contact with the skin for three hours before testing. It can be observed from Fig. 2.15 that only one of the topical formulations, the cream, was active and full anaesthesia, as defined by the maximum instrument reading, required about 5 hours to occur.

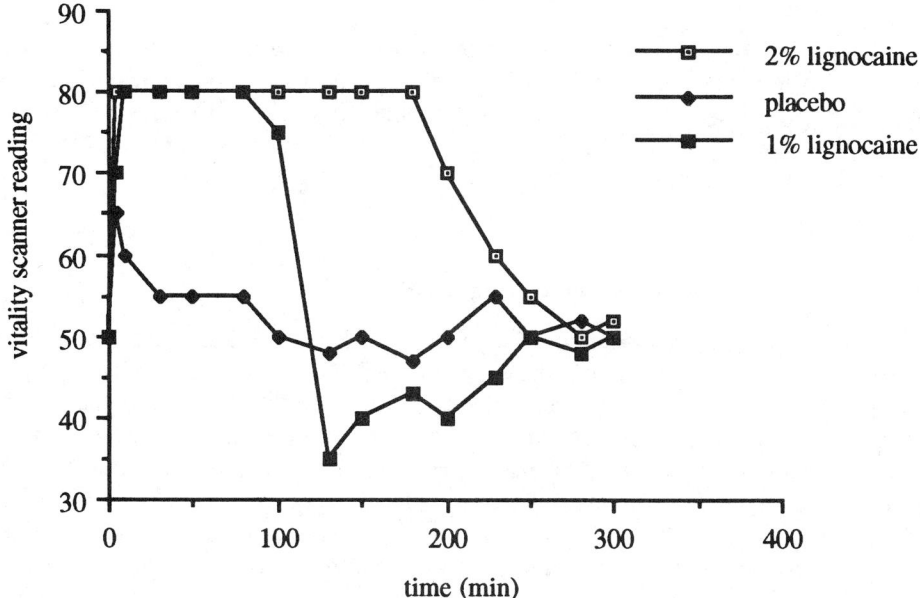

Fig. 2.13 — Measurement of skin anaesthesia, using a Vitality Scanner, following infiltration with a local anaesthetic (modified from Kushla and Katz, 1990)

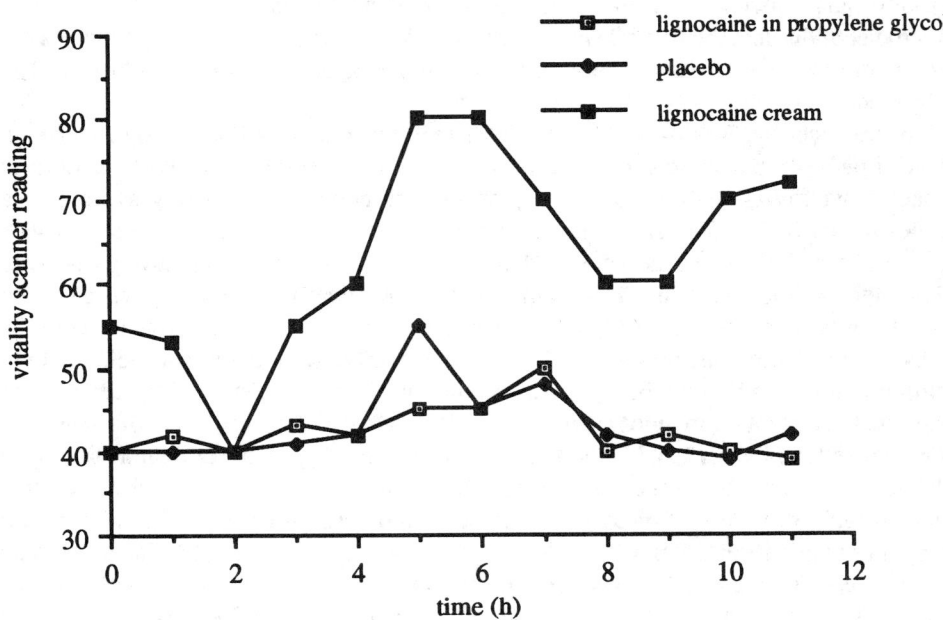

Fig. 2.14 — Measurement of skin anaesthesia, using a Vitality Scanner, following topical application of a local anaesthetic (modified from Kushla and Katz, 1990)

Although the device has the advantage of being a non-invasive technique, the maximum instrument reading may be a limiting factor in its use to discriminate between apparently similar anaesthetic preparations. It would, perhaps, be of interest to compare this method of experimental pain induction with the pin-prick technique using local anaesthesia as a model clinical situation.

2.4 PAIN PERCEPTION IN CHILDREN

Although it was originally thought that very young children (neonates) were incapable of feeling pain since myelinisation of the nerve fibres in neonates is incomplete, there is now substantial evidence that contradicts this theory. Despite the fact that, due to ethical considerations, there is little systematic data on the functional maturity of human neonatal physiology, it would appear that the neonate's spinal cord is intact and the pain receptors are present. However, there is some doubt as to whether or not the interconnections from the nociceptors to the gating mechanism in the substantia gelatinosa are complete. Furthermore, the neonate's motor ability in terms of responding to painful stimuli seems to be limited. Studies involving animals have indicated that there are significant physiological developments related to pain perception after birth. It has been reported that, although C fibres appear to be anatomically and neurochemically developed in young rats, it requires about three weeks after birth before full functional integrity occurs (Fitzgerald and Gibson, 1984). Similarly, Fitzgerald and

Kotzenburg (1986) have shown that the descending inhibitory pathways in the rat which are considered to inhibit the response to pain become functional only between the 9th and 22nd day of life. This may imply that young rats are much more sensitive to pain due to their incomplete inhibitory mechanism. It has been argued that the presence of a high threshold to painful stimuli in neonates would be useful in protecting the infant from pain during the birth process. In contrast, an ability to perceive pain and to respond appropriately could protect the child from potential harm by alerting its parents (Bondy, 1980).

Until comparatively recently it was thought that the infantile response to a noxious stimulus, such as pin-prick, was typified by a whole body motor response. It would require several weeks or months before the development of a localised motor response resulting in specific withdrawal of the affected site (Barr, 1983). Although it might appear initially that neonates do not have the motor ability to react, other than in a general way, to noxious stimuli, more recent research tends to undermine this theory. In a study involving response to heel lance by seventy-seven male and sixty-three female healthy neonates, it was observed that the infants' facial responses to heel rub (swabbing with alcohol soaked tissue) and heel lance (using a 4.9 mm long point microlance) were consistently different. This implies that neonates are quite capable of discriminating, in a specific manner, between comparatively painless and noxious stimuli. Although some differences in response were observed between sexes, it was not considered that these represented strong evidence for behavioural differences in male and female neonates. However, highly significant differences in infant facial activity were observed during the latter phase of blood collection, depending upon which laboratory technician was involved in the collection procedure. This suggests that the infants possessed considerable sensitivity to variations in handling (Grunau and Craig, 1987). In a similar study Franck (1986) examined the response of eight male and two female infants (approximate age 4 hours) to heel lance using photogrammetry. The infants clearly exhibited a dual response to the stimulation which consisted of an immediate withdrawal of both legs (0.12 - 0.7 seconds) followed by crying (1.5 - 2.5 seconds). The latter was often accompanied by vigorous, gross motor activity including facial grimacing and movement of all extremities. This type of two-component response indicates that the infant behaviour following a noxious stimulus is similar to adult reaction to first and second pain.

There have been several reports that there are physiological responses to pain by infants. These include changes in heart rate and pO_2 levels in response to heel prick (stick) and circumcision (Williamson and Williamson, 1983; Owens and Todt, 1984; Beaver, 1987; Johnston, 1989). Various hormonal and metabolic responses to surgery, probably due to pain, have also been reported (Anand and Aynsley-Green, 1985; Anand et al., 1987a,b). Plasma adrenaline, noradrenaline, insulin, glucagon and plasma cortisol responses as well as variations in blood glucose, lactate, pyruvate and alanine were each related to the severity of the surgical stress by means of a five factor stress score (Anand and Aynsley-Green, 1987).

It has also been reported that preterm neonates can experience pain, as shown by a stress response to surgery (Anand and Aynsley-Green, 1985), although it has also been suggested that this group does not respond to painful stimuli (D'Apolito, 1984). Interestingly, a study involving premature neonates in both minimal and intensive care units indicated that they exhibited behavioural and physiological changes to heel prick

(Field and Goldson, 1984). During the study neonates were assigned to one of three sections, namely, healthy term neonates, preterm neonates in minimal care and preterm neonates in intensive care. Each section was further divided into two groups, i.e. control and treated. Infants in the latter group were given a pacifier which was held in the child's mouth for the duration of the procedure. The neonates were observed for two minutes before the heel prick, during the actual procedure and, thereafter, for two further minutes. The following parameters were recorded during the observation period:

(a)   sleep/wake state; deep sleep, active sleep, drowsiness, alertness, active and fussy, crying,

(b)   heart and respiration rate,

(c)   presence of sucking behaviour.

Heart rate and respiration data were monitored only for neonates receiving minimal care or for those in intensive care. Comparatively small changes in heart rate were reported in both treated (i.e. with pacifier) and control neonates in intensive care during heel prick and no change in rate of respiration was observed. In contrast, there was a significant increase in heart and respiration rates for the preterm infants receiving minimal care. It was observed that the use of a pacifier was effective in reducing behavioural distress in both term and preterm neonates during the heel prick procedure, although only the infants receiving minimal care exhibited modified physiological responses when given a pacifier. It is possible that the absence of significant physiological reactions associated with neonates in intensive care may have been due to lack of coherence between physical activity and physiology (Obrist, 1981). The fact that intensive care based infants in the control group were more active behaviourally than the corresponding treated group, although their heart and respiration rates were similar, tends to support this hypothesis. Furthermore, the increase in heart rate, without the concomitant rise in respiration rate found with infants in intensive care, possibly indicates a lack of coordination within the cardiorespiratory system of this group. Respiratory influences on heart rate are markedly greater in infants without medical complications (Porges et al., 1982).

The memory of pain by children is usually illustrated by various anticipatory behavioural responses when, for example, the child sees the approach of a needle or even a person in a white laboratory coat. These anticipatory responses can include crying, defensive and withdrawal actions (Barr, 1983). Defensive actions such as crying, temper tantrums and fighting in anticipation to painful stimuli tend to occur more frequently from 6 months old to about 3 years old. Children younger than approximately 6 months do not exhibit this type of behaviour while in children older than 3 years the frequency of this behaviour decreases (Kassowitz, 1958; Levy, 1960). Although this lack of anticipatory behaviour in children less than 6 months old has been assumed, by some medical personnel, to indicate that pain memory in this group is poor, there is some evidence available that may refute this. In the study undertaken by Franck (1986), where infants' response to a heel lance was investigated, it was noted that the mean latency of withdrawal to the second heel lance was shorter than the first. This could be attributed to a learning process.

The perception of young children to the meaning of pain depends not only on their past experience of pain but also on the level of their cognitive ability. Children between the ages of 2 and 7 years tend to perceive the world in a purely materialistic way rather than in an abstract sense. This can lead to problems when this age group is faced with various medical procedures. For example, if a child attends a surgery for vaccination and subsequently has to revisit for some illness, the child will expect to get an injection. It is also difficult to explain to this group that an injection, which causes pain, is necessary to provide more comprehensive treatment of an illness (Gaffney and Dunne, 1987). Various investigations have been undertaken into the development of children's perception of pain. Gaffney and Dunne (1987) examined 680 children in the age group five to fourteen years where at least 30 children, of each sex, represented each age. These children were presented with a ten item sentence completion task which was designed to allow them to comment on their interpretation of pain under such headings as definition, cause, effect, cure, description and location of pain. The results of the study, in terms of pain-causing factors, were classified into 12 different groups:

(1)   illness, sickness, disease
(2)   malfunction - something was wrong
(3)   trauma
(4)   transgression involving eating
(5)   transgression involving other activities
(6)   transgression of adult rules or carelessness
(7)   health risk behaviours, e.g. smoking
(8)   transgression with the possibility of punishment
(9)   psychological factors, e.g. nervousness
(10)   physical requirements, e.g. hunger
(11)   physiological explanations, e.g. pain as a warning of something else
(12)   contamination, e.g. pain caused by microorganisms.

Approximately half of the children involved in this study described pain causation as originating from transgressions or in some way caused by themselves. It was also observed that more abstract and objective explanations of pain increased with the child's age. Furthermore, the female children put forward psychological reasons more frequently than did males as a basis for causing pain. Children's perception of pain changes gradually with age, i.e. as the child becomes older more abstract and complex concepts are used to define pain although some simplistic descriptions, characteristic of younger children, still remain (Gaffney and Dunne, 1986). An earlier study, involving 994 children aged between five and twelve years, disagreed with the above findings in that they found no age or sex differences as far as pain concepts, definition of pain, pain causality or the potential value of pain as a warning signal were concerned (Ross and Ross, 1984). Although there was no evidence from this study that younger children attributed some pain to punishment for their misbehaviour, virtually all children involved in the project would like a parent present if they were experiencing pain. A possible explanation as to why these studies contradicted each other was that they were all retrospective. Hence, pain perception described after the event might not represent that occurring during the event.

2.5   MEDICALLY INDUCED PAIN IN CHILDREN

It is generally accepted that one of the most difficult forms of paediatric pain to deal with is that inflicted on children during the course of medical treatment. The most frequent response by physicians to the medically induced pain they have caused is to turn away from the child (Neal, 1978). This can be interpreted as a form of denial in so far as some pain is necessary so that the therapy can be successful (McGrath and Unruh, 1987). The most frequent types of medically induced pain arise from routine neonates tests, such as heel pricks, and for immunisation. Heel pricks are used on virtually all children, in the first few hours of life, to collect a small volume of blood for various analyses (e.g. detection of phenylketonuria). It could be argued that the pain caused by these procedures should be acceptable, particularly since they will represent the extent to which most children will be exposed to medically induced pain. However, there are groups of children who receive a much greater exposure to pain caused by medical procedures. For example, children suffering from serious diseases, such as cancer or diabetes, will often have to withstand repeated painful procedures (venepunctures, injections, lumbar punctures, bone marrow aspirations). It has been reported that children undergoing repeated medical procedures that caused pain became sensitised (Katz *et al.*, 1980). Furthermore, it is now well recognised that children can be severely stressed by the process of hospitalisation. This is due to the fact that the child is separated from its normal environment (Blom, 1958). Children under about five years old react to frightening situations by seeking the comfort and protection of their parents and, although the present trend is to facilitate contact between hospitalised child and parent, the latter cannot be present constantly. In an early study involving 143 randomly chosen children undergoing tonsillectomy it was found that the main factors causing anxiety in these children (Figs 2.15 and 2.16) concerned hospitalisation, the operation, needles and anaesthesia (Blom, 1958). It was observed that there was a change in the relative importance of these areas of anxiety with age. For example, the fear of hospitalisation gradually decreased with increasing age (Fig. 2.16) whereas the greatest fear of needles appeared to come from children in the five to seven age group (Fig. 2.15). In a study undertaken by Eland (1981) it was reported that, when 242 hospitalised children (age range four to ten years) were asked which procedure produced the most pain, 49% replied "needles". Furthermore, the fact that injections appear to be a particular source of anxiety to children was highlighted in the Eland study when six of these children, who had undergone at least 25 surgical procedures, also quoted needles as their main painful experience. The authors have found, from their own experience, that young oncology patients became very distressed when receiving repeated venepunctures. In fact, not only were the children stressed but so, also, were the nursing staff, who often had to restrain a struggling child. Although there is less evidence to indicate whether or not infants habituate or sensitise, the impression is that habituation does not occur and that infants may be sensitised to medically induced pain (McGrath and Unruh, 1987).

Various studies have been undertaken to examine the response of children to the pain evoked during immunisation injections. In one such study (Craig *et al.*, 1984) the changes in pain expression in infants receiving routine immunisation injections within the first two years of life were systematically investigated. A system based on behavioural observation was developed which permitted coding of several types of expressive behaviour. In order to properly assess the diverse reactions to needle injections, a series of both vocal and non-vocal expressions, based on clinical experience

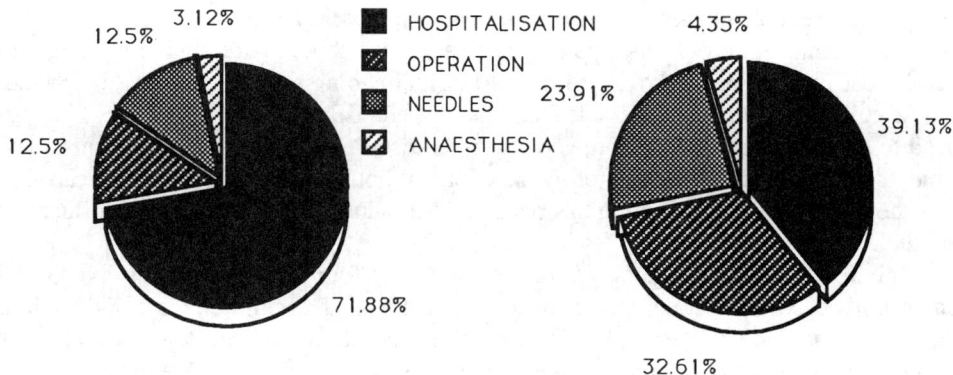

MAIN FOCUS OF ANXIETY
FOR 2-5 YEAR OLDS
(N = 32)

MAIN FOCUS OF ANXIETY
FOR 5-7 YEAR OLDS
(N = 46)

Fig. 2.15 — Main factors causing anxiety in children, aged 2-7 years, undergoing
tonsillectomy (modified from Blom, 1958)

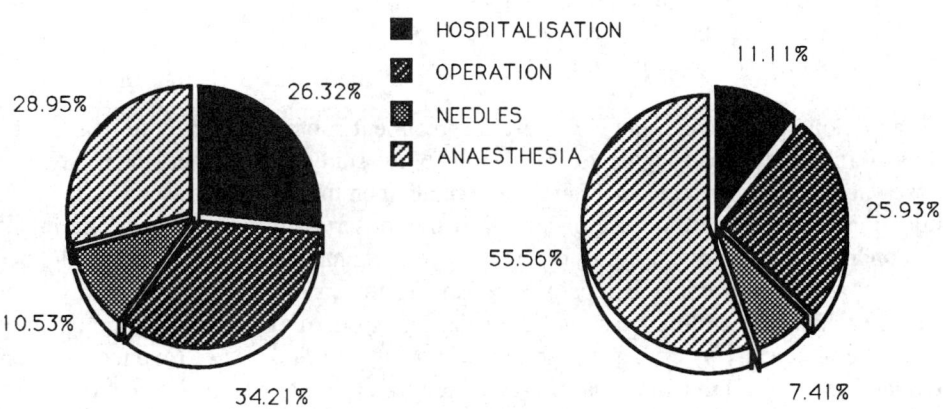

MAIN FOCUS OF ANXIETY
FOR 7-10 YEAR OLDS
(N = 38)

MAIN FOCUS OF ANXIETY
FOR 10-14 YEAR OLDS
(N = 27)

Fig. 2.16 — Main factors causing anxiety in children, aged 7-14 years, undergoing
tonsillectomy (modified from Blom, 1958)

as well as previous research (Cataldo *et al.*, 1979), were selected for observation. It is considered that studies of this type are necessary since children are routinely brought to clinics for immunisation procedures as part of an ongoing preventative health scheme. These children express considerable fear, anxiety and distress during injection, which can lead to avoidance of medical care and a general distaste of medical environments. The study also involved observation of the reactions of both mothers and the nurse carrying out the injection since the children's reaction to a painful stimulus could be influenced by their behaviour.

Children (30), whose age range was two to twenty-four months, were observed, with their mothers, while receiving immunisation injections. The children were divided into four groups according to sex and age so that differences in sex and developmental changes could be investigated. Group 1 included males, age range two to twelve months (mean age six months); group 2 contained females, age range two to twelve months (mean age five months); group 3 included males, age range thirteen to twenty-four months (mean age seventeen months); group 4 contained females, age range thirteen to twenty-four months (mean age fourteen months). The children, their mothers and the nurse were observed via a one-way mirror from the time they entered the treatment room until they left. Each mother was instructed by the nurse to hold their child on her lap and to expose the child's arm and hold it firmly. The various coding categories and summary of the child's, mother's and nurse's responses during the immunisation session are shown in Tables 2.1 and 2.2.

Each session was divided into three sections, which began as follows:

(1)   from the time the child entered the room,
(2)   when the nurse touched the syringe,
(3)   when the needle penetrated the child's skin.

Observation ceased when the child left the treatment room. Each section was further divided into five second segments. The results of the study indicated that the behavioural observation system provided substantial information on the children's responses to needle injections and justified the use of non-obtrusive observation techniques. The infants responded to the painful stimulus of the injection in a manner which would be defined, from an adult perspective, as a pain response. There was considerable diversity in the way in which the children responded to the injection. For example, although most reacted dramatically by crying, screaming, grimacing or writhing, two (one male and one female) did not exhibit the most frequent responses, i.e. crying and screaming. The study also indicated that there were a number of unusual responses to the injection which could be described as idiosyncratic pain behaviour.

There were quite significant development changes in pain expression, with children in groups 3 and 4 (i.e. the older infants of both sexes) crying and screaming for shorter periods. These groups orientated towards the site of the injection and tracked the nurse and their mothers to a greater extent than the other groups. They also protected and touched their limbs more often and exhibited less torso rigidity in reaction to the pain stimulus than the younger infants. The last two groups (the older male and female children) spoke before the injection more frequently than the younger infants. Overall there was little difference in response between male and female children although the latter visually anticipated the injection site whereas the former orientated to the injection site after the procedure had taken place. This lack of marked variation of pain response

Table 2.1 — Infant pain behaviour rating

Category	Sub-category	Definition
Vocal actions	Crying	Vocal expression characterised by high pitched, prolonged rhythmic and perhaps broken manner. Excludes meaningful utterances.
	Pain vocal	Nonverbal expression distinct from crying, i.e. screaming (single high pitched sound), groaning (deep sounds without wailing or sobbing), whining, moaning, gasping, choking, whimpering and sniffling.
	Pain/fear verbal	Use of language to express stress or fear. May include attempts to delay action or expression of physical discomfort indicative of autonomic activity.
	Other	Any verbal-vocal expression that cannot be classified otherwise - defined by exclusion.
Nonvocal - face	Distorted	Departure from neutral facial expression so as to distort facial musculature, i.e. wincing, grimacing. Excludes facial activity associated with crying.
	Eyes: injection	Head and eyes orientated to injection area, implying that it is being watched.
	Eyes: nurse	Head and eyes orientation implies watching nurse or needle.
	Eyes: mother	Head and eyes orientation implies watching mother.
	Eyes: closed	Condition that implies shutting off external input. Must be more than blinking.
Nonvocal - torso	Rigid	Maintenance of stiff posture in the gross torso musculature, i.e. body stiff.
	Withdrawing	Change in body posture so as to have the torso orientated away from the source of pain.
Nonvocal - limbs	Protect/touch	Placement of hand/forearm over injection site as if protecting area, vigorous movement of the arm away from nurse so as to avoid needle penetration or use of hand/arm to push away nurse's effect to insert needle. Rubbing/touching the injection site. Excludes holding the arm.
	Kick/thrash	Flailing of the legs and/or arms.

Reproduced from Craig *et al.* (1984) with permission of the copyright holder, Pergamon Press Ltd

Table 2.2 — Mother and nurse behavioural categories

Category	Sub-category	Definition
Verbal actions to the child	Praise	Statement positively evaluating or approving of prior, ongoing or future actions of the child.
	Criticism	Statements negatively evaluating or disapproving of child's actions.
	Distraction	Statement endeavouring to distract from medical procedure or its sequelae.
	Soothing	Attempt to calm child or alleviate pain.
	Procedural statement	Statements informing about current immunisation procedure.
	Other verbalisation	Those not encompassed by the above.
Verbal actions to another person	About child	Information about child, excluding pain procedure statements.
	Procedural statements	Concerning the injection procedure or the patient's reaction to it.
	Unrelated to child	Statements not encompassed by the above.
	No verbalisation	By exclusion.
Nonverbal behaviour	Pain expression	Any expression of pain or discomfort in face or bodily action.
	Vocal pain	Paralinguistic pain expression such as gasping or sighing.
	Physical distortion	Attempts to divert child's attention from medical procedure or its sequelae.
	Soothing	Attempts to calm the child or alleviate pain by hugging, kissing, bouncing or nursing.
	Physical restraint	Holding the child because of anticipated or real lack of cooperation.

Reproduced from Craig *et al*. (1984) with permission of the copyright holder, Pergamon Press Ltd

between male and female children is very much in contrast to the significant differences in pain expression found in adults of different sexes (Craig and Prkachin, 1983).

Problems associated with interpreting the results from these types of studies include the effect of the mother's behaviour on the overall response of the child to the pain stimulus. In other words, it is likely than the mother's reaction modulated the child's response to pain. Although each mother was effectively asked to restrain her child for the injection, the force used and the vocal and verbal behaviour of the mother would clearly vary from one individual to the next. It was observed that during the immunisation procedure mothers, in general, tended to verbally calm the younger age groups more frequently than the older children. Vocal distraction techniques were more often used for the latter. The effect of this type of variation in the mother's behaviour on the child's response to pain would need to be examined. In contrast, the nurse's interaction with both mothers and children was consistent throughout the four groups.

2.6   MEASUREMENT AND EVALUATION OF PAIN IN CHILDREN

Measuring the degree of pain suffered by children undergoing various medical procedures is much more difficult than in adults. Although adults may express, in verbal terms, the site, quantity and type of pain being experienced, children may be restricted from accomplishing this due to their age, lower cognitive ability and verbal skills, stage of development and lower level of emotional maturity. Although it has been difficult to propose a definition of pain which is universally accepted, the International Association for the Study of Pain has tried to establish a standard definition of pain as "an unpleasant sensory and emotional experience associated with actual or potential tissue damage or described in terms of such damage" (Merskey, 1986). Even with adults pain can be a difficult parameter to measure due to its subjective nature. However, attempts to measure pain can be undertaken in several different ways. For example, individuals can report on their response to the pain stimulus (i.e. subjectively), their behavioural response to pain can be observed and quantified by an independent observer, or their physiological responses to pain can be measured.

Clearly, many factors can influence the child's ability to describe pain. Hence, several researchers have used the behaviour pattern of the preoperational child in the study of painful stimuli (McCaffery, 1972; Hester, 1979). Scientific studies have attempted to establish methods to measure components of pain such as quality, duration, intensity and threshold. One of the most difficult pain parameters to determine in children is quantifying the pain response. Initially most scales and assessment tools used to measure pain in children were based on those developed for adults. However, these were found to be unsatisfactory since children had limited verbal capacity and their body activity did not adequately meet the criteria on the rating scale. A further difficulty associated with the assessment of pain in children, and particularly in young children, is that this group often has had limited experience of pain.

It has been suggested that a distinction should be made between the measurement and assessment of pain. Measurement can be perceived as a quantitative parameter in terms of pain intensity whereas assessment involves the measurement of the interaction of other factors on the experience of pain, such as the the environment in which the child receives the painful stimulus (McGrath and Unruh, 1987). Measurement of children's pain is essential so that appropriate and sufficient pain relief tactics can be employed to adequately control the pain which the child is experiencing. There are many reports in the literature of the use of insufficient postoperative analgesics in children, which can be attributed, at least partly, to the absence of properly validated methods for measuring pain in children. If, for example, there are treatments to obviate or reduce medically induced pain, then appropriate measurement tools are necessary to determine the efficacy of such treatments.

It is possible to divide the concept of the pain event into several different parameters. These include the cognitive or self-report parameter, the behavioural parameter and the physiological parameter. Furthermore, various different measurement strategies can be applied to each parameter. Alternatively, the pain event may be conceptualised as pain sensations and reactions to pain (Melzack, 1983). The choice of a system for measuring pain should be determined by the type of clinical situation involved. For example, the type of measurement tool used to examine medically induced pain (and, perhaps, its alleviation) such as venepuncture would be quite different to that employed to investigate chronic abdominal pain.

2.6.1   Cognitive parameter of pain

The International Association for the Study of Pain has stated that "pain is always subjective" (Merskey, 1986) and, indeed, the cognitive parameter of pain refers to the various emotions, visual, verbal and written reactions of an individual to the experience of pain. The cognitive or self-report parameter of pain has been widely used as a way to measure pain in adults and is becoming increasingly common in the determination of pain in children. However, one of the major difficulties associated with the former is that the way in which the child perceives the question can actually influence the answer given. For example, if children are asked, following an operation, whether or not they are in pain, a negative reply is often provided. This is due to the fact that the admission of pain, as far as the child is concerned, will result in an injection being given. Hence, the children's fear of needles provokes an incorrect response as far as measurement of pain is concerned (Eland and Anderson, 1977). It has also been demonstrated that the person asking the questions can influence the response obtained, i.e. different responses were given, by children, to their mothers when compared to those given to their physicians (Ross and Ross, 1984).

A further problem with the use of the cognitive parameter in children is the difficulty, particularly with very young children, they may have in understanding and, hence, being able to respond sensibly, to the questions. It is important, when attempting to measure children's pain, that specific questions are asked so that the pain perceived can be quantified. Despite this, it has been observed that, even when specific questions have been used, children have overestimated the frequency, intensity and duration of their pain by very substantial margins (Andrasik *et al.*, 1985).

A number of verbal scales have been developed to measure pain in children. Some of these are only suitable for older children who can understand the terminology used and hence describe their pain appropriately (Melzack, 1975). In a study undertaken by Hester (1979) a number of poker chips were used to measure the pain of immunisation in a group of preoperational children whose ages ranged from four years seven months to six years eight months. If children responded that they had not felt hurt during the procedure a zero reading was recorded. However, if, on the other hand, children had been hurt, they were asked to quantity the amount of hurt by choosing 1 to 4 poker chips. Since each poker chip represented a "piece of hurt" the more chips selected the greater the pain felt during immunisation. The reason for using this method was that most children less than eight years old do not know the meaning of pain but do understand the word "hurt" and they tend to use images or symbols to represent abstract concepts such as pain (Mussen, 1973). A modified version of Eland's Projective Tool was also used for comparison purposes. This pain measurement device concerns the use of a series of pictures involving a rabbit, i.e. a rabbit resting on top of a dog house; a rabbit hit on the head by a swing whilst playing; a rabbit falling off the roof of the dog house and bumping its head; a rabbit getting its paw caught in a car door. Each child was asked to rank the pictures from least to most hurt, after which the child was shown a picture of a rabbit getting an injection. The child then had to insert this picture in rank order of pain amongst the others. The results of the study indicated that the poker chip tool was more strongly correlated with vocal and verbal behaviours than was Eland's tool. Interestingly, both tools were negatively correlated with facial expressions. It was possible that this occurred because the latter may be used by children as gating mechanisms to alleviate pain (Melzack and Wall, 1969). An explanation as to why the poker chip tool was better correlated with vocal, verbal and motor behaviours than the Eland tool may have been due to the forced collation nature of the latter. In other words the child had to rank the pain using Eland's tool rather than equate the pain in terms of the number of poker chips. It is likely that the poker chip method would be useful in quantifying the reduction of pain provided by the application of topical percutaneous local anaesthetic formulations.

One of the most popular methods for measuring pain in children, particularly under the age of eight, has been the face scale. Several variations of this technique have been employed in clinical research with young children undergoing medical procedures (Venham and Gaulin-Kremer, 1979; LeBaron and Zeltzer, 1984; Beyer and Aradine, 1987). In face-type scales, five to nine faces depicting expressions ranging from very happy to very distressed are shown to children who then choose the face that best represents their degree of pain (Fig. 2.17). A numerical scoring system can be used in collaboration with the faces. However, it has been suggested there is little evidence available to support the predictive nature of this type of methodology (Carpenter, 1990).

A new method has recently been reported which provides a self-report method for measuring pain and fear in young children. This technique, Children's Global Rating Scale (CGRS), is based on the association of wavy lines radiating from cartoon characters with the depiction of pain or fear (Carpenter, 1990). The wavier the line the greater the pain or fear. A flat line, representing no pain, is followed by four further lines, where each successive line becomes increasingly wavy. Each line has a number (0 - 4) associated with it and this can be used for older children. The advantage of this system is that it is simple to use. For example, if the straight line means no pain or fear then the progressively wavier lines represent increasing pain and fear and the waviest line represents the most pain and fear the child has ever experienced. In the study 145 children, age range four - eight years, were asked to assess their anticipatory fear and pain before a venepuncture procedure required to obtain a blood sample. Medical staff rated the children's distress during the procedure on the basis of whether or not it prolonged the usual time required for treatment. These results were then correlated with those of the children to examine if the CGRS technique was able to predict actual distress during the clinical procedure. The results of this study provided support for the convergent and predictive ability of CGRS. The children's anticipatory CGRS pain scores were significantly correlated with both parents' and clinical observers' measures of the children's anticipatory distress independently taken at the same time. Age, sex or race of the children had no effect on their CGRS score. It may be that this type of technique could be used for children within this age group to assess the modification of their anticipatory fear and pain perceptions about venepuncture when a topical percutaneous local anaesthetic formulation is used prior to such a medical procedure.

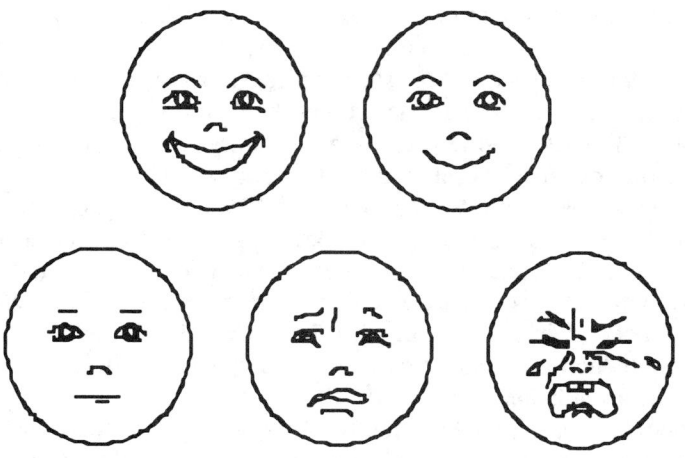

Fig. 2.17 — Typical faces scale for pain assessment in children

Assessment of pain in children in the older age groups becomes less difficult due to their increasing verbal and communicative skills. Therefore, various forms of verbal, as well as visual, pain measurements can be used (Beyer and Wells, 1989; Tesler et al., 1991). Wilkie et al. (1990), in a study undertaken on children from the ages of eight to seventeen years, developed a word list to assess pain quality. Although the results indicated substantial test-retest reliability of the word list scores, the list required both revision and extension to 56 words to produce results relatively free from gender, ethnic and development biases. Since many older children learn to control their facial expression and crying during painful experiences, these indications will not give a reliable assessment of pain. However, physiological determinations such as the Palmar Sweat Index (PSI) may be useful in assessing painful experiences (Gedaly-Duff, 1989). The PSI technique calculates the number of sweating glands in a 4 mm^2 area of a fingertip and studies the patterns and relationships of palmar sweat to painful experience.

2.7 CONCLUSIONS

It is quite clear from the many reports discussed in this chapter that any techniques that will reduce the level of stress in children undergoing invasive medical procedures are to be welcomed. One of the most common of these involves the insertion of a needle. This may be for blood sampling or for providing medication. Since the fear of needles seems to be a major factor in raising the level of apprehension in children, methods which could reduce, or obviate, the pain associated with needles would be of considerable clinical benefit. Furthermore, it has been our experience that, in many cases, the reaction of a child, reacting from both fear and pain, has a stressful effect on medical staff and parents, if they are present. Therefore, one method which would reduce this trauma would be the use of an effective, topically applied percutaneous local anaesthetic. The clinical applications of this specific technique for controlling pain are discussed fully in Chapter 6.

REFERENCES

Adriani, J. and Dalili, H. (1971) Penetration of local anaesthetics through epithelial barriers. *Anesth. Analg.* **50** 834-841.

Anand, K.J.S. and Aynsley-Green, A. (1985) Metabolic and endocrine effects of surgical ligation of patent ductus arteriosus in the human preterm neonate: Are there implications for further improvement of postoperative outcome? *Mod. Probl. Paediatr.* **23** 143-157.

Anand, K.J.S. and Aynsley-Green, A. (1987) Measuring the severity of surgical stress in newborn infants. *J. Pediatr. Surg.* **23** 297-305.

Anand, K.J.S., Sippell, W.G. and Aynsley-Green, A. (1987a) Randomised trial of fentanyl anaesthesia in preterm babies undergoing surgery: Effects on the stress response. *Lancet* **i** 243-247.

Anand, K.J.S., Sippell, W.G. and Aynsley-Green, A. (1987b) Does the newborn infant require anaesthesia during surgery? Answers from a randomised trial of halothane anaesthesia. V World Congress on Pain, Hamburg. *Pain suppl.* **4** S451.

Andrasik, F., Burke, E.J., Attanasio, V. and Rosenblum, E.L. (1985) Child, parent and physician reports of a child's headache pain: Relationships prior to and following treatment. *Headache* **25** 421-425.

Armstrong, D., Jepson, J., Keele, C. and Stewart, J. (1957) Pain producing substance in human inflammatory exudates and plasma. *J. Physiol.* **135** 356-370.

Barr, R. (1983) Variations on the theme of pain: 28A pain tolerance and developmental change in pain perception. In: Levine, M.D., Carey, W.B., Crocker, A.C. and Gross, R.T. (eds) *Developmental behavioural pediatrics.* Saunders, Philadelphia, pp. 505-512.

Bazett, H.C., McGlone, B. and Brocklehurst, R.J. (1930) The temperatures in tissues which accompany temperature sensations. *J. Physiol.* **69** 88-112.

Beaver, P.K. (1987) Premature infants' response to touch and pain: Can nurses make a difference? *Neonatal Network* **6** 13-17.

Beecher, H.K. (1957) The measurement of pain: Prototype for the quantitative study of subjective responses. *Pharmacol. Rev.* **9** 59-209.

Beyer, J.E. and Aradine, C.R. (1987) Patterns of pediatric pain intensity: a methodological investigation of a self report scale. *Clin. J. Pain* **3** 130-141.

Beyer, J.E. and Wells, N. (1989) The assessment of pain in children. *Pediatric Clinics of*

North America **36** 837-854.

Blom, G.E. (1958) The reactions of hospitalised children to illness. *Pediatrics* **22** 590-600.

Bondy, A.S. (1980) Infancy. In: Gabel, S. and Erickson, M.T. (eds) *Child development and development disabilities.* Little Brown, Boston, pp. 3-19.

Bowsher, D. (1979) *Introduction to the anatomy and physiology of the nervous system.* 4th. edn, Blackwell Scientific, London.

Brodal, A. (1981) *Neurological anatomy in relation to clinical medicine.* Oxford University Press, London.

Carpenter, P.J. (1990) New method for measuring young children's self-report of fear and pain. *J. Pain Sympt. Manag.* **5** 233-240.

Cataldo, M.F., Bessman, C.A., Parker, L.H., Pearson, J.E.R. and Rogers, M.C. (1979) Behavioural assessment for pediatric intensive care units. *J. Appl. Behav. Anal.* **12** 83-97.

Campbell, J.N. and LaMotte, R.H. (1983) Latency to detection of first pain. *Brain Res.* **266** 203-208.

Craig, K.D., McMahon, R.J., Moroson, J.D. and Zaskow, C. (1984) Development changes in infant pain expression during immunisation injections. *Soc. Sci. Med.* **19** 1331-1337.

Craig, K.D. and Prkachin, K.M. (1983) Nonverbal measures of pain. In: Melzack, R. (ed.) *Pain measurement and assessment.* Raven Press, New York, pp. 173-179.

D'Apolito, K. (1984) The neonate's response to pain. *Matern. Child Nurs.* **9** 256-257.

Duthie, D.J.R. (1989) The physiology and pharmacology of pain. In: Nimmo,W.S. and Smith, G. (eds) *Anaesthesia.* Blackwell Scientific Publications, London. pp. 60-72.

Eland, J.M. (1981) Minimising pain associated with prekindergarten intramuscular injections. *Issues Compr. Pediatr. Nurs.* **71** 36-40.

Eland, J.M. and Anderson, J.E. (1977) The experience of pain in children. In: Jacox, A.K. (ed.) *Pain: A sourcebook for nurses and other health professionals.* Little Brown, Boston, MA, pp. 453-473.

Elliot, H.C. (1969) *Textbook of neuroanatomy.* 2nd. edn, Lippincott, Philadelphia.

Erlanger, J. and Grasser, H.S. (1937) *The electrical signs of nervous activity.* University of Pennsylvania Press, Philadelphia.

Fields, H.L. (1987) *Pain.* McGraw-Hill, New York.

Field, T. and Goldson, E. (1984) Pacifying effects of non-nutritive sucking on term and preterm neonates during heelstick procedures. *Pediatrics* **74** 1012-1015.

Fitzgerald, M. and Gibson, S. (1984) The postnatal physiological and neurochemical development of peripheral sensory C fibres. *Neuroscience* **13** 933-944.

Fitzgerald, M. and Kotzenburg, M. (1986) The functional development of descending inhibitory pathways in the dorsolateral funiculus of the newborn rat spinal cord. *Development. Brain Res.* **24** 261-270.

Franck, L.S. (1986) A new method to quantitatively describe pain behaviour in infants. *Nurs. Res.* **35** 28-31.

Gaffney, A. and Dunne, E.A. (1986) Developmental aspects of children's definition of pain. *Pain* **26** 105-117.

Gaffney, A. and Dunne, E.A. (1987) Children's understanding of the causality of pain. *Pain* **29** 91-104.

Gedaly-Duff, V. (1989) Palmar sweat index use with children in pain research. *Journal of*

Pediatric Nursing **4** 3-8.

Gracely, R.H. (1989) Methods of testing pain mechanisms in normal man. In: Wall, P.D. and Melzack, R. (eds) *Textbook of Pain*. Churchill Livingstone, New York, pp. 257-268.

Grunau, R.V.E. and Craig, K.D. (1987) Pain expression in neonates: facial action and cry. *Pain* **28** 395-410.

Gybels, J., Handwerker, H.O. and Van Hess, J. (1979) A comparison between the discharges of human nociceptive nerve fibres and the subject's ratings of his sensations. *J. Physiol.* **292** 193-206.

Hallin, R.G. (1974) Blocking effects of a topical anaesthetic composition containing ketocaine on cutaneous C receptors responses in alert man. *Acta Anaesthesiol. Scand.* **18** 306-312.

Hensel, H. and Boman, K.K.A. (1960) Afferent impulses in cutaneous sensory nerves in human subjects. *J. Neurophysiol.* **23** 564-578.

Hensel, H., Iggo, A. and Witt, I. (1960) Quantitative study of sensitive cutaneous thermoreceptors with C afferent fibres. *J. Physiol. (Lond.)* **153** 113-126.

Hester, N.K.O. (1979) The preoperational child's reaction to immunisation. *Nursing Research* **28** 250-255.

Iggo, A. (1957a) Gastrointestinal tension receptors with unmyelinated fibres in the vagus of the cat. *Q. J. Exp. Physiol.* **42** 130-143.

Iggo, A. (1957b) Gastric mucosal chemoreceptors with vagal afferent fibres in the cat. *Q. J. Exp. Physiol.* **42** 398-409.

Iggo, A. (1974) Pain receptors. In: Bonica, J.J., Procacci, P. and Pagni, C.A. (eds), *Recent advances on pain*. C.C. Thomas, Illinois, pp. 3-36.

Iggo, A. (1977) Cutaneous and subcutaneous sense organs. *Brit. Med. Bull.* **33** 97-102.

Iggo, A. (1982) Cutaneous sensory mechanisms. In: Barlow, H.B. and Mollon, J.D. (eds) *The senses*. Cambridge University Press, Cambridge, pp. 369-409.

Johnston, C.C. (1989) Pain assessment and management in infants. *Pediatrician* **16** 16-23.

Juhlin, L., Evers, H. and Broberg, F. (1980) A lignocaine-prilocaine cream for superficial skin surgery and painful lesions. *Acta Derm. Scand.* **60** 544-546.

Kassowitz, K.E. (1958) Psychodynamic reactions of children to the use of hypodermic needles. *Am. Med. Assoc. J. Dis. Child.* **95** 253-257.

Katz, E.R., Kellerman, J. and Siegel, S.E. (1980) Behavioural distress in children with cancer undergoing medical procedures: developmental considerations. *J. Consult Clin. Psychol.* **48** 356-365.

Keele, C.A. (1966) Chemically induced pain. In: DeReuck, A.V.S. and Knight, J. (eds) *Touch, heat and pain*. J. and A. Churchill Ltd., London.

Keele, C.A. and Armstrong, D. (1964) *Substances producing pain and itch*. Edward Arnold, London.

Kohlloffel, L.U.E., Kolzenburg, M. and Handwerker, H.O. (1991) A novel technique for the evaluation of mechanical pain and hyperalgesia. *Pain* **46** 81-87.

Kushla, G.P. and Zatz, J.L. (1990) Evaluation of a noninvasive method for monitoring percutaneous absorption of lidocaine *in vivo*. *Pharm. Res.* **7** 1033-1037.

LeBaron, S and Zeltzer, L. (1984) Assessment of acute pain and anxiety in children and adolescents by self-reports, observer reports and a behaviour checklist. *J. Consult. Clin. Psychol.* **22** 690-701.

Levy, D.M. (1960) The infant's earliest memory of inoculation: a contribution to public health procedures. *J. Genet. Psychol.* **96** 3-46.

Lindahl, O. (1961) Experimental skin pain induced by injection of water-soluble substances in humans. *Acta Physiol. Scand.* **51** 1-89.

Lubens, H.M. and Sanker, J.F. (1964) Anaesthetic skin patch. *Ann. Allergy* **22** 37-41.

McCaffery, M. (1972) *Nursing management of the patient with pain.* J.B. Lippincott, Philadelphia.

McCafferty, D.F., Woolfson, A.D., McClelland, K.H. and Boston, V. (1988) Comparative *in-vivo* and *in-vitro* assessment of the percutaneous absorption of local anaesthetics. *Brit. J. Anaesth.* **60** 164-69.

McCafferty, D.F. and Woolfson, A.D. (1990) The cusum technique: a statistical method for predicting the optimum application time for percutaneous local anaesthesia with a novel formulation. In: Hadgraft, J., Guy, R.H. and Scott, R.C. (eds) *Prediction of Percutaneous penetration: methods, measurements and modelling.* IBC, London, pp. 372-376.

McGrath, P.J. and Unruh, A.M. (1987) *Pain in children and adolescents.* Elsevier, Amsterdam.

Melzack, R. (1972) *The puzzle of pain.* Basic Books, New York.

Melzack, R. (1975) The McGill pain questionnaire: Major properties and scoring methods. *Pain* **1** 277-299.

Melzack, R. (1983) In: Melzack, R. (ed.) *Pain measurement and assessment.* Raven Press, New York, pp. 1-6.

Melzack, R. and Wall, P.D. (1965) Pain mechanisms: A new theory. *Science* **150** 971-979.

Melzack, R. and Wall, P.D. (1969) Pain mechanisms: A new theory. In: Pribram, K.H. (ed.) *Brain and behaviour. Volume 2. Perception and action.* Harmondsworth, Penguin Books, England, pp. 139-158.

Merskey, H. (1986) Classification of chronic pain: description of chronic pain syndromes and definitions of pain terms. *Pain suppl.* **3** S217.

Mongar, J.L. (1955) A study of two methods for testing local anaesthetics in man. *Br. J. Pharmacol.* **10** 240-246.

Mussen, P.H. (1973) *The psychological development of the child.* 2nd edn Prentice-Hall, Englewood Cliffs, N.J.

Neal, H. (1978) *The politics of pain.* McGraw-Hill, New York.

Notermans, S.L.H. (1966) Measurement of the pain threshold determined by electrical stimulation and its clinical application: Part I. Method and factors possibly influencing the pain threshold. *J. Neurology* **16** 1071-1086.

Notermans, S.L.H. (1967) Measurement of the pain threshold determined by electrical stimulation and its clinical application: Part 2. Clinical application in neurological and neurosurgical patients. *J. Neurology* **17** 58-73.

Obrist, P.A. (1981) *Cardiovascular psychophysiology.* Plenum Publishing Corp., New York.

Owens, M.E. and Todt, E.H. (1984) Pain in infancy: Neonatal response to heel lance. *Pain* **20** 77-86.

Petterson, L.O. (1978) Percutaneous anaesthesia for some minor surgical procedures. *Scand. J. Plast. Reconstr. Surg.* **12** 283-287.

Porges, S.W., McCabe, P.M. and Younge, B.G. (1982) Respiratory-heart rate interactions: Psychophysiological implications for pathophysiology and behaviour. In: Cacioppo, J.T. and Petty, R.E. (eds) *Perspectives in cardiovascular psychophysiology.* Guilford Press, New York.

Price, D.D., Hu, J.W., Dubner, R. and Gracely, R.H. (1977) Peripheral suppression of first pain and central summation of second pain evoked by noxious heat pulses. *Pain.* **3** 307-338.

Procacci, P., Della-Corte, M., Zoppi, M., Romano, S., Maresca, M. and Voegelin, M.R. (1974) Pain thresholds measurements in man. In: Bonica, J.J., Procacci, P. and Pagni, C.A. (eds) *Recent advances on pain.* C.C. Thomas, Illinois, pp. 105-148.

Ranson, S.W. and Clarke, S.L. (1959) *The anatomy of the nervous system.* 10th. edn, W.B. Saunders & Co., London.

Ross, D.M. and Ross, S.A. (1984) Childhood pain: the school-aged child's viewpoint. *Pain* **20** 179-191.

Russo, J. (Jnr.), Lipmann, A.G., Comstock, T.J., Page, B.C. and Stephen, R.L. (1980) Lignocaine anaesthesia: Comparison of iontophoresis, injection and swabbing. *Am. J. Hosp. Pharm.* **37** 843-847.

Schmidt, R.F. (1981) Somatovisceral sensibility. In: Schmidt, R.F. (ed.) *Fundamentals of sensory physiology.* 2nd edn., Springer-Verlag, Berlin, pp. 81-126.

Sinclair, D. (1981) *The mechanisms of cutaneous sensations.* 2nd. edn., Oxford University Press, London.

Tesler, M.D., Saveda, M.C., Holzemer, W.L., Wilkie, D.J., Ward, J.A. and Paul, S.M. (1991) The word-graphic rating scale as a measure of children's and adolescents' pain intensity. *Research in Nursing and Health* **14** 361-371.

Venham, L.L. and Gaulin-Kremer, E. (1979) A self-report measure of situational anxiety for young children. *Pediatr. Dent.* **1** 91-96.

Wall, P.D. (1974) Physiological mechanisms involved in the production and relief of pain. In: Bonica, J.J., Procacci, P. and Pagni, C.A. (eds) *Recent advances on pain.* C.C. Thomas, Illinois, pp. 36-64.

Wall, P.D. (1978) The gate control theory of pain mechanisms: A re-examination and re-statement. *Brain* **101** 1-18.

Williamson, P.S. and Williamson, M.L. (1983) Physiologic stress reduction by a local anesthetic during newborn circumcision. *Pediatrics* **71** 36-40.

Wilkie, D.J., Holzemer, W.L., Tesler, M.D., Ward, J.A., Paul, S.M. and Saveda, M.C., (1990) Measuring pain quality: Validity and reliability of children's and adolescents' pain language. *Pain* **41** 151-159.

Zimmermann, M. (1981) Neurophysiology of sensory systems. In: Schmidt, R.F. (ed.) *Fundamentals of sensory physiology.* 2nd edn, Springer-Verlag, Berlin, pp. 31-81.

Zotterman, Y. (1959) Thermal sensations. In: Field, J., Magoun, H.W. and Hall, V.E. (eds) *Handbook of physiology.* Section 1: *Neurophysiology* vol. 1, Washington, pp. 431-458.

3

Local anaesthetics

Local anaesthetics, drugs which reversibly block impulse conduction when applied to nerve tissue, have now been in medical use for more than a century. Percutaneous local anaesthesia, however, represents a new route of absorption, and, consequently, new clinical applications for this class of drugs. Although much has been written about the properties of local anaesthetic drugs, the information is sometimes inappropriate when considering their percutaneous application. After all, it is not so long since the accepted wisdom was that local anaesthetic drugs did not penetrate the skin barrier. Consideration of the topical application of local anaesthetics was then confined to applications made to mucosal epithelia and to damaged or abraded skin where the absorption route was open. It is therefore appropriate, given the knowledge that effective percutaneous anaesthesia of intact skin can now be achieved, to look again at the properties of local anaesthetic drugs. In particular, physicochemical properties, together with anaesthetic potency, toxicity, sensitisation potential and absorption characteristics, are important factors in the selection of candidate local anaesthetics for percutaneous delivery.

3.1 A SHORT HISTORY OF LOCAL ANAESTHETICS

Natives of the Andes Mountains region of Peru were certainly the first known users of a local anaesthetic, albeit in crude drug form. Chewing of the leaves of the *Coca* shrub, *Erythroxylon coca*, an indigenous species in the area, produced both numbness of the tongue and intense central nervous system stimulation. The extraction of the active principle from the leaves of *Erythroxylon coca* yielded the alkaloids erythroxylon, identified by Gaedcke in 1855, and cocaine (Fig. 3.1) , reported by Niemann (1860).

The local anaesthetic properties of cocaine were first noted almost a decade after its

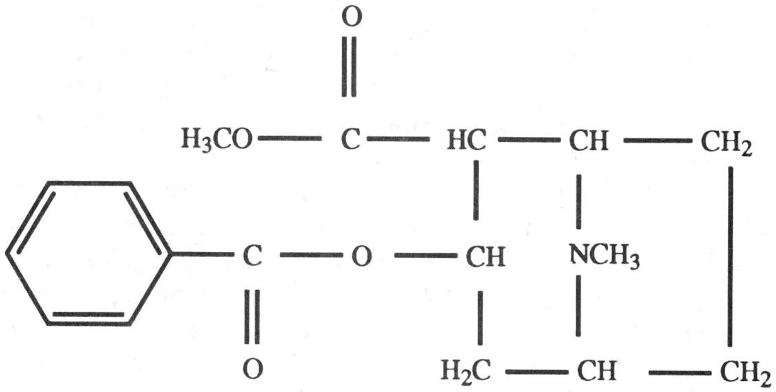

Fig. 3.1 — Structure of cocaine

introduction by a Peruvian army surgeon, who also recorded the less attractive properties of the drug. Von Anrep, in 1880, infiltrated the drug subcutaneously, and recognised its potential as a local anaesthetic. Recognition of the clinical importance of the drug is now usually ascribed to Koller (Becker, 1963) who, having been introduced to the properties of cocaine by Freud (Freud, 1884), instilled it into the eye. The resulting insensitivity of the cornea lasted for about ten minutes. This led to the widespread use of cocaine as an ophthalmic anaesthetic.

By the beginning of the twentieth century administration of cocaine by injection could produce effective peripheral nerve blockade. The drug was also used for infiltration and spinal anaesthesia. As was the case with many other classes of drugs, enthusiasm for the initial discovery was reduced by an increased awareness of the side effects of cocaine, notably its acute systemic toxicity and the chronic problems resulting from physical addiction to the drug. The molecular structure of cocaine was therefore used as a progenitor of new, synthetic drugs designed to enhance the local anaesthetic properties of cocaine, and to reduce or eliminate undesirable side effects.

Cocaine is an ester of benzoic acid. Changing the esterifying alcohol was a relatively simple chemical procedure and led to the rapid discovery of the first members of the ester class of local anaesthetics. Benzocaine was synthesised in 1890, and is still in clinical use today. In 1905, Einhorn introduced the first para-aminobenzoic acid derivative, procaine (Einhorn and Uhlfelder, 1909). Procaine had a significantly more favourable therapeutic ratio than cocaine, leading to its use both for regional blockade and infiltration anaesthesia. Other para-aminobenzoic acid derivatives rapidly followed the introduction of procaine, and all of these agents are still in common clinical use. Amethocaine, the most lipophilic and, consequently, the most potent para-aminobenzoic acid derivative, was reported in 1929 (Eisler, 1929) with chloroprocaine, a less toxic but also less potent drug, following about twenty years later.

Hypersensitivity reactions following sensitisation to the ester group of local anaesthetics were a feature of their early use. How many such reactions were true allergic responses, and how many were due to impure synthetic compounds, or application to sensitive or damaged areas, remains a subject of debate. Nevertheless, the need for an alternative class of agents was established. Thus, the synthesis of cinchocaine, a toxic but long-lasting local anaesthetic, was reported by Uhlmann (1929), an accidental discovery following a study on the antipyretic activity of acetanilides. Interestingly, this drug was originally named percaine. Confusion with the similarly named procaine led to several fatal episodes, and the drug was therefore renamed. Cinchocaine was an amide rather than an ester, and was thus the forerunner of the second major group of local anaesthetics.

In 1948 the synthesis of lignocaine, another amide with local anaesthetic properties, was reported (Lofgren and Lundqvist, 1948). Again, as with cinchocaine, serendipidity played a significant part in the discovery of lignocaine. Although many such amides with local anaesthetic properties had been synthesised, lignocaine was of particular significance in that, unlike earlier members of this class, it caused little irritation on injection. It is now generally accepted that the amide local anaesthetics also cause fewer allergic reactions than members of the ester group. The difference in the linkage (ester or amide) between the aromatic group and the sidechain also has important consequences for drug stability and, thus, for metabolic deactivation.

Following the synthesis of lignocaine, which itself established a pre-eminence for Sweden in the whole area of local anaesthesia, a range of other amide local anaesthetics have been produced, offering the clinician a choice in potency, duration of action, toxicity and route of application. The most recent edition of The Extra Pharmacopoeia (Martindale, 1989) lists almost forty different local anaesthetic agents, not all of which fit the ester or amide classification. Wildsmith and Strichartz (1984) have considered many of these agents from a historical perspective. Despite the number of local anaesthetic drugs that have been discovered, the search continues for new molecular structures with conduction blockade properties, but with superior therepeutic and toxicological profiles (Covino, 1982). For example, the local anaesthetic properties of ropivacaine, a new amino-amide drug similar in activity to bupivacaine, but with reduced toxicity, have recently been reported (Akerman *et al.*, 1988; Concepcion *et al.*, 1990). The discovery of a new route of administration for existing local anaesthetics, via percutaneous absorption, represents a further significant stage in the clinical history of these agents.

3.2   CLASSIFICATION

Drugs used specifically for their local anaesthetic properties may be conveniently classified into four main groups. These are the amino-esters, amino-amides, amino-ketones and amino-ethers, of which the first two groups are of greatest significance. The chemical structures of important local anaesthetics in each class are given in Fig. 3.2.

As with all classifications of this type, many exceptions occur. A diverse range of compounds possess some degree of local anaesthetic activity, but are not normally used clinically for this property. These include benzyl alcohol, menthol, phenol and some members of the following pharmacological groups: antihistamines, beta-adrenergic blocking agents, anti-arrhythmic drugs.

3.2.1   Nomenclature

The confusion that is often apparent in the naming of drugs also applies to the local anaesthetics. The British Approved Name (BAN), United States Adopted Name (USAN) and International Non-Proprietary Name (INN), or their modified versions, are sometimes

AMINO-ESTER LOCAL ANAESTHETICS

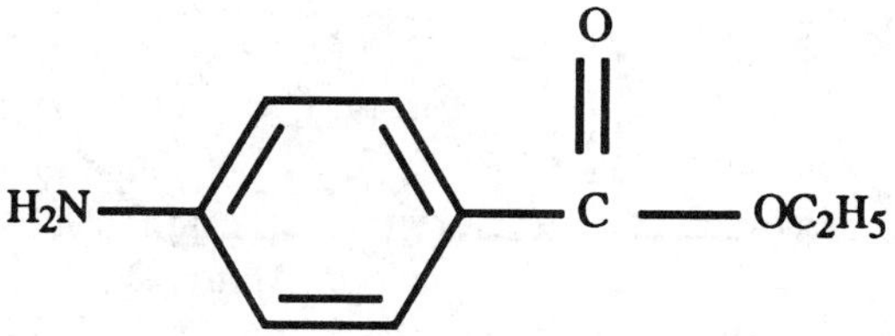

benzocaine {ethyl 4-aminobenzoate}

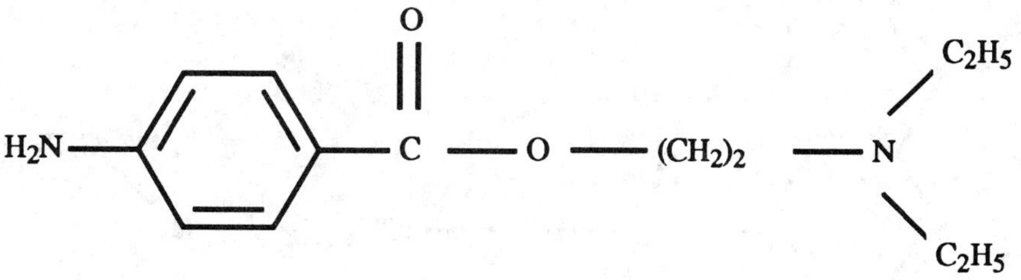

procaine {2-diethylaminoethyl 4-aminobenzoate}

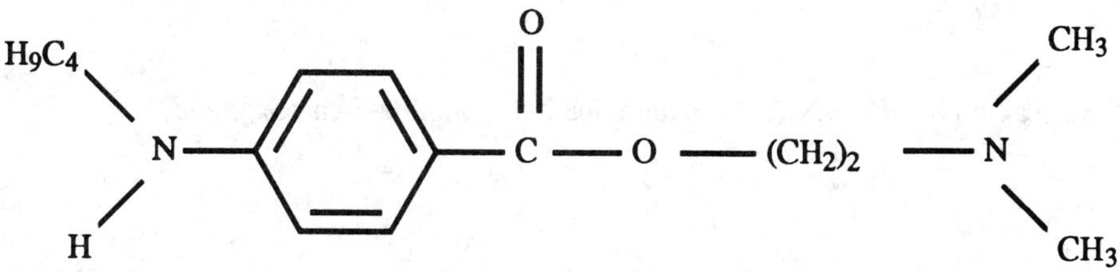

amethocaine {2-dimethylaminoethyl 4-butylaminobenzoate}

Fig. 3.2 — Representative chemical structures of the four main classes of local anaesthetics (1)

AMINO-AMIDE LOCAL ANAESTHETICS

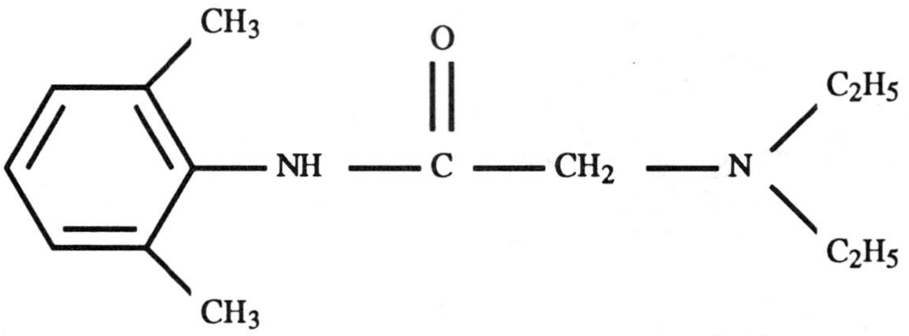

lignocaine {2-diethylaminoaceto-2',6'-xylidide}

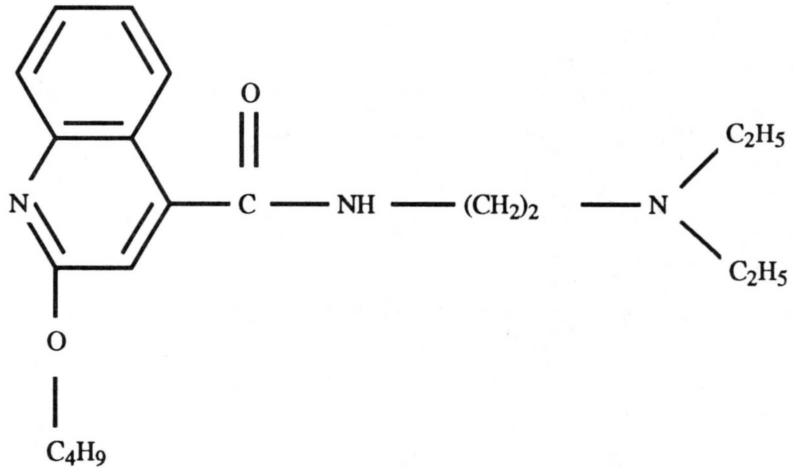

cinchocaine {2-butoxy-N-(2-diethylaminoethyl)quinoline-4-carboxamide}

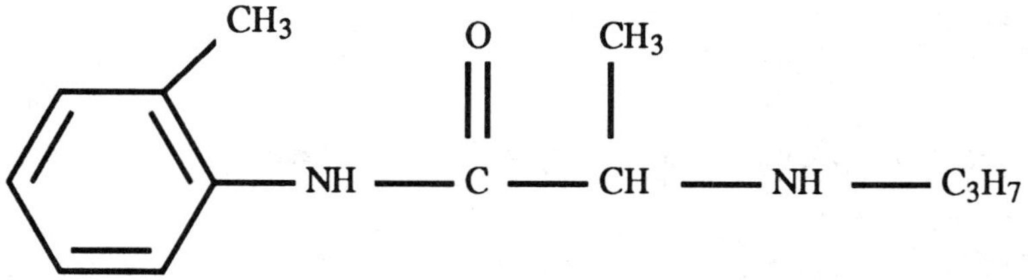

prilocaine {2-propylaminopropiono-o-toluidide}

Fig. 3.2 — Representative chemical structures of the four main classes of local anaesthetics(2)

AMINO-KETONE LOCAL ANAESTHETIC

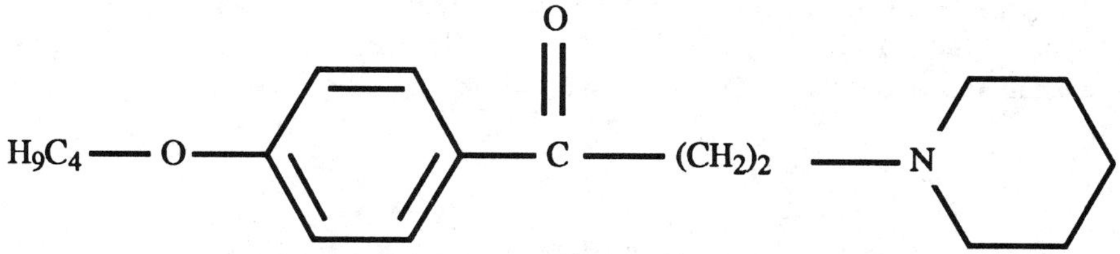

$$H_9C_4 - O - \langle \bigcirc \rangle - C - (CH_2)_2 - N \langle \bigcirc \rangle$$

dyclonine {4'-butoxy-3-piperidinopropiophenone}

AMINO-ETHER LOCAL ANAESTHETICS

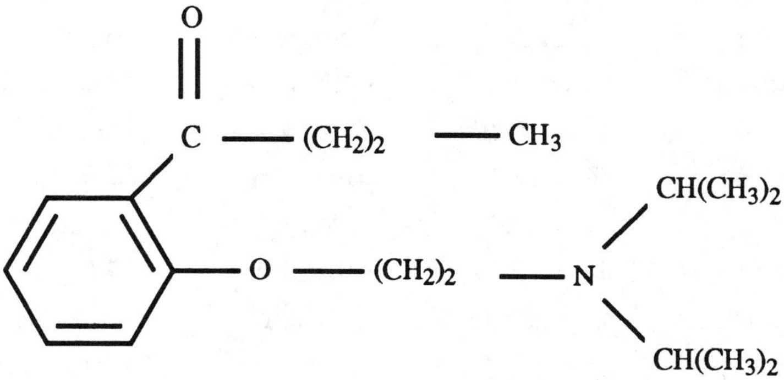

ketocaine {2'-(2-di-isopropylaminoethoxy)butyrophenone}

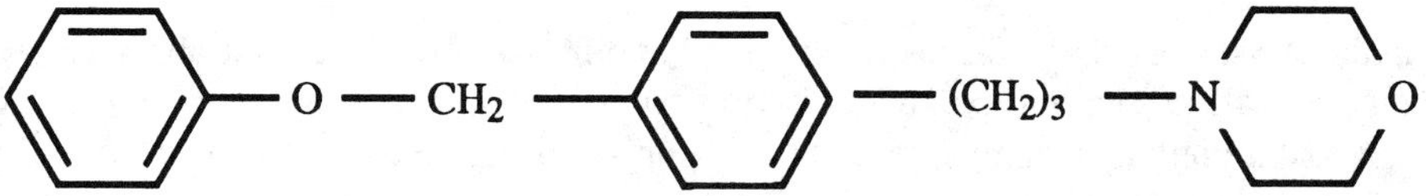

fomocaine {4-[3-(α-phenoxy-p-tolyl)propyl]morpholine}

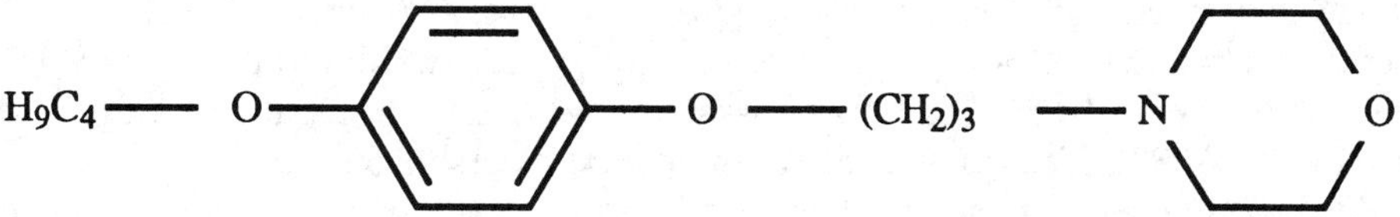

pramoxine {4-[3-(4-butoxyphenoxy)propyl]morpholine}

Fig. 3.2 — Representative chemical structures of the four main classes of local anaesthetics (3)

at variance. A further complication is the tendency to use a proprietary name in place of
the drug name. An example of this is the use of Xylocaine for lignocaine (BAN) or
lidocaine (USAN, INN). In this book local anaesthetic drugs are named according to
their BAN. Table 3.1 gives the BAN, USAN and INN for some of the more important
local anaesthetics, together with their common or proprietary names as used in the UK
or USA.

Table 3.1 — Nomenclature for local anaesthetics

BAN	USAN	INN	common or proprietary name
amethocaine	tetracaine	tetracaine	Pontocaine (USA)
benzocaine	benzocaine	benzocaine	Americaine (USA)
bupivacaine	bupivacaine	bupivacaine	Marcain (UK)
—	chloroprocaine	chloroprocaine	Nesacaine (USA)
cinchocaine	dibucaine	cinchocaine	Nupercaine (UK, USA)
etidocaine	etidocaine	etidocaine	Duranest (USA)
lignocaine	lidocaine	lidocaine	Xylocaine (UK)
mepivacaine	mepivacaine	mepivacaine	Carbocaine (USA)
prilocaine	prilocaine	prilocaine	Citanest (UK, USA)

3.3   STRUCTURAL CHARACTERISTICS

The main classes of local anaesthetic drugs all exhibit a similar structural pattern. An
intermediate alkyl chain separates a hydrophobic and a hydrophilic moiety. The
hydrophobic moiety is generally an aromatic group derived from benzoic acid or, in the
case of para-aminobenzoate derivatives, from aniline. The link between the aromatic
moiety and the intermediate alkyl chain is via an ester, amide, ketone or ether group.
The hydrophilic moiety is a tertiary or, less commonly, a secondary amine. Fig. 3.3
emphasises the common structural characteristics amongst all the major classifications
of local anaesthetics. The pharmacological functions associated with the various
structural components of a local anaesthetic drug are now well known, and have been
summarised by Lofstrom (1970), Takman (1975) and Foussard-Blandpin and
Quevauviller (1982). These functions are summarised in Table 3.2.

With a knowledge of the function of the various chemical units comprising the
generalised local anaesthetic structure, the effects of altering one or more of these
components can be readily predicted. An increase in the length of the intermediate alkyl
chain results in an increase in the overall lipophilicity of the molecule. This produces
an increase in anaesthetic potency, though too great an increase in the chain length
eventually leads to a reduction in potency as lipophilicity is increased beyond the

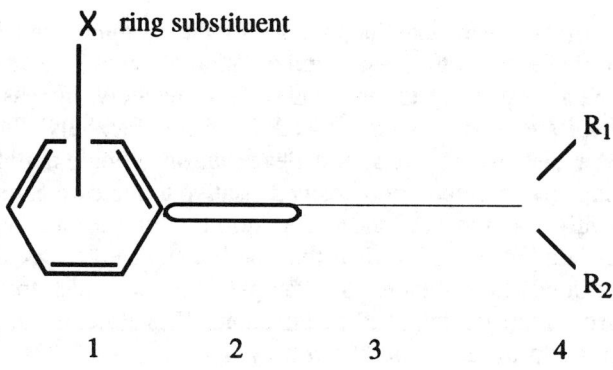

1   HYDROPHOBIC (AROMATIC) SECTION
     X = RING SUBSTITUENT

2   LINKING GROUP (AMIDE, ESTER, KETONE, ETHER)

3   INTERMEDIATE CHAIN

4   HYDROPHILIC SECTION

Fig. 3.3 — Structural pattern for a local anaesthetic

Table 3.2 — Relationship between local anaesthetic structure and pharmacological
function

chemical group	description	function
aromatic ring	lipophilic	required for diffusion through lipid substrates
substituted amine/ heterocyclic ring	hydrophilic	confers aqueous solubility
ester, amide, ketone or ether	link between alkyl chain and aromatic ring	reactive pivot - promotes alignment at receptor
alkyl chain	link between reactive pivot and hydrophilic group	alignment at receptor

optimum value. Similarly, an increase in the lipophilicity of the aromatic ring by addition of further alkyl groups increases both potency and duration of action, the latter by increasing the protein binding capacity of the molecule. Unfortunately, increased lipophilicity and increased potency are often directly related to increased toxicity. This may be due to an increased resistance to metabolic deactivation. For example, chloroprocaine, in which the halogen is in the ortho position relative to the carboxylate group, is hydrolysed more rapidly than procaine and is therefore less toxic, but is also less potent and has a shorter duration of action than the non-halogenated molecule. Conversely, amethocaine has a slower rate of hydrolysis than procaine and is therefore a more potent and more toxic drug when administered by injection. This effect is due to substitution of the para nitro group by the lipophilic n-butyl moiety. The effect of substitution at various points in the procaine molecule is illustrated with respect to potency and toxicity in Table 3.3. The structural characteristics of classical local anaesthetic drugs have been reviewed by Buchi and Perlia (1971).

The structural characteristics of local anaesthetic molecules are of some concern with respect to their potential application as percutaneous anaesthetics. Lipophilicity and aqueous solubility, potency, duration of action and toxicity are all vital factors which determine the ability of the drug to reach its site of action by absorption through the stratum corneum, and to safely produce a sufficient degree of anaesthesia at the treated site.

Table 3.3 — Effect of substitution on the relative potency and toxicity of procaine analogues

anaesthetic	R_1	R_2	R_3	R_4	R_5	Relative potency	Relative toxicity
procaine	NH_2	H	H	C_2H_5	C_2H_5	1	1
chloro-procaine	NH_2	H	Cl	C_2H_5	C_2H_5	< 1	< 1
propoxy-caine	NH_2	H	$O.C_3H_7$	C_2H_5	C_2H_5	42	10
oxybupro-caine	NH_2	$O.C_4H_9$	H	C_2H_5	C_2H_5	140	24
phenacaine	$NH.C_4H_9$	H	OH	C_2H_5	C_2H_5	105	13

3.4   PHYSICOCHEMICAL PROPERTIES

A typical local anaesthetic agent is, chemically, a weak base with a pK_a (negative logarithm of the acid dissociation constant) between about 7.5 and 9. The property of basicity is conferred on the molecule by the nitrogen atom of the substituted aliphatic amine. When a para amino group is present on the aromatic ring, this will give rise to a second, lower pK_a. The nitrogen atom in this group cannot be readily protonated due to interaction with the conjugated aromatic system.

Aqueous solubility is normally conferred on local anaesthetic bases by forming a salt with the substituted aliphatic amine. Typically, hydrochlorides are formed but other salts, such as sulphates, may also be used. Aqueous solubility is a prerequisite for administration of local anaesthetics by injection. However, when considering the topical or percutaneous routes (the distinction between the terms refers to drug penetration through damaged skin/mucous membranes or intact skin, respectively), aqueous solubility is not required. In fact, a significant degree of aqueous solubility is contra-indicated for the percutaneous delivery of local anaesthetics. Local anaesthetics that cannot form a water-soluble salt are suitable only for topical application. This applies, notably, to benzocaine, with a pK_a of 2.78. The pK_a values of some other common local anaesthetic drugs are given in Table 3.4.

Table 3.4 — pK_a Values of some local anaesthetic drugs

local anaesthetic	pK_a
amethocaine	8.39
benzocaine	2.78
bupivacaine	8.10
cinchocaine	8.30
lignocaine	7.86
mepivacaine	7.70
prilocaine	7.89
procaine	8.80

The percentages of local anaesthetic in the free base and water-soluble ionised forms varies quite dramatically with pH when the pH is close to the pK_a of the drug. This observation is significant when formulating local anaesthetics for percutaneous delivery, where the free base form is essential, and also in terms of the mechanism of conduction blockade exerted by these drugs (Menczel *et al.*, 1977; Menczel and Goldberg, 1978). If the pK_a value of the local anaesthetic is known, the percentage of drug in the ionised form may be readily calculated from eqn (3.1).

$$\text{percentage of drug ionised} = 100 / \{1 + \text{antilog} (pH - pK_a)\} \quad (3.1)$$

Equation (3.1) is a modified version of the Henderson-Hasselbach equation. Table 3.5 shows, for various pH values, the percentage of drug in the ionised form for typical examples of the ester and amide local anaesthetic groups.

Table 3.5 — Percentage ionisation of typical ester and amide local anaesthetics - variation with pH

pH	percent ionised amethocaine	percent ionised lignocaine
7	96.1	87.9
8	71.1	42.0
9	19.7	6.8
10	2.4	0.7

Whereas the salts of local anaesthetics are well-defined, stable crystalline materials, local anaesthetic free bases are either oils or amorphous solids. The free bases all have reduced chemical stability when compared to the equivalent salts. There is, however, a marked difference between the esters and the other local anaesthetic classifications in respect of the stability of the free bases. This difference resides in the nature of the link between the aromatic ring and the intermediate chain. Whereas the amide, ketone and ether linkages are quite stable, the ester group in local anaesthetics such as procaine is subject to hydrolytic cleavage. This results in liberation of the constituent acid and alcohol components of the free base. The effect of substituents on the molecule, particularly on the aromatic ring, can substantially alter the rate of the hydrolysis. Thus, amethocaine, with a para n-butyl substituent, hydrolyses at a much slower rate than procaine. Nevertheless, the comparatively poor stability of local anaesthetic ester free bases is a problem for the formulator, since it is this form of the drug which is required for percutaneous delivery. The hydrolysis of ester local anaesthetics is also significant for drug metabolism, since this represents a major pathway for breakdown of the drugs by plasma pseudocholinesterase. The difference in systemic toxicity between procaine and amethocaine is partly due to the reduced rate of hydrolysis and increased plasma half-life of the latter.

Clearly, an awareness of local anaesthetic pK_a, together with the pH of the candidate delivery system, are of major importance in the percutaneous delivery of the drug. The other physicochemical factor of significance is the lipophilicity of the free base. Lipophilicity is a prime indicator of the intrinsic ability of the drug to penetrate lipid membranes. This property therefore determines the ability of the anaesthetic free base to penetrate the stratum corneum, which can be regarded as primarily a lipid barrier (see Chapter 4). Lipophilicity is most readily judged by reference to the partition coefficient (P) of the local anaesthetic. Partition coefficient is closely related to solubility and is derived from consideration of the partitioning of a solute between two immiscible liquid phases. Although a rigorous definition of P involves the relative activities of the solute in each of the phases, in practice molar concentrations are used. Thus, P may be defined as the ratio of the molar lipid phase concentration to the molar aqueous phase concentration.

P is determined by equilibrating the solute between the two phases, each of which has been pre-saturated with the other, and analysing for the drug, preferably in each phase. The aqueous phase is usually a buffer at physiological pH, to prevent changes in drug solubility in the aqueous phase due to changes in pH following initial dissolution of the drug.

When considering the partition coefficients of local anaesthetics, literature compilations of data unfortunately present a confusing picture. The pH of the aqueous buffer chosen for the measurement is not always the same. Of greater concern is the variation in the choice of lipophilic (oil) phase. The use of n-octanol as representative of the partitioning characteristics of a biological lipid membrane is widespread, particularly in quantitative drug structure-biological activity relationships. The choice of n-octanol is based on its apolar nature and an ability to dissolve limited amounts of water (Leo et al., 1971). The choice may not necessarily be a good one, since n-octanol has a considerable tendency for hydrogen bonding, which can significantly influence the dissolution characteristics of some drugs. However, the use of n-octanol does allow meaningful inter- and intra-class comparisons of P to be made. Unfortunately, P values for local anaesthetics are not quoted primarily with n-octanol as the lipid phase. Such phases as oleylalcohol and n-heptane have been used, or no lipid phase has been specified in tabulated data. Thus, tabulated values of P for local anaesthetics are of limited use.

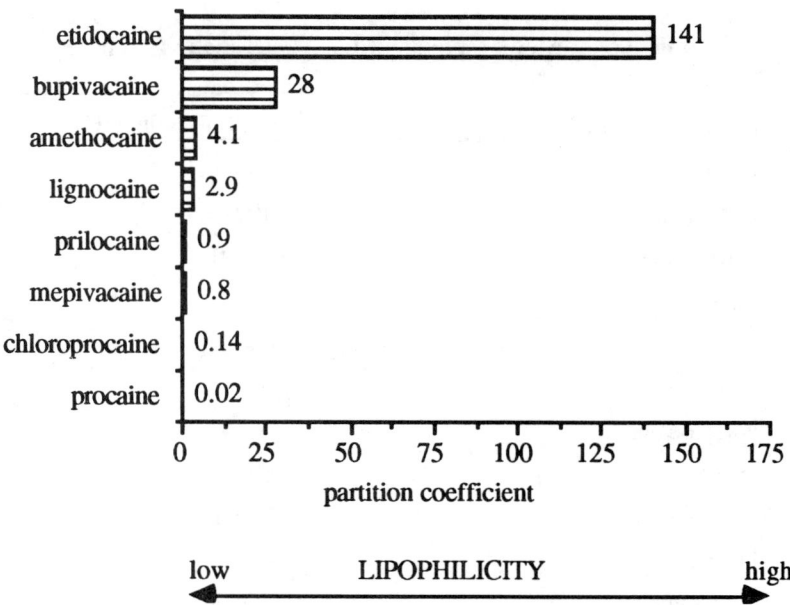

Fig. 3.4 — Lipophilicity range of major local anaesthetic agents, as determined by their partition coefficients between n-heptane and pH 7.4 aqueous buffer solution. Data from Wood (1990)

Rather, a banding of the drugs into low, medium and high lipophilicities may be preferable, as shown in Fig. 3.4.

Since the percutaneous delivery of a local anaesthetic requires the use of the anaesthetic free base, lipophilicity and pK_a are physicochemical pointers towards the selection of a suitable drug, or drug combination. Solubility of the free base is a related and important factor. Solubility considerations are not limited purely to water, or to aqueous buffers, but must also involve solubility in pharmaceutical water-miscible solvents, such as propylene glycol. The solubility in the oil phase of a formulation is of considerable importance, since this will determine, to some extent, the available concentration of the drug with respect to skin penetration and, ultimately, activity at the nerve receptor. The solubility characteristics for local anaesthetic free bases are not readily available in the literature. Values are usually quoted for the more commonly used local anaesthetic salts. Thus, it is often necessary to make individual solubility measurements for the anaesthetic bases.

The poor crystallinity of the anaesthetic free bases is reflected in lower melting points for the bases compared to their equivalent salts. In some cases, the free base exists only as an oil, rather than an amorphous solid. Percutaneous absorption of a local anaesthetic free base requires the drug to be in liquid form, present either as a solution or an oily liquid. Thus, the melting point of the free base is another useful indicator of the potential for percutaneous absorption of any local anaesthetic base. A lower melting point indicates reduced crystallinity, and more promising formulation possibilities. Table 3.6 gives the melting points for some anaesthetic free bases. Those that exist as oily liquids, or have melting points below 100°C, are of particular relevance for percutaneous delivery.

Table 3.6 — Melting points of local anaesthetic free bases

local anaesthetic base	melting point (°C)
mepivacaine	150-151
bupivacaine	107-108
benzocaine	88-90
lignocaine	68-69
cinchocaine	64
procaine	61
amethocaine	42-46
prilocaine	37-38
amylocaine	liquid
butacaine	liquid
*ketocaine	liquid

Data compiled from *The Merck Index. 10th. edn.*, Merck & Co., New Jersey.
* determined in the authors' laboratory

3.5 MECHANISM OF CONDUCTION BLOCKADE

Local anaesthetics produce a reversible conduction blockade in the peripheral nervous system. A peripheral nerve fibre consists of the axon, which may be regarded as a projection of the originating neurone, and a surrounding sheath, the Schwann cell. The nature of the Schwann cell sheath yields two distinct classes of peripheral nerves. Unmyelinated nerves, notably the very fine C fibres responsible for reflex actions and some pain transmission, involve outgrowths from a single Schwann cell surrounding several axons. The thicker, myelinated nerves have a single axon surrounded by the outgrowth from a single Schwann cell. The thicker diameter of a myelinated nerve is due to the Schwann cell outgrowths spiralling around the axon, thus forming an outer, cylindrical phospholipid membrane known as the myelin sheath. Each Schwann cell extends along the axon for about 1 mm, interlinking with the next such cell at a junction, the node of Ranvier.

3.5.1 Nerve depolarisation

The membrane of a nerve axon is a semi-permeable structure. It consists of a phospholipid bilayer whose polar groups are in contact with inter- or intracellular fluid. The semi-permeable nature of the membrane refers to the passage of sodium and potassium ions across the structure. Protein molecules forming part of the axonal membrane act as channels for these ions, forming, in the case of sodium ions, a "gate" mechanism which controls the entry of sodium into the axoplasm.

In the non-stimulated or resting condition the inside of a nerve axon has a negative charge compared to the outside. This causes a potential difference (the resting potential) across the membrane of about -70 mV. The source of the internal negative charge is the movement of potassium ions out of the axoplasm and across the membrane. Since, normally, each positive ion will have a counterbalancing anion, removal of the cation results in a net negative internal charge on the membrane. Potassium can diffuse readily out of the axon along a concentration gradient. In the resting condition an equilibrium is established in which the driving force for potassium diffusion out of the axon, the concentration gradient, is counterbalanced by the electrical gradient caused by the increased negative charge on the internal side of the membrane. Thus, potassium ions move back across the membrane into the axoplasm as the negative membrane potential increases. The two-way movement of potassium ions is thus responsible for maintenance of the resting membrane potential.

When the nerve is in the resting condition it can be regarded as polarised, that condition in which there is charge separation across the membrane. If the internal negative charge is eliminated by the influx of positive sodium ions across the axonal membrane, the nerve is said to be depolarised. In the depolarised state there is a net surplus of sodium ions on the internal side of the axonal membrane, yielding a membrane potential of approximately +20 mV. Influx of sodium ions into the axoplasm across a sodium concentration gradient is permitted by the sudden opening of sodium channels in the membrane. When the "gate" of these channels is closed, as in the resting condition, the membrane is impermeable to sodium ions. The control mechanism of the sodium channels is thought to be influenced by the presence of calcium ions (Strichartz, 1980). The normal outward leakage of positive charge in the form of potassium ions is overwhelmed by the sudden inflow of sodium ions. However, as is the case with establishment of the equilibrium condition for potassium ions and consequent maintenance of the resting potential, the driving force for sodium ion diffusion along its concentration gradient is opposed to an increasing extent by the electrical gradient brought about by the increasing positive charge on the internal side of the axonal membrane. This causes closure and temporary inactivation of the sodium channels across the membrane (Agnew, 1984). Potassium ions, which, unlike sodium, have unhindered passage across the membrane, can now leak outwards, thus removing the excess positive charge and restoring the normal internal negative charge on the membrane. Thus, in less than 2 ms, the axonal membrane potential moves through approximately 180 mV, from -70 mV to +20 mV and back to the resting condition. This sudden change in potential, which is known as the action potential, occurs initially at the nerve endings as a result of a physiological stimulus such as pain, temperature change, touch, or pressure.

When a stimulus of sufficient magnitude is received, the initial opening of the sodium channels in the nerve membrane will produce sufficient ingress of sodium ions to generate an action potential and subsequent conduction of the impulse along the nerve. A stimulus of insufficient magnitude will not trigger sufficient ingress of sodium ions to overcome the balancing outflow of positive charge in the form of potassium cations. In these circumstances, a full action potential will not be generated and conduction of the impulse will not take place. Strichartz and Ritchie (1987) have given a detailed account of the action of local anaesthetics on ion channels.

3.5.2   Impulse conduction

When an action potential is generated at a nerve ending a short length of the axon has a positive charge on the axoplasm side of the membrane. The adjacent region, which is still at the resting potential, has a negative charge. Thus, positive ions from the depolarised region are attracted towards the negative electrical field adjacent to them. This flow of ions along the internal side of the axonal membrane constitutes an electric current. As each adjacent region of the axon, along its length, becomes in turn positively charged, the sodium channels in that region are opened and an action potential is generated (Catterall, 1984, 1987). Thus, the initial impulse is conducted along the length of the nerve.

A question arises as to the unidirectional nature of impulse conduction along the axon. Following the initial stimulus of the nerve ending, a depolarised section of axon is, in effect, conducted along the nerve. This means that, as conduction proceeds, the length of axonal membrane with a positive charge on the axoplasm side is sandwiched between two adjacent, polarised regions at their resting potential, that is, with a negative charge on the internal side of the membrane. There must be a mechanism to prevent the conducted current flowing backwards towards the nerve ending, as well as the desired forward flow of the current along the axon. It appears that depolarisation of the axonal membrane causes a subsequent refractory period in the sodium channels. These cannot immediately open again and, by the time the channel has returned to its normal state, the depolarised region has passed further along the axon (Strichartz and Ritchie, 1987). Interestingly, an isolated nerve stimulated at a low frequency and then exposed to a local anaesthetic exhibits a lesser degree of conduction blockade than one stimulated initially at a higher frequency. This is known as phasic (use- or frequency-dependent) blockade. A resting nerve is still less sensitive to a local anaesthetic (resting or tonic blockade), but such effects may be of limited clinical significance (Hille, 1980).

Nerve fibres are classified into three main groups, A, B and C fibres (Table 3.7). The A group is further subdivided into Aα, Aβ, Aγ and Aδ fibres. The classification is based on nerve fibre thickness, conduction velocity and function. The nerve thickness is itself dictated by the diameter of the myelin sheath. In the case of the thinnest group, C fibres, the myelin sheath is absent. The greater the thickness of the nerve fibre, the greater is the concentration of local anaesthetic required for effective conduction blockade. This is significant with regard to percutaneous administration of local anaesthetic drugs, where the limiting factor with respect to efficacy is, in practice, the ability to produce a sufficient concentration of drug molecules at the nerve. However, the cutaneous sensory network of myelinated Aδ fibres and unmyelinated C fibres, which penetrate into the stratum granulosum and respond to temperature and pain stimuli, are thin structures. They therefore require a lesser concentration of anaesthetic for effective conduction blockade.

Table 3.7 — Classification of nerve fibres

nerve fibre and type	diameter (µm)	conduction velocity (m s^{-1})	function
Aα (myelinated)	15-20	70-120	motor
Aβ (myelinated)	5-12	30-70	touch and pressure
Aγ (myelinated)	5-10	30-70	proprioception
Aδ (myelinated)	2-5	12-30	pain and temperature
B (myelinated)	1-4	3-15	preganglionic autonomic
C (unmyelinated)	0.5-1	0.5-2.0	pain and temperature

Reproduced from Wood (1990) with permission of the copyright owner, Williams and Wilkins, Baltimore

The speed of impulse conduction is also related to nerve thickness, being greater in the Aδ fibres, and slowest in the unmyelinated C fibres. The depolarisation process travels as a wave along unmyelinated nerve fibres, but moves in increments of about 1 mm along the myelinated fibres, between each node of Ranvier. This process, known as saltatory conduction, accounts for the more rapid transmission of impulses along myelinated fibres, compared with unmyelinated nerves (see section 2.1).

3.5.3   Reversible impulse blockade

Postulating an all-embracing mechanism by which external chemical substances block impulse conduction along the axon is complicated by the realisation that chemicals other than classical local anaesthetics can interfere with the conduction process. Benzyl alcohol, for instance, has local anaesthetic properties but bears little family resemblance to the typical local anaesthetic chemical structure. It seems likely, therefore, that two independent, but possibly complementary mechanisms are in operation (Mrose and Ritchie, 1978). One mechanism can be regarded as non-specific (Trudell *et al.*, 1975; Vanderkooi and Adade, 1986) whereas the other involves a specific interaction between a drug and a membrane protein acting as a receptor in the sodium channel (Greenberg and Tsong, 1982; Lin *et al.*, 1988).

The key factor in the action of local anaesthetic drugs is an appreciation of the equilibrium that exists between the two forms of most of these drugs, the water-soluble salt and the water-insoluble free base (Hille, 1980). Here, a difference arises between the classical routes of administration for local anaesthetics, by injection or by topical application to mucosa or damaged skin, and the percutaneous route. The latter involves drug penetration of a lipid barrier, the stratum corneum. The former routes present no appreciable absorption problems. Thus, for administration by injection or normal topical application, a local anaesthetic drug is presented as the water-soluble salt. For percutaneous absorption, the drug must be presented as the water-insoluble free base. However, at physiological pH (7.4) the relative percentages of available free base and ionised quaternary amine will be dictated by the pK_a of the drug, irrespective of the original form in which the local anaesthetic was administered. Thus, from the data in Table 3.4, and applying equation (3.1), it can be easily calculated, for example, that 9.3% amethocaine and 25.8% lignocaine are available in the free base form at physiological pH. However, the apparent pK_a of a local anaesthetic bound to a protein receptor is not necessarily the same as the pK_a of the same drug in aqueous solution (Chernoff and Strichartz, 1990). This may further influence the rates of binding to, and dissociation from, the sodium channel receptors.

Impulse blockade due to local anaesthetics is brought about by blockage of the sodium channels in the axonal membrane, thus preventing generation of an action potential. This process almost certainly involves interaction between the local anaesthetic and a specific protein receptor in the sodium channel. However, in order for the drug to reach the sodium channel it must first penetrate into the axonal membrane, which is lipophilic in nature. This penetration can only be achieved to any appreciable extent by the lipophilic form of the local anaesthetic. In this sense, an analogous situation exists between penetration of the lipid stratum corneum barrier during percutaneous absorption of local anaesthetic drugs and penetration of the phospholipid-rich axonal membrane. Once the drug has reached the axoplasm, equilibrium between the ionised and unionised forms of the local anaesthetic is again established under the influence of physiological pH in an aqueous environment. Thus, most of the available drug in the sodium channels is in the cationic form, following "back diffusion" from the axoplasm into the channels. Experiments on isolated nerves have clearly demonstrated that it is the local anaesthetic cation which is the active entity responsible for significant conduction blockade.

The theory of local anaesthetic conduction blockade by a specific receptor interaction, resulting in blockage of the sodium channels and prevention of action potential generation, does not fit the physicochemical profile of benzocaine, or compounds with impulse blocking properties such as benzyl alcohol. For these compounds, a second, non-specific blockade mechanism may operate. Benzocaine, with a pK_a of less than 3, is almost 100% unionised at physiological pH. This drug, and other non-specific agents, may, due to their lack of aqueous solubility, concentrate in the lipid-rich axonal membrane. Consequently, the membrane, essentially a lipid matrix, may swell and distort, blocking the sodium channels by a purely physical mechanism.

The free base form of a conventional local anaesthetic, such as amethocaine or lignocaine, may also exert some direct blocking activity by disruption of the axonal membrane. Although this has traditionally been regarded as of minor significance compared to the specific receptor interaction mechanism, more recent studies have focused on the interaction of certain local anaesthetics, notably amethocaine, with model lipid membranes. Amethocaine has been shown to reduce the stability of the lamellar structure in mixed glycolipid bilayers (Auger *et al.*, 1989). Glycolipids are common components of the myelin sheath. Of greater significance, perhaps, are the numerous studies (Coster *et al.*, 1981; Boulanger *et al.*, 1981; Kelusky and ·Smith, 1984) by nuclear magnetic resonance and X-ray diffraction which have clearly demonstrated the ability of amethocaine to partially intercalate into the lipid bilayer in model phospholipid membranes. More specifically, amethocaine has been shown to partition into a model membrane system consisting of a multilamellar aqueous dispersion of two phosphatidylserine derivatives. In this system the drug concentrates in the environment close to the membrane-water interface and interacts electrostatically with the lipid head group (Auger *et al.*, 1990). All of these model interactions are dependent on the form in which the local anaesthetic is present. Mertz *et al.* (1990) have identified no less than five separate forms of amethocaine in solution. These were the neutral free base, monocation, dication (formed when the secondary aromatic amine is protonated), hydrogen-bonded and aggregated species. How relevant this is to the physiological environment is not clear. Neither is the relevance of studies on model phospholipid membrane systems fully established. Nevertheless, for a long established class of drugs, the exact mode of action of local anaesthetics is still a subject of active research and debate.

3.6   CLINICAL CHARACTERISTICS OF LOCAL ANAESTHETICS

From a clinical perspective the fundamental characteristics of local anaesthetic drugs may be regarded as the potency, speed of onset and duration of anaesthesia. These factors, which are influenced to some extent by the vasoactivity of local anaesthetics, are normally assessed by examining the effect of the drug in an isolated nerve preparation. In the practical situation, when the drug is administered percutaneously, such information is often misleading, or even irrelevant. Therefore, given the limited, and relatively slow, percutaneous absorption of local anaesthetic drugs, it is necessary to assess again their previously accepted clinical properties.

3.6.1   Potency

Lipid solubility appears to be of prime importance in determining the intrinsic potency of a local anaesthetic drug (Covino, 1986). A highly lipophilic agent will more readily penetrate the lipoprotein matrix of the nerve membrane. The relationship between lipophilicity and potency is apparent for both the ester and amide classifications. Thus, the more lipophilic amethocaine has a greater anaesthetic potency than procaine. Similarly, amide local anaesthetics such as prilocaine and mepivacaine are less lipophilic, and therefore less potent, than bupivacaine and etidocaine. However, potency in this respect is quoted with reference to the effect of the drugs on an isolated nerve *in vitro*. The relationship is less clear *in vivo*. Lignocaine, with a greater anaesthetic potency than prilocaine *in vitro*, has a similar potency *in vivo*. The available drug concentration of lignocaine at the nerve is reduced as a result of its greater vasodilator properties, resulting in its more rapid redistribution into the vasculature (Covino and Vassallo, 1976). Similarly, the *in vitro* potency relationship between the very lipophilic etidocaine and bupivacaine is reversed *in vivo*, with the latter being more potent *in vivo*. Again, the effective concentration of etidocaine at the nerve is reduced, the very high lipophilicity of the drug favouring its redistribution into adipose tissue (Scott *et al.*, 1980).

The intrinsic potencies of the commonly used local anaesthetics have been determined *in vitro* from their relative abilities to produce a fixed percentage reduction in the magnitude of the action potential, under standard conditions, in the isolated frog sciatic nerve preparation (Covino and Vassallo, 1976). The classification of local anaesthetic potencies by this means is shown in Fig. 3.5.

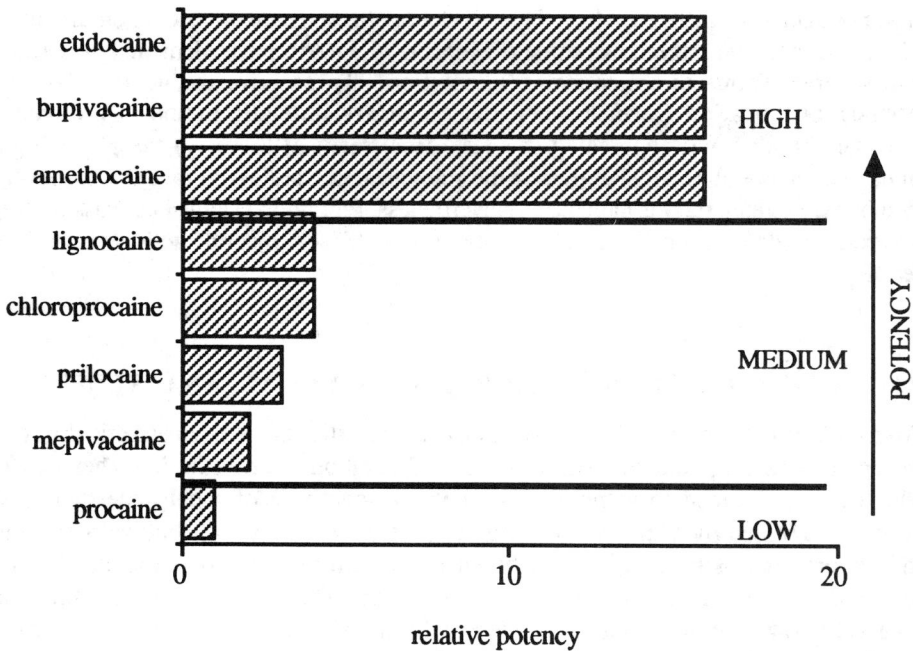

Fig. 3.5 — Relative anaesthetic potencies of some commonly used local anaesthetics, determined under standard conditions in an isolated nerve preparation. Data from Covino and Vassallo (1976)

The standard assessment of intrinsic potency is a fixed response technique in which the most potent agent is that which achieves the required response with the minimum drug concentration. The relative potencies of local anaesthetics determined by this means relate very well to their lipophilic properties. This is not surprising, given the nature of the potency assessment. The most lipophilic drug will penetrate the axonal membrane most readily, and thus a lesser number of molecules, that is, a lower drug concentration, will be necessary to elicit the fixed pharmacological response.

When a local anaesthetic is applied to intact skin with an effective barrier to drug absorption, the relative potencies of the drugs become rather less important. This route of application represents a new situation in which, for the first time, a local anaesthetic is not being delivered directly to its site of action, either by injection or direct application to a surface site. Now, penetration of the axonal membrane is not the only factor determining potency. It is also influenced, to an even greater degree, by the ability of the drug to actually reach the nerve ending. Percutaneous absorption of local anaesthetics is partially determined by the lipophilicity of the drug but, unlike the situation in an isolated nerve preparation, increasing lipophilicity does not necessarily mean increased ease of absorption. Drug solubility and crystallinity also determine the bioavailability of the agent from percutaneous delivery, since these factors influence the formulation of the percutaneous anaesthetic preparation. Thus, although higher potency (more lipophilic) agents are generally more suitable for percutaneous delivery, the choice of drug is not a simple one. The desired clinical characteristics for a percutaneous local anaesthetic, the influence of physical properties on drug bioavailablity at the site of action, and the increased toxicity that often accompanies increased potency, must all be considered in the overall design of the final dosage form.

3.6.2   Speed of onset

In the *in vitro* situation, speed of onset of anaesthesia is largely dictated by the amount of available unionised drug at the nerve. This, in turn, is dependent on the pK_a of the drug. From Table 3.4, it is readily seen that lignocaine, prilocaine and mepivacaine, all with pK_a values less than 8, have a substantial percentage of drug (about 25%) available in the free base form. Local anaesthetics such as amethocaine, with a pK_a greater than 8, have about 10% or less available free base at physiological pH. Since penetration of the lipophilic nerve membrane involves drug diffusion along a concentration gradient, it follows that those drugs with lower pK_a values, and a greater availability of free anaesthetic base, will penetrate into the axoplasm more rapidly. Therefore, a more rapid onset of conduction blockade should occur. However, this relationship between onset of anaesthesia and drug pK_a is complicated by differences in the lipophilicities of the free bases, which results in different inherent abilities to penetrate the nerve membrane. Thus, onset speed is really dictated by the amount of free base available at the nerve and the lipophilicity of that base. A comparison of the onset speeds of some commonly used local anaesthetics is given in Fig. 3.6.

The speed of onset of conduction blockade is derived from a standard test on frog sciatic nerve. The latency period before onset of anaesthesia is determined as that concentration of drug required to produce a 50% reduction in the height of the sheathed frog sciatic nerve action potential within ten minutes (Covino and Vassallo, 1976). However, some care needs to be taken when considering onset times determined in this way in the context of percutaneous local anaesthesia. The situation is similar to that governing the potency of local anaesthetics in that the influence of drug availability by the percutaneous route is paramount, greatly outweighing the significance of what might conveniently be termed the pharmacological onset time. Typically onset times for percutaneous local anaesthesia are in the region of thirty minutes to one hour

(McCafferty *et al.*, 1989). This latency period is almost entirely due to the time required for the drug to diffuse through the skin barrier. The pharmacological onset time, therefore, has little relevance. Thus, amethocaine, with a much slower pharmacological onset time than either lignocaine or prilocaine, actually produces onset of percutaneous anaesthesia in about half the time required for a eutectic mixture of the two amides to produce a similar effect (McCafferty *et al.*, 1989). This is due to the better cutaneous penetration properties of amethocaine, when suitably formulated, compared to that of the amides (McCafferty *et al.*, 1988).

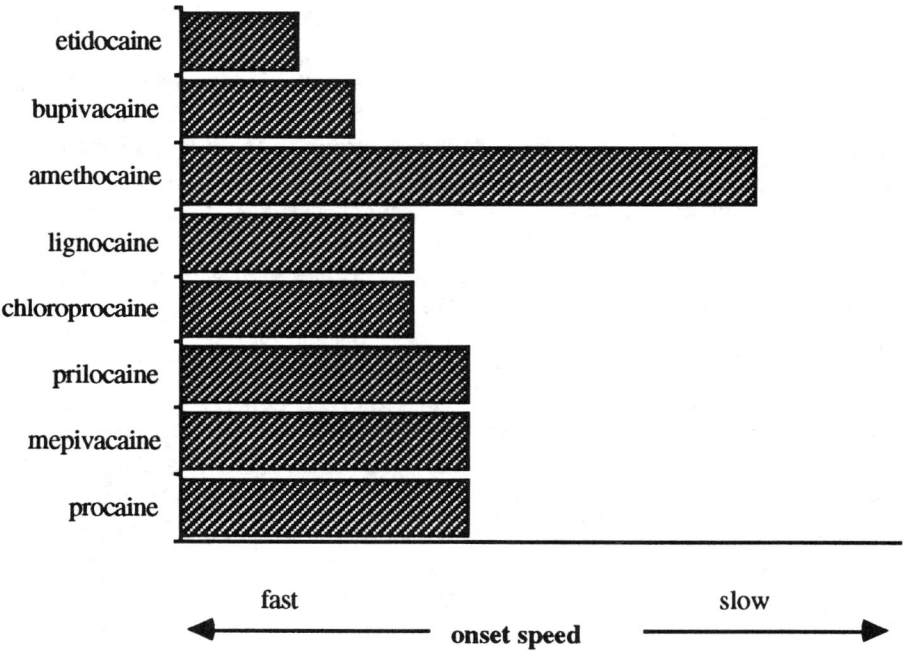

Fig. 3.6 — Relative onset speeds of anaesthesia for some commonly used local anaesthetic agents, determined under standard conditions in an isolated nerve preparation. Data from Covino and Vassallo (1976)

3.6.3   Duration of anaesthetic effect

There is an accepted correlation between duration of local anaesthesia and the protein binding capacity of local anaesthetic agents. Those agents which are highly plasma protein bound tend to produce the longest duration of anaesthesia (Fig. 3.7). This is thought to be due to an equivalent ability to bind more firmly to the proteinaceous receptor sites in the sodium channels. Maintenance of the drug at the receptor for longer periods directly correlates with an increased duration of activity. Drugs that are strongly bound to the receptor, such as amethocaine or etidocaine, are less readily washed out from isolated nerve preparations than short acting, weakly protein-bound agents such as procaine (Wildsmith *et al.*, 1985). The difference in duration of anaesthesia between procaine and amethocaine is directly attributable to substitution of the para nitro group in the shorter acting drug by a butylamino residue in amethocaine, thus increasing lipophilicity, potency and duration of anaesthesia in the latter, but at the price of greater systemic toxicity.

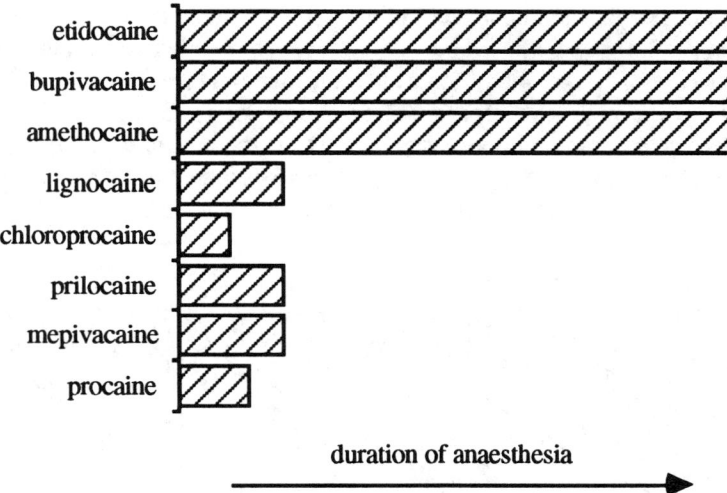

duration of anaesthesia

Fig 3.7 — Relative durations of anaesthesia for some commonly used local anaesthetic agents, determined under standard conditions in an isolated nerve preparation. Data from Covino and Vassallo (1976)

In contrast to speed of onset and potency of anaesthesia, the pharmacological property of duration of action is not substantially modified by either the time taken for percutaneous absorption of the drug, or reduced bioavailability from this route. Thus, an amethocaine percutaneous anaesthetic preparation will produce effective skin anaesthesia for at least 3 hours, and the formulation can be "tailored" to produce up to 12 hours of profound conduction block (McCafferty *et al.*, 1989). The strong protein binding capacity of amethocaine may produce some depot effect in the epidermal region, further enhancing duration of effect, though this may be counterbalanced by plasma protein binding reducing the available drug concentration at the nerve. The importance of protein binding in determining the duration of anaesthesia seems to outweigh the greater ease of metabolic breakdown of the amino-esters compared to the chemically more stable amino-amides (Woolfson *et al.*, 1990a).

3.6.4 Vasoactivity

Local anaesthetic drugs are intrinsically vasoactive. Although this activity is relatively weak compared to such compounds as methyl nicotinate (Guy *et al.*, 1983), it can nevertheless influence the clinical profile of the drug. In particular, when a local anaesthetic is administered via the percutaneous route, vasoactive effects can influence the interpretation of possible sensitisation reactions. Thus, it is necessary to be aware of the vasoactive properties of local anaesthetics and the effects these can have on the skin surface following application of percutaneous anaesthetic preparations.

Amino-amide local anaesthetics, at low concentrations, possess vasoconstrictor properties (Reynolds *et al.*, 1976). However, these drugs appear to exert a biphasic effect on vascular smooth muscle, producing vasoconstriction at higher concentrations. In contrast, the amino esters, procaine and amethocaine, produce vasodilation at all concentrations when administered intradermally to human volunteers (Willatts and Reynolds, 1985). An exception to this is cocaine, which produces a marked vasoconstriction by direct inhibition of noradrenaline uptake (Muscholl, 1961). On the skin surface, the practical effect of these properties is to produce localised colour changes, which are transient and reversible. Blanching (Smith *et al.*, 1990) or erythema at the site may be observed (Fig. 3.8). Erythema is sometimes accompanied by a brief, localised oedema, particularly with amethocaine.

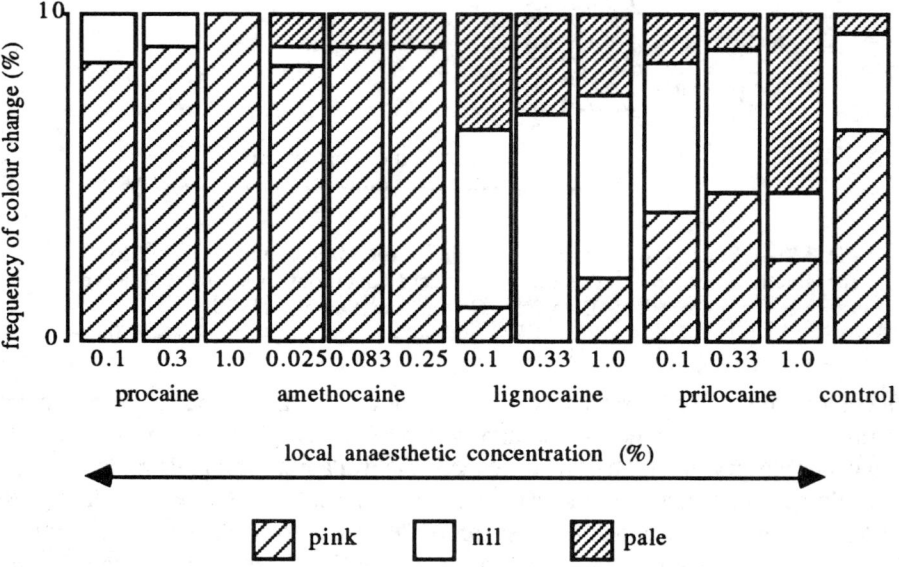

Fig. 3.8 — Frequency of localised skin colour changes observed following intradermal injections of procaine, amethocaine, lignocaine or prilocaine. Modified from Willats and Reynolds (1985) with permission of the copyright owner

The vasodilator properties of local anaesthetics can enhance their vascular absorption. For certain applications, including nerve blocks, they are often formulated with a vasoconstrictor such as adrenaline. This inhibits wash-out of the drug from the nerve and prolongs the duration of anaesthesia. Systemic absorption of the drug is also reduced (Vickers *et al.*, 1984). However, animal studies have, in some cases, indicated an increase in toxicity associated with local anaesthetic and adrenaline mixtures (Taylor and Dorris, 1989).

When a local anaesthetic is delivered percutaneously, a much lower effective concentration is achieved at the nerve. Most of the dose is not absorbed, but simply acts to establish a large concentration gradient across the skin. This is well illustrated by the observation that a eutectic mixture of lignocaine and prilocaine produces a marked blanching of the skin at the application site, an effect seen only with low concentrations of amide local anaesthetics. The total concentration of the drugs in the dosage form is relatively high, but the amount reaching the cutaneous nociceptors is small (McCafferty *et al.*, 1989).

Vasodilation has been observed following the percutaneous delivery of amethocaine (Woolfson *et al.*, 1990b). From a total of 1241 recorded applications of a 4% w/w amethocaine percutaneous anaesthetic preparation, 6.3% of these applications resulted in mild, transient erythema of the site. A further 0.6% of the applications produced oedema, a qualitatively similar pattern to that seen with intradermal delivery of amethocaine. These reactions were not repeated on a subsequent exposure of the same individual to the preparation. This, together with the increased blood flow in the cutaneous microcirculation monitored by laser-Doppler velocimetry (Woolfson *et al.*, 1989), confirmed that vasodilation, rather than an overt hypersensitivity reaction, was responsible for the changes observed on the skin surface. Clearly, it is necessary to exercise care in interpreting such skin reactions when local anaesthetics are applied to healthy, intact skin. Incorrect interpretation of skin surface symptoms could easily lead to identification of a hypersensitivity reaction where none actually exists.

3.7 SYSTEMIC TOXICITY

The main pharmacological activity of interest exhibited by local anaesthetic drugs is the ability to produce reversible conduction blockade of nerve impulse transmission. The underlying mechanism by which this property is achieved unfortunately renders these drugs potentially toxic. However, the toxicity of local anaesthetics is almost exclusively associated with their clinical misuse. Such adverse reactions to local anaesthetic agents are usually due to rapid, inadvertent intravenous injection, administration into a highly vascular anatomical site, or the extravascular administration of an excessive amount of drug (Covino, 1978). For example, 300 mg of lignocaine administered for lumbar epidural anaesthesia would yield a peak plasma level of approximately 3 mg ml^{-1}. Toxic responses to such relatively small doses of local anaesthetics are rare. Inadvertent administration of the same dose of lignocaine into a peripheral vein would, however, be likely to produce a blood level high enough for symptoms of central nervous system toxicity to be apparent.

The use of local anaesthetic preparations specifically formulated to facilitate percutaneous absorption carries little risk of systemic toxicity, provided such preparations are used as intended, that is, for application to intact, healthy skin. The permeability of skin to an applied drug can, of course, be altered by an underlying disease state or other physical damage (Behl *et al.*, 1980). Drug absorption from the skin takes place through the microcirculation in the dermis. Since the epidermis has no direct blood supply, no drug absorption occurs in this region. The slow rate of drug penetration through the epidermal layers means a correspondingly slow entry into the systemic circulation from the dermal sink. Most of the drug, in fact, remains in the formulation on the skin surface. Thus, the blood level of a local anaesthetic absorbed from the percutaneous route is unlikely to approach a toxic concentration. However, if very large areas of the body were to be covered, for example in the harvesting of several split skin grafts, caution would be advisable, as would an awareness of the danger in inadvertently leaving such large areas covered by a percutaneous anaesthetic preparation for excessive periods, perhaps several hours.

Several studies have confirmed the low systemic absorption of local anaesthetics following percutaneous delivery. Ketocaine, a highly lipophilic amino-ether local anaesthetic, has been shown to produce effective percutaneous anaesthesia when presented to the skin surface as a 10% saturated solution in a solvent mixture containing isopropanol, glycerol and water (Akerman, 1978). The blood concentrations of the drug were determined by mass fragmentography immediately following removal of the drug solution from the site, and again some 3 hours later. The application time for the procedure, which was carried out prior to the harvesting of split skin grafts, varied between 1 and 10 hours. The drug solution was applied as a soaked pad, with the skin area covered determined by the number of pads. The blood levels of ketocaine found (Table 3.8) were in the ng ml^{-1} range.

Table 3.8 — The blood concentrations (ng ml^{-1}) of ketocaine in 84 patients following percutaneous absorption of ketocaine. Numbers in parentheses are values found at three hours after removal of the drug solution from the skin surface. The number of patients per category is denoted by n

no.of pads used	duration of application (h)						
	1-2 n=9	2-3 n=39	3-4 n=17	4-5 n=8	5-6 n=9	6-7 n=1	9-10 n=1
8, n=1			416 (138)				
6, n=1		506 (844)					
4, n=3		106.0 (136.5)	539 (331)				
3, n=8	119 (23)	232.5 (93)	250.0 (106.5)		207.0 (161.7)		
2, n=34	111.7 (38.0)	92.5 (63.0)	108.4 (85.5)	239.2 (111.2)	329.3 (151.70)		
1, n=37	55.4 (30.0)	70.6 (40.4)	73.5 (72.0)	195.5 (79.0)	44.0 (40.0)	147 (139)	91 (7)

Reproduced from Ohlsen and Englesson (1980) with permission of the copyright owner

Studies on the blood levels of lignocaine and prilocaine, following application of a eutectic mixture of the two drugs for percutaneous anaesthesia (Engberg *et al.*, 1987; Manner *et al.*, 1987), again showed very low concentrations of the local anaesthetics in the systemic circulation. Blood samples were taken from a cannula inserted at the application site and, simultaneously, from the opposite extremity (Table 3.9). In the latter case the lignocaine concentration was below the limit of detection by high performance liquid chromatography with ultra-violet spectroscopic detection at 210 nm.

Table 3.9 — Mean ($\pm$ s.d.) serum lignocaine concentrations (mg ml^{-1}) after percutaneous application of a lignocaine-prilocaine eutectic mixture to children

pilot study (n=4)	application site		
10 min	0.65 ± 0.4		
20 min	0.24 ± 0.04		
60 min	0.21 ± 0.1		
90 min	0.24 ± 0.1		
control study (n=6)	application site	antecubital fossa	contralateral extremity
0 min	0.39 ± 0.4	–	–
15 min	0.10 ± 0.1	0.05 ± 0.04	0
25 min	0.06 ± 0.1	0.03 ± 0.04	0
40 min	0.12 ± 0.1	0.03 ± 0.04	0
90 min (n=2)	0.08 ± 0.1	0.02 ± 0.03	0

Reproduced from Manner *et al.* (1987) with permission of the copyright owner.

A study (Woolfson and McCafferty, 1991) on the percutaneous absorption of amethocaine *in vitro* through human stratum corneum further confirmed the view that percutaneous delivery of local anaesthetics through intact skin presents little risk of systemic toxicity. The maximum predicted blood concentration of amethocaine was 24 ng ml^{-1} following a 30 minute application of a typical application to a venepuncture site. This figure would be substantially lower *in vivo*, since this study was designed on a worst case scenario in which it was assumed that all drug penetrating beyond the stratum corneum would reach the systemic circulation. Given the slow rate of drug penetration and the effects of protein binding and metabolism, this is unlikely. Studies *in vivo* in the authors' laboratory have indicated that, following application of an amethocaine percutaneous anaesthetic, approximately 75% of the drug is recoverable from the preparation.

The main danger arising from the percutaneous delivery of local anaesthetics is inadvertent application to mucosal epithelia, or to diseased or abraided skin, particularly open wounds where the barrier to absorption is missing or damaged. This point is well illustrated by a case report (Daya *et al.*, 1988) in which a five year old boy developed grand mal seizures following treatment with topical tetracaine (0.5%), adrenaline (1:2000) and cocaine (11.8%) solution (TAC). A pad soaked in 2 ml of TAC was applied to a 1 cm laceration of the buccal mucosa. The pad subsequently became inadvertently lodged in the posterior pharynx, and although removed promptly, seizures onset within ten minutes, necessitating clinical intervention. Similar occurrences have been noted previously (Adriani and Campbell, 1956; Balamoutsos and Alevizou-Christophoridou, 1979; Meyers, 1980; Dailey, 1986). Since percutaneous anaesthetic preparations are specifically designed to be highly penetrative in order to overcome the skin barrier, it is quite possible for potentially toxic blood concentrations to be achieved by their inadvertent or incorrect application to highly vascular sites. Although the less toxic amino-amides, such as lignocaine and prilocaine, have a safety advantage over esters such as amethocaine in this respect, it is really preferable to avoid use of percutaneous anaesthetics other than on intact, healthy skin. In fact, where the skin barrier is not intact, existing formulations of local anaesthetic salts are perfectly adequate for topical application, and should be used in preference to those formulations designed specifically to promote drug penetration through the stratum corneum. Since the risk of unexpected complications is always present, however, as it is with all pharmaceutical products, it is necessary to be aware of the potential systemic toxicity of local anaesthetic drugs. The point is well illustrated by a report of severe lignocaine intoxication following application of a 5% topical formulation for the treatment of painful, erosive skin lesions where the skin barrier was no longer intact (Lie *et al.*, 1990). The patient displayed progressive abnormalities culminating in an episode of cardiorespiratory arrest and consequent fatality.

3.7.1   Systemic   reactions

Toxic reactions due to accumulation of a local anaesthetic drug in the systemic circulation involve primarily the central nervous system (CNS) and the cardiovascular system. CNS symptoms tend to parallel the blood level of the drug, a higher level producing more profound symptoms (de Jong, 1978). Thus, a progression of toxic effects can be seen starting with drowsiness, a ringing in the ears, peripheral numbness and double vision. At still higher blood levels fine tremors of hand and face muscles are seen, leading to clonic convulsions and, if the blood level of the drug rises still further, depression of respiration and consciousness (Vickers *et al.*, 1984). Thus, the recommended dose of a local anaesthetic is partly based on the necessity of avoiding CNS toxicity (Moore *et al.*, 1977). These recommended doses, however, have little relevance when the drug is given percutaneously. For lignocaine, a blood level in excess of 5 mg ml^{-1} is usually required to produce signs of systemic toxicity. A single epidural injection of no less than 500 mg would be required to produce a level approaching this value (Covino, 1978), a situation far removed from that possible with percutaneous delivery of the drug through intact skin.

Cardiovascular toxicity, if it occurs, usually onsets subsequent to the appearance of CNS symptoms. It is characterised by bradycardia and hypotension, leading ultimately to cardiac arrest if clinical intervention is not made. The highly lipophilic agents, bupivacaine and etidocaine, which are also among the most potent local anaesthetics, have been primarily associated with cardiotoxicity in laboratory studies (Marx, 1984) but such observations are rare in clinical practice.

A measure of the cardiotoxicity of local anaesthetics is the CC/CNS ratio (Wood, 1990), which is the ratio of dosage or blood levels required to produce irreversible cardiovascular collapse to the dosage or blood levels required to elicit convulsions (CNS toxicity). Cardiotoxicity, if it occurs, always follows the onset of CNS symptoms, which therefore act as a warning of possible further complications. This is a reflection of the higher blood concentration of a local anaesthetic necessary to cause cardiovascular symptoms. The CC/CNS ratio for lignocaine, as determined in animal studies, is about 7.0 (Morishima *et al.*, 1981) whereas the corresponding figure for bupivacaine is 2.7 (Morishima *et al.*, 1985). The electrophysiological effects on the heart of both of these drugs at lower, therapeutic (in the case of lignocaine) concentrations has been demonstrated by Clarkson and Hondeghem, 1985). Although acute systemic toxicity following the use of local anaesthetic drugs is unlikely if such drugs are properly administered in safe dosages, it is still necessary to have an emergency treatment regimen available in the event that complications arise (Abadir, 1975).

3.8   LOCAL ADVERSE REACTIONS

Local anaesthetics infiltrated below the skin surface produce no significant local tissue damage as compared to saline controls (de Jong, 1978). There is certainly no evidence that these drugs have any effect on subsequent wound healing (Nilsson and Wanderberg, 1957), an important consideration when such drugs are given percutaneously, for instance, prior to the harvesting of split skin grafts. Rather, the main concern is an immediate hypersensitivity reaction following an initial exposure (sensitisation) to a local anaesthetic allergen.

It is undoubtedly true that local anaesthetics have received a "bad press" with respect to hypersensitivity reactions. An extreme example of this is the comment of one dermatologist that "the relief provided (by local anaesthetics) does not justify the risk of dermatitis resulting from allergic sensitivity" (Wilson, 1966). In fact, true allergic responses to local anaesthetics are extremely rare (de Jong, 1978; AMA, 1986). Such type 1 IgE mediated reactions to local anaesthetics probably represent less than 1% of the total of all adverse reactions to these drugs (Somerfield, 1990).

In common with most drug molecules local anaesthetics are, comparatively, low molecular weight compounds. They are therefore too small to be sensitising allergens (immunogens) and must bind via irreversible covalent bonds to a carrier protein molecule in order to induce an immune response. Such a response may result in the synthesis of specific immunoglobulins, of which IgE is responsible for immediate hypersensitivity reactions. Specifically, sensitised lymphocytes may also be produced in addition to, or in place of, the immunoglobulins (Bundgaard, 1990). Although the influence of local anaesthetic lipophilicity has not been investigated specifically with regard to sensitisation potential, it has been shown for 2,4-dinitro phenylprotein conjugates that increasing lipophilicity was directly correlated with increasing sensitisation potential (Roberts *et al.*, 1983). This may reflect an increase in the protein-binding capacity of the more lipophilic derivatives and could be of significance when considering the sensitisation potentials of, for example, procaine and the more lipophilic amethocaine.

Covino and Vassallo (1976) have pointed out that a diagnosis of hypersensitivity reactions to local anaesthetics is often made when no obvious alternative explanation is available for an adverse effect following exposure to a drug in this class. An anaphylactic type of reaction, although very rare, can occur but requires systemic absorption of the drug following either parenteral or topical administration. The more common symptoms, however, which are often ascribed to a hypersensitivity reaction, are associated with topical application of local anaesthetics. The presence of rash, urticaria and oedema have all been noted, and contact dermatitis following repeated exposure to local anaesthetics amongst health professionals has long been known (Wilson, 1958). However, topical applications of local anaesthetics have often been made to sensitive areas of the body, such as the ano-genital area. Frequently, such an application has been for the treatment of a pre-existing inflammatory condition such as pruritis (Wilson, 1966). This must raise doubts as to the reliability of many reports of topical hypersensitivity reactions involving the appearance of rashes and related symptoms.

The use of local anaesthetics to produce profound anaesthesia of intact, healthy skin represents not only a new use for these drugs but also, perhaps, an opportunity to look again at the true extent of adverse cutaneous symptoms. Previously, the only data available involving intact, healthy skin came from patch testing. Such tests tend to concentrate on the ester class of local anaesthetics since almost all reports of skin rashes and contact dermatitis involve the para-amino benzoic acid derivatives, such as procaine, benzocaine and amethocaine. In a sample of three thousand patients undergoing patch tests with a mixture of benzocaine, amethocaine hydrochloride and a non para-aminobenzoic acid derivative, cinchocaine, 2.8% of the subjects were classed as exhibiting an allergic response to the mixture (Beck and Holden, 1988). Interestingly, despite the well-known cross-sensitivity in the ester group, 52.5% of a sample of 40 allergic patients reacted to amethocaine or cinchocaine, but not to benzocaine. This probably reflects the limited use of benzocaine in the UK, thereby reducing the number of patients initially sensitised to the drug. By comparison, hypersensitivity to the amides, including cross-sensitivity within the group, is even rarer than with the esters, but has nevertheless been reported (Goransson, 1976; Fregert et al., 1979; Curley et al., 1986; Black et al., 1990).

3.9   METABOLISM

The balance between the rate of destruction in the body due to drug metabolism and the rate of drug absorption is a major factor in determining the potential systemic toxicity of a local anaesthetic administered by injection. When administration of the drug is by the percutaneous route, the rate of absorption into the systemic circulation is greatly exceeded by the rate of metabolism. There is also the possibility of drug metabolism occurring in the cutaneous tissues (see Chapter 4).

The eventual site of metabolic destruction for all local anaesthetic drugs is in the liver. However, the amino-esters are also significantly metabolised in plasma by the enzyme pseudocholinesterase (butyrylcholinesterase). Procaine is comparatively rapidly metabolised by plasma pseudocholinesterase to diethylaminoethanol and para-aminobenzoic acid. Amethocaine is the most slowly metabolised of the amino-ester local anaesthetics (Foldes et al., 1965), yielding dimethylaminoethanol and para-(butylamino)benzoic acid by the same route (Fig. 3.9). Further metabolism of para-(butylamino)benzoic acid in the liver produces the primary metabolite, para-

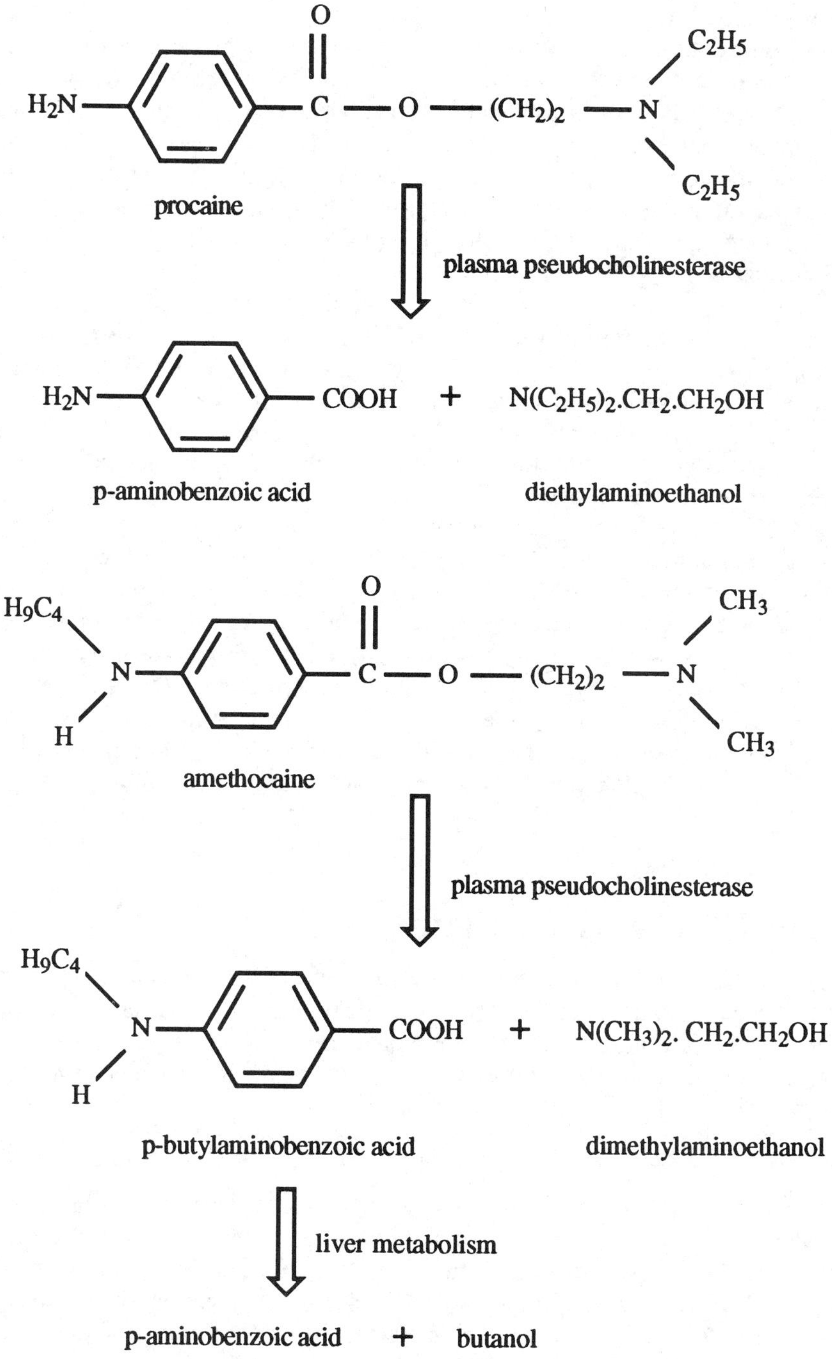

Fig 3.9 — Metabolic routes for the amino-ester local anaesthetics, procaine and amethocaine

aminobenzoic acid, thought to be the source of the allergic phenomena occasionally associated with these drugs.

The metabolism of the amino-esters is only likely to be of significance in respect of their use as percutaneous anaesthetics in those patients with atypical pseudocholinesterase. In such cases the enzyme is known to have a lower affinity than normal for the ester substrate (Valentino *et al.*, 1981). This may lead to a reduction in the rate of metabolism of amethocaine and the other amino esters (Foldes *et al.*, 1963). However, given the limited and slow penetration of these drugs through the stratum corneum (Woolfson and McCafferty, 1991), it is unlikely that this will prove to be a serious clinical problem.

Amino-amide local anaesthetics have more complex metabolic pathways than the esters, and that for lignocaine is now well established (Keenaghan and Boyes, 1972, Narang *et al.*, 1978). The only point of potential concern on the metabolism of percutaneously administered amino-amides centres on prilocaine. Prilocaine is metabolised in the liver to yield, amongst other products, ortho-toluidine. This compound can induce the formation of methaemoglobin, from the oxidation of haemoglobin, in man (Olson and McEvoy, 1981; Duncan and Kobrinsky, 1983). Methaemoglobin, unlike haemoglobin, is not an efficient oxygen carrier. Although methaemoglobin is normally formed in erythrocytes it is immediately reduced again to haemoglobin, a reaction catalysed by the enzyme NADH-dehydrogenase. In adults, a high blood level of prilocaine is necessary to produce sufficient ortho-toluidine to interfere with this process. In infants, however, NADH-dehydrogenase activity is not fully established and they are therefore more susceptible to the influence of comparatively small doses of prilocaine in respect of its metabolite. It is possible to achieve this situation even through the percutaneous absorption of prilocaine (Jakobson and Nilsson, 1985), and it is probably best to completely avoid the use of this drug in infants.

3.10   ROUTES OF ADMINISTRATION

Percutaneous local anaesthesia may be regarded as a specialised application of topical local anaesthesia. It may equally well be thought of as an alternative to local infiltration. To put the percutaneous route, considered in Chapter 4, into a proper context, it is necessary to appreciate the alternative methods that are available for local anaesthetic administration.

3.10.1   Nerve block

Peripheral nerve block is achieved by direct injection of a local anaesthetic solution into, or immediately adjacent to, an individual nerve or nerve plexus. This type of block is used prior to specific surgical procedures, for example, sciatic and femoral nerve blocks for surgery distal to the knee. Peripheral block of a sensory nerve with lignocaine typically onsets quite rapidly, in about three minutes, and these techniques are therefore very useful for outpatient surgical procedures.

Central neural blocks represent the other main applications of regional block techniques and include epidural and spinal anaesthesia. Epidural anaesthesia, widely used in obstetrics, requires the needle to be inserted between the vertebrae. The injection of local anaesthetic is then made directly into the epidural space. For spinal anaesthesia, the drug must be injected intrathecally, that is, into the cerebrospinal fluid of the subarachnoid space, producing anaesthesia of the abdominal and pelvic regions. These local anaesthetic techniques require the specialist skills of the anaesthetist (anesthesiologist).

3.10.2 Local infiltration

When a local anaesthetic solution is injected directly into the tissue that is to receive a pain stimulus, rather than into a specific nerve, the technique is known as infiltration anaesthesia. Infiltration anaesthesia can be applied to deeper organs and is, of course, routinely used in dentistry. Subcutaneous or intradermal infiltration is frequently used to achieve local anaesthesia of the skin, particularly for plastic surgery procedures such as the harvesting of split skin grafts. Prior to the availability of effective percutaneous drug delivery, the only alternative to local infiltration for these procedures was general anaesthesia, with all its attendant risks, particularly for the elderly patient.

Local infiltration requires relatively large amounts of drug if effective anaesthesia of the site is to be achieved. For non-superficial applications to deeper sites infiltration anaesthesia, although feasible, tends to be avoided since toxic levels of local anaesthetic would be approached. Even for superficial sites, such as donor skin grafts, multiple infiltration is generally required. The problem with this is simply that infiltration is itself a painful procedure (McKay et al., 1987; Morris et al., 1987; Martin, 1990). The discomfort due to the injection of a local anaesthetic is often the worst aspect of commonly undertaken minor procedures such as the suturing of small wounds, insertion of venous and arterial cannulae, and surgical excisions (Morris and Whish, 1984). When repeated several times around a large site, the benefit of eventual pain prophylaxis is substantially reduced by the initial discomfort. Clearly, the painless, single application of a percutaneous local anaesthetic preparation has significant advantages in this respect. Frequently, local infiltration anaesthetic solutions contain a vasoconstrictor, usually

Table 3.10 — Recommended doses of local anaesthetic agents by infiltration

agent	% solution	plain solutions			
		max. adult dose (mg)	max dose (mg kg^{-1})	max. adult dose (mg)	max dose (mg kg^{-1})
procaine	1-2	800	11	1000	14
lignocaine	0.5-1	300	4	500	7
mepivacaine	0.5-1	300	4	500	7
prilocaine	0.5-1	500	7	600	8
bupivacaine	0.25-0.5	175	2.5	225	3

adrenaline, in order to prolong the duration of anaesthesia at the site. This also allows a larger dose of the local anaesthetic to be given (Table 3.10).

Local infiltration techniques usually involve extravascular injection of the drug at the site. A variation on local infiltration is intravenous regional anaesthesia (intravascular anaesthesia; Bier Block), used for surgery on part of a limb, such as the hand or lower limb. The injection is made into a vein from which blood has been removed, usually by simple drainage under gravity. The upper part of the limb is occluded with a tourniquet to prevent removal of the drug during the surgical procedure.

3.10.3 Topical (surface) anaesthesia

In the authors' experience there is a certain degree of confusion between the terms topical and percutaneous anaesthesia. The word topical in this sense implies an application of a pharmaceutical product to an external region of the body. This may not necessarily mean the body surface. For example, a drug application made to the oral epithelium would be considered as a topical form of administration. In addition to creams, gels and ointments, topical preparations can also include sprays, gargles, lozenges, suppositories and dusting powders (Adriani et al., 1985).

Unlike the other forms of regional anaesthesia, topical anaesthetic preparations are widely available without prescription. Therefore, this route of application is certainly the most widely used, as well as the oldest, form of local anaesthesia. Topical anaesthesia is effective on mucous membranes and on open skin wounds such as suture lines. It can be used to relieve the pain of sunburn, localised skin abrasions and pruritis, as well as localised damage due to, for example, insect bites and stings (Adriani et al., 1985). These are relatively trivial applications, most frequently made with over-the-counter remedies. Benzocaine is often a common component of such preparations. As an essentially water-insoluble drug, its only application as a local anaesthetic is for topical use. The low water solubility of the drug means that there is little risk of absorption from, for instance, cut skin.

A topical anaesthetic preparation is ineffective on intact skin since the drug cannot normally penetrate the stratum corneum to act on the underlying nociceptors, unless specifically formulated as a percutaneous anaesthetic (Hanks and White, 1988). Due to this important distinction, it is preferable to regard percutaneous local anaesthesia as a separate regional technique, rather than as another application of topical anaesthesia.

3.11   LOCAL ANAESTHETICS FOR PERCUTANEOUS ABSORPTION

With research on the subject now stretching back over thirty years, it is perhaps surprising that only four drugs have been clearly shown to produce effective percutaneous local anaesthesia. These are amethocaine, ketocaine, and lignocaine/prilocaine as a eutectic mixture. Lignocaine itself has also produced some degree of skin anaesthesia, but only at a high concentration. To formulate a clinically useful percutaneous anaesthetic product requires the correct choice of drug or drugs, together with appropriate pharmaceutical processing. It is likely that other local anaesthetics, if properly formulated, could yield significant advances in this area.

The list of available local anaesthetic drugs is large but there is limited information available on the anaesthetic free bases. A comprehensive review of all the individual local anaesthetic drugs is outside the scope of this volume. However, the properties of those drugs known to be effective by the percutaneous route, and those that may have promise as percutaneous anaesthetics, should be considered.

3.11.1   Amethocaine

Amethocaine is a long-acting, potent local anaesthetic. Its comparatively slow onset time when administered by injection is not relevant to the percutaneous route. The drug is poorly soluble in water, but solubility increases dramatically with a reduction in pH. Amethocaine, being an ester, has poor aqueous stability except in acidic solutions. The drug is soluble in ethanol (1:5). For extraction and analytical purposes, amethocaine base is readily soluble in organic solvents such as ether and dichloromethane. Amethocaine is a low-melting, waxy solid. Storage should therefore be in dry, cool conditions, and the drug should be protected from light. In this situation amethocaine free base will have a shelf life of approximately five years.

The main uses for amethocaine are for spinal anaesthesia, as the hydrochloride, and for surface anaesthesia, including anaesthesia of the eye. Amethocaine base is formulated as both an ointment (U.S.P.) and an ophthalmic ointment (U.S.P.). Ointment formulations of the free base, which use a hydrophobic vehicle, offer enhanced stability since hydrolytic cleavage of the ester group cannot take place in a non-aqueous system. However, ointment bases do not promote absorption through the stratum corneum and are unsuitable for percutaneous anaesthetic formulations of amethocaine.

Amethocaine is particularly effective as a local anaesthetic on mucous membranes. Therefore, it can be used, as the hydrochloride, on such areas as the rectum and anus, the oral mucosa, and for anaesthesia of the tracheo-bronchial area prior to passage of an endoscope. In the latter case the rapid systemic absorption of the drug can give rise to fatal systemic reactions, particularly when a large surface area is covered by aerosol application.

The recommended maximum doses, for topical application to areas capable of substantial absorption of amethocaine, are 300 mg for an adult and 75 mg for a child per 24 hour period (AMA, 1986). The figures must be interpreted sensibly when the drug is used for percutaneous application since only a small portion of the actual drug content of the formulation is absorbed through intact, healthy skin. By comparison, the recommended maximum dose for spinal anaesthesia is 15 mg (AMA, 1986). Here, all of the drug is administered directly as a bolus rather than being very slowly absorbed, and comparatively rapidly metabolised, as in the case of percutaneous application. In the authors' experience applications of amethocaine in a percutaneous anaesthetic formulation have frequently been made to adults prior to the harvesting of split skin grafts (Small *et al.*, 1988). Such applications tend to cover an area of about 300 cm^2, contain approximately 400 mg of amethocaine, and remain in place for a minimum of one hour. No systemic reactions, even with quite elderly patients, have been observed.

Amethocaine is a highly suitable agent for percutaneous anaesthesia on the basis of its lipophilicity, potency and physicochemical properties. The disadvantages of the drug are its perceived potential toxicity and its linkage with contact hypersensitivity reactions.

3.11.2   Lignocaine

Lignocaine is poorly absorbed through intact skin (Martindale, 1989) but, as its hydrochloride salt, it is an effective local anaesthetic for wounds and mucous membranes. It is the most widely used of all the local anaesthetic agents, being of medium potency and duration. Perhaps because of this, much effort has been expended on making effective percutaneous anaesthetic preparations based solely on lignocaine, ignoring the fact that the drug has the wrong characteristics for this application. Lipophilicity and potency are too low, and melting point is too high. Some limited success has been reported clinically with percutaneous lignocaine, but only at unrealistically high concentrations of the drug, such as 30% lignocaine base in a cream formulation (Lubens et al., 1974).

In addition to topical anaesthesia the main uses of lignocaine are for infiltration and certain regional nerve blocks. Up to 1.75 g of the free base can be applied as an ointment to broken skin (AMA, 1986). In this respect the drug has a better toxicity profile than amethocaine. As an amide, contact hypersensitivity reactions are extremely rare. Unfortunately, potency and duration of effect reflect the lower lipophilicity of the drug compared to amethocaine, making it a marginal choice as the sole drug for percutaneous anaesthesia.

3.11.3   Prilocaine

Prilocaine has a similar pharmacological profile to lignocaine but is more rapidly metabolised and excreted. This substantially reduces its toxicity compared to lignocaine, making it the agent of choice for intravenous regional anaesthesia. The recommended maximum adult dose by injection is 600 mg per two hours. Given that the drug is metabolised to ortho-toluidine, methaemoglobinaemia is a potential problem at higher doses or in infants.

Prilocaine is not used on its own as a topical anaesthetic. However, prilocaine and lignocaine bases in admixture form a lower melting point entity, a eutectic mixture. This oily eutectic mixture, formulated as a cream, is an effective percutaneous anaesthetic with good skin penetration properties. The eutectic mixture is formed from the two anaesthetics, each at a concentration of 2.5% w/w (Ehrenstrom Reiz and Reiz, 1982). The importance of proper formulation procedures is therefore emphasised in that, although neither lignocaine nor prilocaine bases are suitable themselves for percutaneous anaesthesia, their combination yields an effective product.

3.11.4   Ketocaine

Ketocaine, an amino ether, is a potent, highly lipophilic local anaesthetic, synthesised originally in Italy. The pharmacological properties of ketocaine have been reported by Setnikar (1966). The drug is not widely available and is not official in either the United States or British Pharmacopoeias. In Italy ketocaine is available as Vericaina (Recordati SpA, Milan).

The main interest in ketocaine is its reported formulation (Ohlsen and Englesson, 1980) to produce effective percutaneous anaesthesia suitable for the harvesting of split skin grafts. Unfortunately, subsequent trials demonstrated quite severe local adverse reactions, and the drug is no longer used for this purpose. Since the concentration used was quite high (10% w/V), and the solvent mixture employed contained isopropanol and acetic acid, it may be that local skin reactions were, at least in part, due to the formulation. Further investigation of ketocaine for percutaneous anaesthesia is probably warranted, but is undoubtedly curtailed by commercial and financial considerations in that the drug is not registered in most western markets.

3.11.5   Miscellaneous agents

In addition to those drugs that have been shown to produce effective percutaneous anaesthesia, a number of other agents are worthy of some further study for delivery by this route. Generally, these drugs tend to be less well-known than the major local anaesthetics and are often not registered in all major markets. A further complication is that, in all cases, the free base form must be precipitated from an aqueous solution of its salt. The free bases, unfortunately, are not commercially available and there is minimal information on their physicochemical properties.

The amino-ketone, dyclonine, has a potency similar to cocaine. It has been used topically as the hydrochloride salt to anaesthetise both the oral and anogenital mucosa, and as a 0.5% or 1% aqueous solution for broken skin (AMA, 1986). A gel formulation of dyclonine hydrochloride is official in the United States Pharmacopoeia. The limited aqueous solubility of the salt restricts the use of the drug to topical applications. No information is available on the free base but the topical activity of the salt suggests that it may offer formulation possibilities for percutaneous delivery.

Pramoxine is an amino-ether which, like dyclonine, is used as a topical agent in the form of its hydrochloride. Pramoxine hydrochloride may be used for anaesthesia of minor skin wounds and the relief of haemorrhoids and other anorectal disorders. The drug is an ingredient of many proprietary topical products, and the U.S.P. has official cream and gel formulations. Unfortunately, again, like dyclonine, little is known on the properties of the free base, but the potency of the hydrochloride has been likened to that of benzocaine (AMA, 1986).

Fomocaine, an amino-ether, is also a morpholine derivative in common with pramoxine (Oelschlager, 1959). It may be a more promising agent than pramoxine in that it has greater potency and substantially reduced toxicity (Temple, 1977). The drug is indicated for general applications in dermatology as a 4% cream or ointment. A proprietary preparation is available in Germany. No studies are presently available on the skin penetration properties of fomocaine.

REFERENCES

Abadir, A. (1975) Use of local anaesthetics in dermatology *J. Derm. Surg.* **1:2** 65-70.

Adriani, J. and Campbell, D. (1956) Fatalities following topical application of local anesthetics to mucous membranes. *J. Am. Med. Ass.* **162** 1527-1530.

Adriani, J., Beuttler, W.A., Brihmadesam, L. and Naraghi, M. (1985) Topical anesthetics: use and misuse. *South. Med. J.* **78** 1224-1229.

AMA Drug evaluations, 6th. edn. (1986) American Medical Association, Philadelphia, pp. 275-289.

Agnew, W.S. (1984) Voltage-regulated sodium channel molecules. *Annu. Rev. Physiol.* **46** 517-530.

Akerman, B. (1978) Percutaneous local anaesthesia: problems-solutions. *Acta Anaesthesiol. Scand.* **Suppl. 70** 90-91.

Akerman, B., Hellberg, I.B. and Trossvik, G. (1988) Primary evaluation of the local anaesthetic properties of the amino amide agent ropivacaine (LEA 103). *Acta*

Anaesthesiol. Scand. **32** 571-578.

Auger, M., Smith, I.C.P. and Jarrell, H.C. (1989) Interactions of the local anesthetic tetracaine with glyceroglycolipid bilayers: a ^{2}H NMR study. *Biochim. Biophys. Acta* **981** 351-357.

Auger, M., Smith, I.C.P., Mantsch, H.H. and Wong, P.T.T. (1990) High pressure infrared study of phosphatidylserine bilayers and their interactions with the local anesthetic tetracaine. *Biochemistry* **29** 2008-2015.

Balamoutsos, N.G. and Alevizou-Christophoridou, F. (1979) Survival following 1000 mg of amethocaine. *Br. J. Anaesth.* **51** 469-470.

Beck, M.H. and Holden, A. (1988) Benzocaine - an unsatisfactory indicator of topical anaesthetic sensitisation for the U.K. *Br. J. Dermatol.* **118** 91-94.

Becker, H.K. (1963) Carl koller and cocaine. *Psychoanal. Quart.* **32** 309-373.

Behl, C., Flynn, G., Kurihara, T., Smith, W. and Higuchi, W. (1980) Permeability of thermally damaged skin: 1. Influence of 60°C scalding on hairless mouse skin. *J. Invest. Dermatol.* **75** 340-345.

Black, R.J., Dawson, T.A.J. and Strang, W.C. (1990) Contact sensitivity to lignocaine and prilocaine. *Contact Dermatitis* **23** 117-118.

Boulanger, Y., Schreier, S. and Smith, I.C.P. (1981) Molecular details of anesthetic-lipid interaction as seen by deuterium and phosphorous-31 nuclear magnetic resonance. *Biochemistry* **26** 6824-6830.

Buchi, J. and Perlia, X. (1971) Structure-activity relations and physicochemical properties of local anaesthetics. In: Lechat, P. (ed.) *Local Anaesthetics, Vol 1. International encyclopoedia of pharmacology and therapeutics, Section 8.* Pergamon Press, Oxford, pp. 39-130.

Bundgaard, H. (1990) Drug allergy: chemical and pharmaceutical aspects. In: Florence, A.T. and Salole, E.G. (eds) *Formulation factors in adverse drug reactions.* Wright, London, pp. 23-55.

Catterall, W.A. (1984) The molecular basis of neuronal excitability. *Science* **223** 653-661.

Catterall, W.A. (1987) Common modes of drug action on sodium channels: local anesthetics, antiarrhythmics, and anticonvulsants. *Trends Pharmacol. Sci.* **8** 57-65.

Chernoff, D.M. and Strichartz, G.R. (1990) Kinetics of local anesthetic inhibition of neuronal sodium currents. *Biophys. J.* **58** 69-81.

Clarkson, S.W. and Hondeghem, L.M. (1985) Mechanism for bupivacaine depression of cardiac conduction: fast block of sodium channels during the action potential with slow recovery from block during diastole. *Anesthesiology* **62** 396-405.

Concepcion, M., Arthur, R., Steele, S.M., Bader, A.M. and Covino, B.G. (1990) A new local anaesthetic, ropivacaine. *Anesth. Analg.* **70** 80-85.

Coster, H.G.L., James, V.J., Berthet, C. and Miller, A. (1981) *Biochim. Biophys. Acta* **641** 281-285.

Covino, B.G. and Vassallo, H.G. (1976) *Local Anaesthetics. Mechanism of Action and Clinical Use.* Grune and Stratton, New York.

Covino, B.G. (1978) Systemic toxicity of local anaesthetic agents. *Anesth. Analg.* **57** 387-388.

Covino, B.G. (1982) New developments in the field of local anaesthetics and the scientific basis for their clinical use. *Acta Anaesthesiol. Scand.* **26** 242-249.

Covino, B.G. (1986) Pharmacology of local anaesthetic agents. *Br. J. Anaesth.* **58** 701-716.

Curley, R.K., MacFarlane, A. and King, C. (1986) Contact sensitivity to the amide anaesthetics: lidocaine, prilocaine and mepivacaine. Case report and review of literature. *Arch. Dermatol.* **122** 924-926.

Dailey, R.H. (1986) Fatality secondary to misuse of topical TAC solution. *Ann. Emerg. Med.* **17** 59-160.

Daya, M.R., Burton, B.T., Schleiss, M.R. and Diliberti, J.H. (1988) Recurrent seizures following mucosal application of TAC. *Ann. Emerg. Med.* **17** 646-648.

de Jong, R.H. (1978) Toxic effects of local anesthetics. *J. Am. Med. Ass.* **239** 1166-1173

Duncan, P.G. and Kobrinsky, N. (1983) Prilocaine-induced methemoglobinemia in a newborn infant. *Anesthesiology* **59** 75-76.

Ehrenstrom Reiz, G.M.E. and Reiz, S.L.A. (1982) EMLA - a eutectic mixture of local anaesthetics for topical anaesthesia. *Acta Anaesth. Scand.* **26** 596-598.

Einhorn, A. and Uhlfelder, E. (1909) Ueber den p-aminobenzoesaurediathylester. *Liebigs Ann.* **371** 131-142.

Eisler, O. (1929) β-Dimethylaminoethyl ester of p-butylaminobenzoic acid. U.S. Patent 1,889,645.

Engberg, G., Danielson, K., Henneberg, S. and Nilsson, A. (1987) Plasma concentrations of prilocaine and lidocaine and methaemoglobin formation in infants after epicutaneous application of a 5% lidocaine-prilocaine cream (EMLA). *Acta Anaesthesiol. Scand.* **31** 624-628.

Foldes, F.F., Foldes, V.M., Smith, J.C. and Zsigmond, E.K. (1963) The relation between plasma cholinesterase and prolonged apnea caused by succinylcholine. *Anesthesiology* **24** 208-216.

Foldes, F.F., Davidson, G.M., Duncalf, D. and Kuwabara, S. (1965) The intravenous toxicity of local anesthetic agents in man. *Clin. Pharmacol. Ther.* **6** 328-335.

Foussard-Blandpin, O. and Quevauviller, A. (1982) A propos des relations "structure-activite" dans le domaine des anesthetiques locaux. I. Amino-esters et amino-ethers. *Ann. Pharm. Franc.* **40** 133-143.

Fregert, S., Tenge, E. and Thalsi, I. (1979) Contact allergy to lidocaine. *Contact Dermatitis* **5** 185-188.

Freud, S. (1884) Uber coca. *Zentralbl. Ges. Ther.* **2** 289-314.

Goransson, K. (1976) Hypersensitivity to prilocaine. *Dermatologica* **152** 158-160.

Greenberg, M. and Tsong, T.Y. (1982) Binding of quinacrine, a fluorescent local anesthetic probe, to mammalian axonal membranes. *J. Biol. Chem.* **257** 8964-8971.

Guy, R.H., Wester, R.C., Tur, E. and Maibach, H.I. (1983) Non-invasive assessment of the percutaneous absorption of methyl nicotinate in humans. *J. Pharm. Sci.* **72** 1077-1079.

Hanks, G.W. and White, I. (1988) Local anaesthetic creams. *Br. Med. J.* **297** 1215.

Hille, B. (1980) Theories of anesthesia: general perturbations versus specific receptors. In: Fink, B.(ed.) *Molecular mechanisms of anesthesia*, Vol. II. Raven Press, New York, pp. 1-5.

Jakobson, B. and Nilsson, A. (1985) Methemoglobinemia associated with a prilocaine-lidocaine cream and trimethoprim-sulphamethoxazole. A case report. *Acta Anaesthesiol. Scand.* **29** 453-455.

Keenaghan, J.B. and Boyes, R.N. (1972) The tissue distribution, metabolism and excretion of lidocaine in rats, guinea pigs, dogs and man. *J. Pharmacol. Exp. Ther.* **180** 454-463.

Kelusky, E.C. and Smith, I.C.P. (1983) Characterisation of the binding of the local anaesthetics procaine and tetracaine to model membranes of phosphatidylethanolamine. A nuclear magnetic resonance study. *Biochemistry* **22** 6011-6017.

Leo, A., Hansch, C. and Elkins, D. (1971) Partition coefficients and their uses. *Chem. Rev.* **71** 525-616.

Lie, R.L., Vermeer, B.J. and Edelbroek, P.M. (1990) Severe lidocaine intoxication by cutaneous absorption. *J. Am. Acad. Dermatol.* **25** 1026-1028.

Lin, C.T., Williamson, L.N., Chyan, Y.G. and Marques, A.D.S. (1988) Deprotonation dynamics of local anesthetics in hydrophobic media: dibucaine HCl in water/alcohol or surfactant mixtures. *Photochem. Photobiol.* **48** 733-740.

Lofgren, N.M. and Lundqvist, B.J. (1948) Alkylglycinanilides. *U.S. Patent* 2,441,498.

Lofstrom, B. (1970) Aspects of the pharmacology of local anaesthetic agents. *Br. J. Anaesth.* **42** 194-206.

Lubens, H.M., Ausdenmoore, R.W., Shafer, A.D. and Reece, R.M. (1974) Anesthetic patch for painful procedures such as minor operations. *Am. J. Dis. Child* **128** 192-194.

Manner, T., Kanto, J., Iisalo, E., Lindberg, R., Vunamaki, O. and Scheinin, M. (1987) Reduction of pain at venous cannulation in children with a eutectic mixture of lidocaine and prilocaine (EMLA cream): comparison with placebo cream and no medication. *Acta Anaesthesiol. Scand.* **31** 735-739.

Martin, A.J. (1990) pH-adjustment and discomfort caused by the intradermal injection of lignocaine. *Anaesthesia* **45** 975-978.

Martindale. The Extra Pharmacopoeia (1989) *Local anaesthetics.* Pharmaceutical Press, London, pp. 1205-1227.

Marx, G.F. (1984) Cardiotoxicity of local anesthetics: the plot thickens *Anesthesiology* **60** 3-5.

McCafferty, D.F., Woolfson, A.D., McClelland, K.H. & Boston, V. (1988) Comparative *in vitro* and *in vivo* assessment of the percutaneous absorption of local anaesthetics. *Brit. J. Anaesth.* **60** 64-69.

McCafferty, D.F., Woolfson, A.D. & Boston, V. (1989) *In-vivo* assessment of percutaneous local anaesthetic preparations. *Brit. J. Anaesth.* **62** 17-21.

McKay, W., Morris, R. and Mushlin, P. (1987) Sodium bicarbonate attenuates pain on skin infiltration with lidocaine, with or without epinephrine. *Anesth. Analg.* **66** 572-574.

Menczel, E., Yacobi, A., Paran, I. and Lustig, A. (1977) Comparative subcutaneous absorption of local anesthetics: lidocaine, procaine and tetracaine. *Arch. Int. Pharmacodyn.* **225** 330-342.

Menczel, E. and Goldberg, S. (1978) pH effect on the percutaneous penetration of lignocaine hydrochloride. *Dermatologica* **156** 8-14.

Mertz, C.J., Marques, A.D.S., Williamson, L.N. and Lin, C.T. (1990) Photophysical studies of local anesthetics, tetracaine and procaine: drug aggregations. *Photochem. Photobiol.* **51** 427-437.

Meyers, E.F. (1980) Cocaine toxicity during dacrocystorhinostomy. *Arch. Ophthalmol.* **98** 842-843.

Moore, D.C., Bridenbaugh, L.D. and Thompson, G.E. (1977) Factors determining dosages of amide-type local anesthetic drugs. *Anesthesiology* **47** 263-268.

Morishima, H.O., Pederson, H., Finster, M., Sakuma, K., Bruce, S.L., Gutsche, B.B., Stark, R.I. and Covino, B.G. (1981) Toxicity of lidocaine in adult, newborn and foetal sheep. *Anesthesiology*, **55** 57-61.

Morishima, H.O., Pederson, H., Finster, M., Hiraoka, H., Tsuiji, A., Feldman, H.S., Arthur, G.R. and Covino, B.G. (1985) Bupivacaine toxicity in pregnant and nonpregnant ewes. *Anesthesiology* **63** 134-139.

Morris, R.W. and Whish, D.K.M. (1984) A controlled trial of pain on skin infiltration with local anaesthetics. *Anaesth. Intens. Care* **12** 113-114.

Morris, R.W., McKay, W. and Mushlin, P. (1987) Comparison of pain associated with intradermal and subcutaneous infiltration with various local anesthetic solutions. *Anesth. Analg.* **66** 1180-1182.

Mrose, H. and Ritchie, J.M. (1978) Local anesthetics: do benzocaine and lidocaine act at the same single site? *J. Gen. Physiol.* **71** 223-225.

Muscholl, E. (1961) Effect of cocaine and related drugs on the uptake of noradrenaline by heart and spleen. *Br. J. Pharmacol. Chemother.* **16** 352-359.

Narang, P.K., Crouthamel, W.G., Carliner, N.H. and Fisher, M.L. (1978) Lidocaine and its active metabolites. *Clin. Pharm. Ther.* **24** 654-662.

Niemann, A. (1860) Sur l'alcoloide de coca. *J. Pharmacol.* **34** 474-475.

Nilsson, E. and Wanderberg, B. (1957) Effect of local anaesthetics on wound healing. *Acta Anaesthesiol. Scand.* **2** 87-89.

Oelschlager, H. (1959) Preparation of the amino ether N-{3-[4-(phenoxymethyl)-phenyl] propyl} morpholine with local anaesthetic properties. *Arzneim. Forsch.* **9** 313-321.

Ohlsen, L. and Englesson, S. (1980) New anaesthetic formulation for epicutaneous application tested for cutting split skin grafts. *Br. J. Anaesth.* **52** 413-417.

Olson, M.L. and McEvoy, G.K. (1981) Methemoglobinemia induced by local anesthetics. *Am. J. Hosp. Pharm.* **38** 89-93.

Philip, B.K. (1990) Local anaesthetics. In: White, P.F. (ed) *Outpatient anaesthesia.* Churchill Livingstone, New York, p. 264

Reynolds, F., Bryson, T.H.L. and Nichols, A.D.G. (1976) Intradermal study of a new local anaesthetic agent, aptocaine. *Br. J. Anaesth.* **48** 347-354.

Roberts, D.W., Goodwin, B.F.L., Williams, D.L., Jones, K., Johnson, A.W. and Alderson, J.C.E. (1983) Correlations between skin sensitisation potential and chemical reactivity for p-nitrobenzyl compounds. *Food Chem. Toxicol.* **21** 811-813.

Scott, D.B., McClure, J.H., Giasi, R.M., Seo, J. and Covino, B.G. (1980) Effects of concentration of local anaesthetic drugs in extradural block. *Br. J. Anaesth.* **52** 1033.

Setnikar, I. (1966) Ortho-substituted β-phenoxyethyl-amino derivatives. *Arzneim. Forsch.* **16** 1025.

Small, J., Wallace, R.G.H., Woolfson, A.D. and McCafferty, D.F. (1988) Pain-free cutting of split skin grafts by application of a percutaneous local anaesthetic cream. *Brit. J. Plastic Surgery* **41** 539-543.

Smith, M., Gray, B.M., Ingram, S. and Jewkes, D.A. (1990) Double-blind comparison of lignocaine-prilocaine cream (EMLA) and lignocaine infiltration for arterial cannulation in adults. *Br. J. Anaesth.* **65** 240-242.

Somerfield, S.D. (1990) Local anaesthetic allergic reactions. *N.Z. Med. J.* **103** 545.

Strichartz, G.R. and Ritchie, J.M. (1987) Action of local anesthetics on ion channels of excitable tissues. In: Strichartz, G.R. (ed.) *Handbook of experimental pharmacology, Vol. 81: Local anaesthetics.* Springer-Verlag, Heidelberg, pp. 21-52.

Strichartz, G.R. (1980) Use-dependent conduction block produced by volatile general anesthetic agents. *Acta Anaesthesiol. Scand.* **24** 402-406.

Takman, B.H. (1975) Chemistry of local anaesthetic agents: classification of blocking agents. *Br. J. Anaesth.* **47** 183-190.

Taylor, S.E. and Dorris, R.L. (1989) Modification of local anesthetic toxicity by vasoconstrictors. *Anesth. Prog.* **36** 79-87.

Temple, C.F. (1977) Studies on the stability and disposition of 1-(3-phenoxymethylphenyl)-methylmorpholine, a new local anaesthetic agent. *PhD. Thesis.* Johann Wolfgang Goethe Universitat, Frankfurt am Main, Germany.

Trudell, J.R., Payou, D.G., Chiu, J.H. and Cohen, E.N. (1975) The antagonistic effect of an inhalation anesthetic and high pressure on the phase diagram of mixed dipalmitoyl-dimyristoylphosphatidylcholine bilayers. *Proc. Natl. Acad. Sci. USA* **72** 210-213.

Uhlmann, F. (1929) Percaine - a new local anaesthetic. *Arch. Intern. Pharmacodynamie* **36** 253-271.

Valentino, R.J., Lockridge, O., Eckerson, H.W. and La Du, B.N. (1981) Prediction of drug sensitivity in individuals with atypical serum cholinesterase based on *in vitro* biochemical studies. *Biochem. Pharmacol.* **30** 1643-1649.

Vanderkooi, G. and Adade, A.B. (1986) Stoichiometry and dissociation constants for the interaction of tetracaine with mitochondrial ATPase as determined by fluorescence. *Biochemistry* **25** 7118-7124.

Vickers, M.D., Schnieden, H. and Wood-Smith, F.G. (1984) *Drugs in anaesthetic practice.* Butterworths, London, pp. 209-205.

Wildsmith, J.A.W. and Strichartz, G.R. (1984) Local anaesthetic drugs - an historical perspective. *Br. J. Anaesth.* **56** 937-939.

Wildsmith, J.A.W., Gissen, A.J., Gregus, J. and Covino, B.G. (1985) Differential nerve blocking activity of amino ester local anaesthetics. *Br. J. Anaesth.* **57** 612.

Willatts, D.G. and Reynolds, F. (1985) Comparison of the vasoactivity of amide and ester local anaesthetics. *Br. J. Anaesth.* **57** 1006-1011.

Wilson, H. (1958) Streptomycin dermatitis in nurses *Br. Med. J.* **i** 1378-1382.

Wilson, H. (1966) Dermatitis from anaesthetic ointments. *Practitioner* **197** 673-677.

Wood, M (1990) Local anesthetic agents. In: Wood, M. and Wood, A.J. (eds) *Drugs and anesthesia.* Williams and Wilkins, Baltimore, pp. 319-345.

Woolfson, A.D., McCafferty, D.F. & McGowan, K. E. (1990a) The metabolism of amethocaine by porcine and human skin extracts: influence on percutaneous anaesthesia. *Int. J. Pharm.* **62** 9-14.

Woolfson, A.D., McCafferty, D.F. and Boston, V. (1990b) Clinical experiences with a novel percutaneous amethocaine preparation: prevention of pain due to venepuncture in children. *Br. J. Clin. Pharmac.* **30** 273-279.

Woolfson, A.D. and McCafferty, D.F. (1991) Influence of application time and predicted systemic absorption with a novel tetracaine percutaneous anaesthetic preparation. *Pharmacotherapy.* **11** 271.

4

Percutaneous absorption of local anaesthetics

The administration of chemical agents to the skin surface has long been practised, whether for healing, protective or purely decorative or cosmetic reasons. Topical drug therapy involves the localised administration of medicinal formulations to the skin, generally when the skin surface has been breached by disease or infection and a route of drug absorption into the deeper cutaneous layers has consequently been opened. Historically, the skin was thought to be totally impervious to exogenous chemicals. Topical drug administration was therefore usually restricted to those situations where skin lesions were apparent. However, once it was realised that the skin was really a semi-permeable membrane rather than a totally exclusive barrier (Homalle, 1853), new possibilities were apparent both for drug therapy of the skin and drug delivery through it.

4.1 PERCUTANEOUS ABSORPTION AND TRANSDERMAL DRUG DELIVERY

There is currently much interest in using the skin as a port of entry for drugs into the systemic circulation. This has led to the development of many novel transdermal drug delivery systems (Nimmo, 1990). Transdermal drug delivery refers to the delivery of the drug across intact, healthy skin and into the systemic circulation. The diffusive process by which this is achieved is known as percutaneous absorption, meaning, literally, absorption through the skin. Thus, classical topical formulations can be distinguished from those intended for transdermal drug delivery in that, whilst the former are generally applied to a broken, diseased or damaged integument, the latter are used exclusively on healthy skin where the barrier function is intact.

A further application of percutaneous drug absorption, in addition to transdermal drug delivery, can also be identified. This is the application to healthy, intact skin of a drug formulation designed to produce a local effect by acting on specific targets or receptors within the underlying cutaneous tissues. Such an effect is achieved by a limited form of percutaneous absorption, insufficient to lead to any significant systemic drug absorption. Indeed, such a formulation must be specifically designed to preclude, as far as is possible, this occurrence. Thus, percutaneous absorption does not necessarily constitute a process leading to transdermal drug delivery, since this latter term is used exclusively in connection with the achievement of a therapeutic drug concentration in the systemic circulation. Percutaneous local anaesthesia, in which the skin is anaesthetised via the percutaneous absorption of one or more local anaesthetic drugs, constitutes perhaps the best example of local drug delivery, via the percutaneous route, to specific target receptors in the skin (Woolfson and McCafferty, 1989).

4.2 SKIN ANATOMY: SIGNIFICANCE FOR PERCUTANEOUS ABSORPTION

The skin, effectively the largest organ of the body, is a multi-purpose, non-homogeneous membrane with a complex structure (Fig. 4.1). It contains and protects the internal body organs and fluids, and exercises environmental control over the body in respect of temperature and, to some extent, humidity. In addition, the skin is a

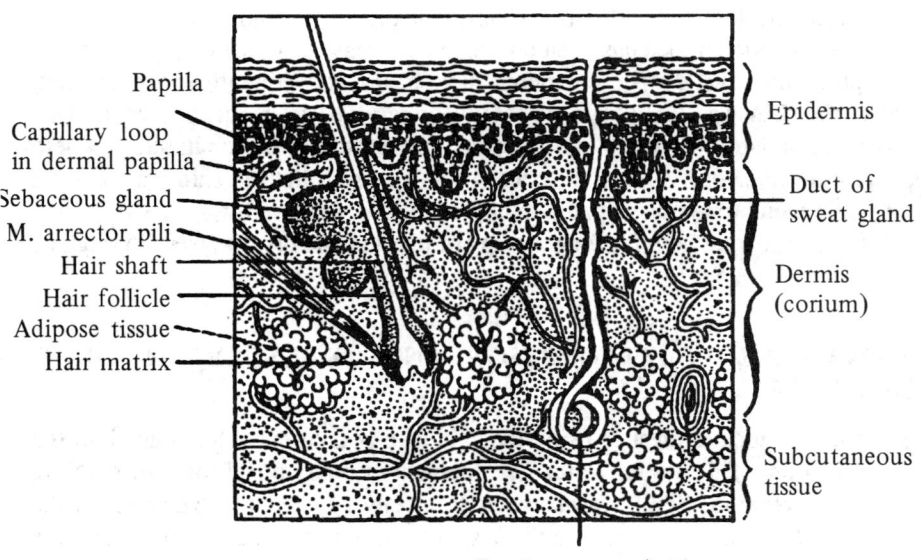

Fig. 4.1 — General structure of the skin and appendages. Reprinted with permission from Rosen *et al. The nurses atlas of dermatology*, Little, Brown and Co., Boston, 1983

communicating organ, relaying the sensations of heat, cold, touch, pressure and pain to the central nervous system. The intervention of a percutaneous local anaesthetic into the normal regime of skin function is specifically designed to reduce or abolish the ability of the skin to detect and transmit the sensation of pain.

As with all organs of the body, the skin can exhibit a wide variety of disease states, acute and chronic, minor and life-threatening (Flynn, 1979). Since it forms the body's interface with the external environment, the skin must additionally cope with the hazards of cuts, abrasions and other mechanical damage. Sometimes, these are inflicted as a medical necessity, and it is in these situations that local anaesthesia of the skin is indicated.

It is fortuitous for all of us that the skin is a self-repairing organ. Both this ability, and the barrier protective properties associated with the integument, are direct functions of skin anatomy. Therefore, in order to formulate a percutaneous local anaesthetic system, or, indeed, deliver any other drug locally to the skin, it is necessary to be aware of how skin anatomy can either facilitate or constrain the percutaneous absorption of exogenously applied chemicals.

4.2.1 The epidermis

The multilayered nature of human skin can be resolved into three distinct layers. These are the outermost layer, the epidermis, beneath which lies the much larger dermis and, finally, the deepest layer, the subcutis. The nociceptors, which are the target site of action for a percutaneous local anaesthetic, are located at or near the dermo-epidermal junction (Iggo, 1982). Therefore, any drug administered via this route must first overcome the epidermal barrier in order to exert its pharmacological action.

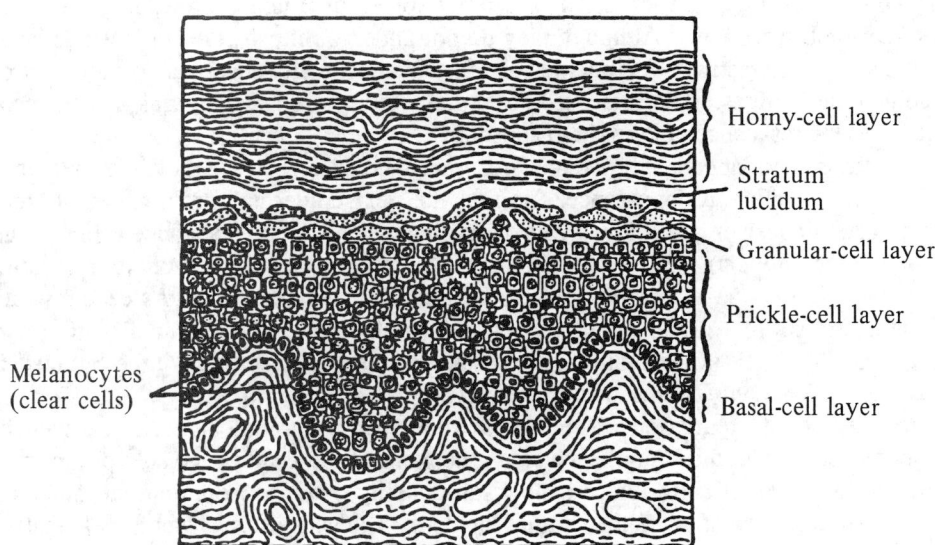

Fig. 4.2 — Stratified epithelium of the epidermis. Reprinted with permission from Rosen *et al. The nurses atlas of dermatology*, Little, Brown and Co., Boston, 1983

The epidermis, which is essentially a stratified epithelium (Fig. 4.2), lies directly above the dermo-epidermal junction. This provides mechanical support for the epidermis and anchors it to the underlying dermis. The junction itself is a complex glycoprotein structure about 50 nm thick. The dermo-epidermal junction does possess barrier properties to the passage of exogenous chemicals into the dermis, but only in respect of very large molecules with molecular weights probably in excess of 40,000 (Schreiner and Wolff, 1969). Thus, no barrier will be offered to the passage of a much smaller local anaesthetic molecule that may penetrate to this depth, and, should this occur, the drug will be absorbed into the systemic circulation via the vascular dermis. Of course, the lack of an effective barrier function at the dermo-epidermal junction is necessary since nutrients must pass into the epidermis from the dermal blood supply via this route.

Directly above the undulating ridges of the dermo-epidermal junction lies the basal layer of the epidermis, the stratum germinativum. This layer is single-cell in thickness with columnar-to-oval shaped cells, which are actively undergoing mitosis. As the name implies, the stratum germinativum generates replacement cells to counterbalance the constant shedding of dead cells from the skin surface. In certain disease states, such as psoriasis, the rate of mitosis in this layer is substantially raised in order to compensate for a diminished epidermal barrier, the epidermal turnover time being as fast as four days. Such conditions, where the rate of drug uptake is both rapid and unpredictable, necessarily preclude the use of percutaneous local anaesthesia. With normal skin, however, the epidermal cells are completely renewed about every four weeks (Jarrett, 1973).

As the cells of the basal layer gradually move upwards through the epidermis, they undergo rapid differentiation, becoming flattened and granular. The ability to divide by mitosis is lost. Directly above the stratum germinativum is a layer, several cells in thickness, in which the cells are irregular and polyhedral in shape. This layer is the stratum spinosum, and each cell has distinct spines or prickles protruding from the surface in all directions. Although they do not undergo mitosis, the cells of this layer are metabolically active. The prickles of adjacent cells interconnect via desmosomes or intercellular bridges. The increased structural rigidity produced by this arrangement increases the resistance of the skin to abrasion.

As the epidermal cells migrate upwards towards the skin surface they become flatter and more granular in appearance, forming the next epidermal stratum, the stratum granulosum, consisting of a few layers of granular cells. Their appearance is due to the actively metabolising cells producing granular protein aggregates of keratohyalin. Keratohyalin may be a precursor of keratin (Reaven and Cox, 1965). As cells migrate through the stratum granulosum, cell organelles undergo intracellular digestion and disappear. The cells of the stratum granulosum die due to degeneration of the cell nuclei, and metabolic activity ceases towards the top of this stratum.

A further differentiation of cells above the stratum granulosum can be seen in sections taken from thick skin, such as on the palm of the hand or the sole of the foot. This distinct layer of cells, which is now substantially removed from nutrients supplied via the dermal circulation, is the stratum lucidum. The cells of this layer are elongated, translucent and anuclear.

The outermost skin stratum is the horny layer or stratum corneum. Keratin, a fibrous protein, is the main constituent of the cells in this layer. The stratum corneum is, in effect, the outer envelope of the body, most of which is covered by a layer 15 to

20 cells in thickness. Those areas where the stratum lucidum is apparent, however, have a much thicker stratum corneum designed to cope with the effects of weight support and pressure. Overall, the epidermis in these regions, such as the palms and soles, can be up to 800 μm in thickness, compared to 75 to 150 μm elsewhere.

The stratum corneum is an unusually dense tissue, which swells in water to several times its own thickness. The elongated cells, approximately 1 μm in thickness, form a close-packed array of interdigitated cells stacked in vertical columns (Mackenzie and Linder, 1973). Interdigitation between adjacent cells allows the formation of cohesive laminae. Each cell is contained by a largely proteinaceous envelope rather than the conventional lipid bilayer cell membrane (Bissett, 1987). An individual horny cell is approximately one micron thick with a surface area of between 700 and 1200 μm^2. There are approximately 10^5 cells to each 1 cm^2. The mechanical strength of the horny layer is largely due to the nature of the proteinaceous envelope together with the disulphide bonds of the intracellular keratin (Matoltsy, 1976). This is further enhanced by the closely packed anatomical structure with desmosome bridges linking cells that are embedded in an intercellular lipoidal matrix.

The intracellular and intercellular components of the stratum corneum are readily distinguished. Protein is present in both phases, whereas lipid is largely concentrated in the intercellular phase, which constitutes some 30% by volume of the stratum corneum (Elias and Leventhal, 1980). The intercellular lipids have a lamellar structure, with phospholipid components being largely absent (Elias, 1981).

The water content of the stratum corneum varies across the layer, being higher on the inner section in those cells nearer the stratum granulosum, and falling off as the external interface is approached. The water content of the stratum corneum is also influenced by the external environment. Anderson and Cassidy (1973) have estimated a stratum corneum water content of 40% by weight in an environment with a relative humidity of between 33 and 50%, and have further shown that the layer has a typical chemical composition, by weight, of 40% protein, largely keratin, 40% water and 15 - 20% lipid. The main lipid components of the stratum corneum are ceramides, unesterified sterols and fatty acids (Elias, 1981). These bipolar lipids, occupying the intercellular space in the stratum corneum, originate from a variety of sources including the discharged lamellae of membrane-coating granules, intercellular cement and the keratinocyte cell envelope (Stuttgen, 1982).

Unlike other body organs, the stratum corneum constantly sheds its outermost layer, a process known as desquamation. The daily loss of flakes from the horny layer of healthy skin is typically between 0.5 and 1g (Goldschmidt and Kligman, 1964). Desquamation must necessarily involve cleavage of the intercellular bridges or desmosomes suggesting that, although the stratum corneum is a dead layer in the conventional sense, some metabolic activity and regulatory control of the desquamation and replacement processes are ongoing. However, this view is not universally accepted and, in general, the desquamation process is not fully understood (Wertz and Downing, 1989).

The anatomical nature of the stratum corneum indicates that, despite its lack of depth (only 10 μm in the non-hydrated state), this layer is responsible for the rate-limiting barrier function of the skin with respect to the percutaneous absorption of exogenous chemicals (Blank and Scheuplein, 1969; Knutson *et al.*, 1985). In particular, the presence of alternating hydrophilic and lipophilic regions has important implications for the percutaneous absorption of local anaesthetics and other drug molecules (Wiechers, 1989).

4.2.2   The dermis

This region, also known as the corium, underlies the dermo-epidermal junction and varies in thickness from 1000 to 4000 μm. Collagen, a fibrous protein, is the main component of the dermis and is responsible for the tensile strength of this layer. Elastin, also a fibrous protein, forms a network between the collagen bundles and is responsible for the elasticity of the skin and its resistance to external deforming forces. These protein components are embedded in a gel composed largely of mucopolysaccharides. The skin appendages such as the sebaceous and sweat glands, together with hair follicles, penetrate this region. Since these open to the external environment they present a possible entry point into the skin.

The dermis has a rich blood supply extending to within 0.2 mm of the skin surface and derived from the arterial and venous systems in the subcutaneous tissue. This blood supply consists of microscopic vessels and does not extend into the epidermis. Thus, a drug reaching the dermis through the epidermal barrier will be rapidly absorbed into the systemic circulation, with the effective drug concentration in the dermis falling to zero through the upper 200 μm of this layer. The presence of this dermal sink thus ensures a maximum drug concentration gradient across the epidermis (Barry, 1983a).

The dermis is the effective target for a transdermal drug delivery system, since any drug molecule reaching into the cutaneous tissues to this depth will be absorbed via the dermal microcirculation into the systemic circulation. In percutaneous local anaesthesia, however, the drug targets are the pain receptors (nociceptors) that are located at or just above the dermo-epidermal junction. Therefore, skin anatomy dictates that the penetration characteristics of a percutaneous local anaesthetic preparation must be controlled in a manner that allows diffusion across the stratum corneum, a long residence time in both the epidermis and at the nerve receptors, and very slow penetration into the dermis in order that the systemic drug concentration never approaches the significant levels achieved with a typical transdermal delivery system. This adds an additional design parameter, over and above those normally associated with transdermal systems, to be considered by the formulator of percutaneous anaesthetic systems.

4.2.3   Skin appendages

The skin appendages comprise the hair follicles and associated sebaceous glands, together with the eccrine and apocrine glands. Hairs are formed from compacted plates of keratinocytes, with the hair shaft housed in a hair follicle formed as an epidermal invagination. Associated flask-like sebaceous glands are formed as epidermal outgrowths. They secrete an oily material, sebum, onto the skin surface This mixture of lipids acts as a plasticiser for the stratum corneum and maintains an acid mantle of about pH 5 on the skin surface. Of importance to the percutaneous absorption process is the observation that hair follicles occupy only a fraction of the human skin surface estimated as only about 10^{-3} of the total skin area (Scheuplein, 1967). The role and nature of hair has been comprehensively reviewed by Ebling and Rook (1979).

The eccrine glands have temperature control as their principal function. This is achieved by secretion and evaporation of sweat, a dilute, hypotonic solution of salts. These glands occupy an estimated fractional surface area of only 10^{-4} (Scheuplein, 1967).

Secretion is stimulated by an increase in the external temperature and, due to innervation of the glands by the autonomic nervous system, by emotional factors. The glands extend well into the dermis (Woodburne, 1965).

The eccrine sweat glands are widely distributed over the body. However, the apocrine glands are found only at specific locations, notably in the axillae and anogenital regions although, like the eccrine glands, they do extend into the dermis. The milky secretions are of uncertain purpose, and the apocrine glands are generally regarded as secondary sexual characteristics.

4.3 POSSIBLE ROUTES TO PERCUTANEOUS LOCAL ANAESTHESIA

There are three potential routes (Scheuplein, 1967) by which a topically applied local anaesthetic drug can reach the underlying nociceptors. The location of the target site for percutaneous local anaesthesia is depicted in Fig 4.3, with the possible routes to the target shown in Fig. 4.4.

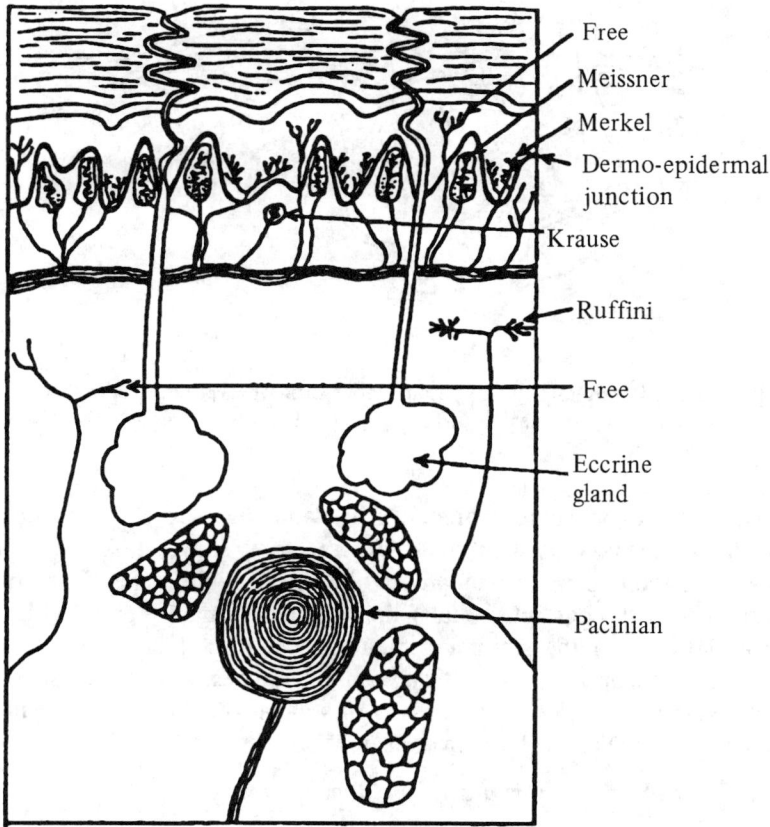

Fig. 4.3 — Location of the cutaneous sensory network. Modified from Miller in
Montagna (ed.) *Advances In Biology of the Skin Vol 1 Cutaneous Innervation* (1960)
with permission of the copyright holder

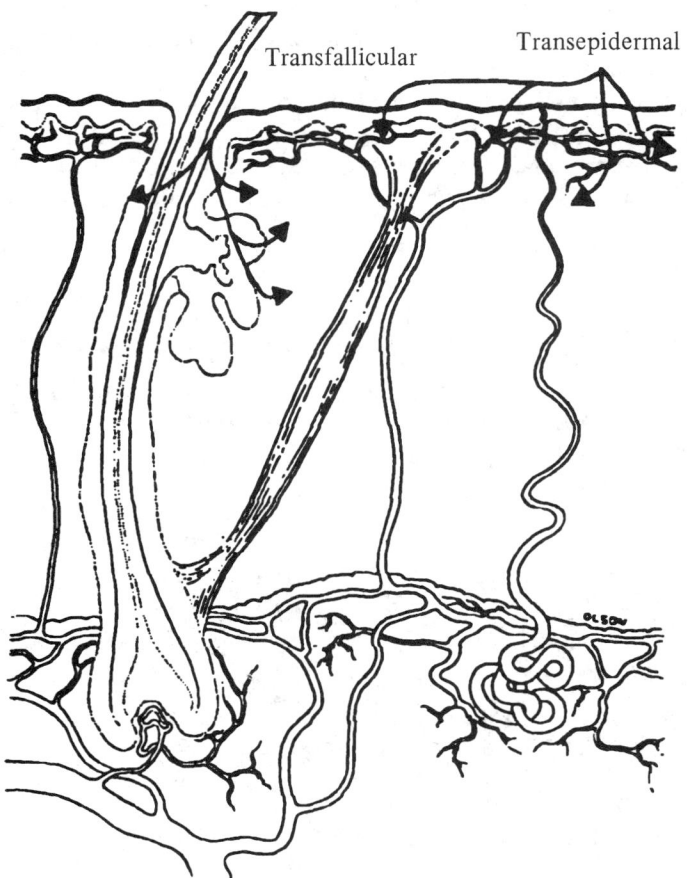

Fig. 4.4 — Possible routes of percutaneous drug absorption. Reproduced from Flynn (1979). With permission of the copyright holders, Marcel Dekker, New York

The most rapid route available is certainly via the skin appendages. This is sometimes known as the shunt route. Alternatively, slower diffusion of drug molecules across the stratum corneum can proceed by two possible routes. The drug may diffuse predominantly through intercellular lipid, or may primarily partition in multiple steps across the cells of the stratum corneum, the transcellular route. The design of a successful percutaneous anaesthetic preparation is dependent on a knowledge of the likely route favoured by the drug, which is in turn dictated by its physicochemical properties and the way in which the local anaesthetic is presented to the skin.

4.3.1　Models of percutaneous absorption

An elegant model for the percutaneous absorption of a topically applied drug has been proposed by Flynn (1979). An analogy is made between the flow of electrons in an electrical circuit through series and parallel resistors, and the passive diffusional flow of a drug through the resistances offered by the various skin components. The current flow is driven by an electrical potential gradient whereas the diffusional drug flow is driven by a concentration gradient across the skin.

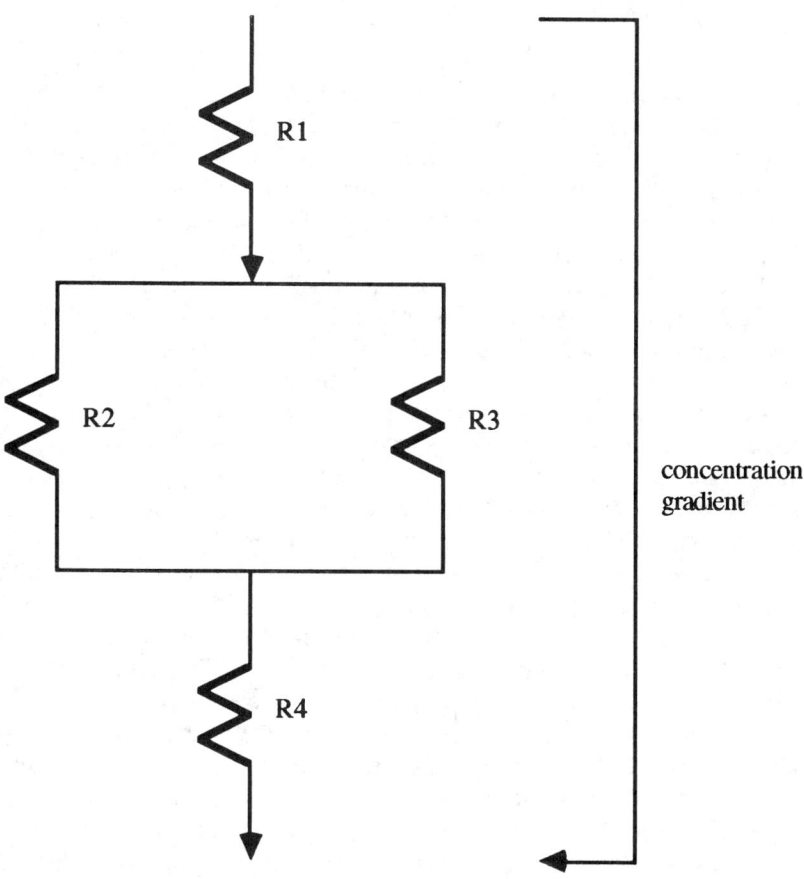

concentration
gradient

R1 = vehicle resistance
R2 = appendageal resistance
R3 = stratum corneum
R4 = viable tissue resistance

Fig. 4.5 — Series and parallel resistances to percutaneous drug penetration. Modified from Flynn (1979). With permission of the copyright holders, Marcel Dekker, New York

Skin diffusional resistances can be thought of as the transepidermal and transappendageal routes, in parallel (Fig. 4.5). The transepidermal resistance is essentially that offered by the stratum corneum. As with the ohmic magnitude of an electrical resistance, the chemical magnitude (R) of a membrane resistor with respect to drug diffusion through that membrane can be expressed as

$$R = \frac{h}{F\,D\,K}$$

(4.1)

where h is the thickness of the resistor membrane, F is the fractional area of the route (where there is more than one pathway involved), D is the diffusion coefficient of the drug through that resistor (the ease of movement of the drug through the tissue) and K represents the capacity of a particular tissue for the drug (in effect, the partition coefficient of the drug between one tissue phase and that immediately preceding it). It follows that the rate of skin penetration of a given drug is inversely proportional to the total diffusional resistance due to the various skin layers and components.

The transepidermal route has a fractional area approaching unity. In the percutaneous absorption process the total diffusional resistance offered by this route would consist of the sum of resistances due to the stratum corneum, viable epidermis and dermis. However, in the case of percutaneous local anaesthesia, where the target is relatively close to the skin surface, any diffusional resistance due to the dermis can be neglected. Indeed, since it is desired to minimise systemic absorption of the local anaesthetic, diffusional resistance offered by the dermis can be regarded beneficially.

The stratum corneum is a narrow layer, hence the value of h in (4.1) is small, thus tending to reduce the diffusional resistance of this layer. However, the main factor to consider is the densely packed, organised anatomical characteristics of this layer, ensuring that its overall resistance to chemical penetration is substantial, notwithstanding the reduced thickness of the horny layer compared to that of the viable epidermis.

The transappendageal route has a very low fractional area (Scheuplein and Blank, 1971). Shunt diffusion of penetrants through the skin appendages appears to be of significance only during the initial phase following application of the drug. The higher diffusion coefficients through the appendages compared to the stratum corneum (Scheuplein and Blank, 1971) leads to an excess initial penetration via this route, with an exponential relationship to time compared to the linear time dependency of drug penetration which characterises the establishment of steady state diffusion. Thus, although the transappendageal route may be important initially, its small fractional area suggests that it is of no great significance in the overall percutaneous penetration of most topically applied drugs (Scheuplein, 1976).

Given the tortuous nature of the skin ducts and glands, and the upwards flow of material towards the skin surface opposing the downwards diffusion of an applied drug, it is not surprising that the shunt route is unimportant in steady state drug diffusion through the skin (Blank, 1965). However, the initial build-up of drug achieved by rapid diffusion along the appendageal route, probably the hair follicles, prior to the establishment of steady state transepidermal diffusion, may explain the appearance of vasoactive phenomena associated with the percutaneous application of local anaesthetics (Woolfson *et al.*, 1989). This represents a similar situation to that existing with nicotinates (erythema) and steroids (skin blanching), both effects rapidly following topical administration of these agents (Stoughton, 1972).

Since the transappendageal route can be neglected as a major contributor to the overall penetration of non-electrolytes such as local anaesthetics, the overall resistance to the drug reaching its target site of action can be seen as analogous to the flow of current through electrical resistors in series. Thus, the total resistance (R) of the skin to the percutaneous absorption of a local anaesthetic can be described by

$$R = \frac{h}{F_{sc} D_{sc} K_{sc}} + \frac{h}{F_e D_e K_e}$$

(4.2)

where the denominator subscripts refer to the stratum corneum and viable epidermis respectively.

The stratum corneum has been shown to have approximately 10^3 times greater resistance to water penetration than the dermis, and is thus even more resistant to the passage of polar solutes (Scheuplein, 1972). For non-polar lipophilic solutes such as local anaesthetic bases the stratum corneum has a lower resistance than to the passage of water. Although the viable epidermis and the dermis are more resistant to the passage of non-polar compared to polar materials, as might reasonably be expected, this effect is relative and minimal with only 4% of the total skin resistance being ascribed to these viable layers (Scheuplein, 1972). It is clear, therefore, that the passage of the drug through the stratum corneum is the rate-limiting step for the percutaneous absorption of both polar and non-polar molecules. The decreased resistance of the horny layer to lipophilic drugs dictates, in the case of the percutaneous absorption of local anaesthetics, the use of the lipophilic anaesthetic free bases rather than their water-soluble salts.

Although numerous mathematical models are available to describe the process of percutaneous absorption (Osborne, 1986), that proposed by Flynn et al. (1974) provides a good description of the overall process involved in the percutaneous absorption of a drug. Where that drug is a local anaesthetic, and where the target site of action is located at or near the dermo-epidermal junction, the model can be considerably simplified. Thus, the resistance to drug penetration of the dermis can be neglected since it is beyond the target site. The transappendageal route is largely insignificant, and the resistance due to the viable epidermis is so small compared to that due to the stratum corneum that it approaches zero. Thus, the stratum corneum fractional area can, in this case, be taken as unity. When steady state diffusion of the drug across the stratum corneum barrier has been established, the amount of material passing through the barrier per unit area of vehicle coverage per unit time, i.e. the drug flux, J, is given by

$$J = \left(\frac{D_{sc} K_{sc/w}}{h_{sc}} \right) \Delta C$$

(4.3)

where $K_{sc/w}$ represents the partition coefficient between the stratum corneum and the formulation vehicle and ΔC is the drug concentration gradient across the stratum corneum, which, assuming sink conditions, is the effective drug concentration in the vehicle. This equation, which is essentially Fick's first law for steady state diffusion (Brown and Langer, 1988), can be simplified to

$$J = P (\Delta C)$$

(4.4)

where P is the permeability coefficient of the drug through the skin. P is described by the term in brackets in (4.3).

Equation (4.3) provides a guide to those factors which can be acted upon to maximise the efficiency of the percutaneous absorption of a local anaesthetic drug through the stratum corneum barrier. Clearly, little can be done to reduce the value of h, the barrier thickness, unless an adhesive tape stripping technique were to be employed (Blank, 1965). The barrier thickness may be reduced in the event of an existing clinical disease state, and of course it will vary depending on the site of application for the anaesthetic, but otherwise it may be regarded as a constant.

The drug diffusivity in the stratum corneum, as measured by D_{sc}, is a physicochemical parameter of the chosen drug or drug combination. Although the barrier characteristics may be altered by the use of a chemical penetration enhancer such as Azone® (Wiechers and De Zeeuw, 1990), the relative values of D_{sc} for different local anaesthetics will retain their same comparative ranking. An increase in the value of $K_{sc/w}$, the vehicle/stratum corneum partition coefficient, therefore represents the best available means to ensure that an adequate concentration of local anaesthetic can penetrate to the target nociceptors within an acceptable time period. The vehicle composition is therefore of paramount importance in the percutaneous absorption of local anaesthetics and many other drugs (Ostrenga *et al.*, 1971). This approach is considered in Chapter 5 and must be combined with a formulation that maximises the value of ΔC, the total drug concentration when sink conditions are assumed to operate. However, the extent to which ΔC can be increased is limited by toxicological considerations. Thus, a percutaneous anaesthetic patch containing 30% w/w lignocaine base (Lubens and Sanker, 1964) provides an example of achieving the desired pharmacological response by relying solely on achieving a very large drug concentration gradient across the barrier. Such a high drug concentration, though, would now be considered unacceptable.

Equation (4.3) is based on the assumption that steady state diffusion is operating. Although this may be true in *in vitro* experimentation, in most *in vivo* cases steady state diffusion will not occur. For a more complex transdermal drug delivery to the dermis and systemic circulation a more rigorous model based on Fick's second law of diffusion would be required (Scheuplein, 1967). In practice the typical drug penetration profile through a given skin barrier with respect to time can be seen in Fig. 4.6. With all drug delivery processes by passive percutaneous diffusion, there is a measurable time period, the lag time (t_l), before steady state diffusion is established. The lag time is related to membrane thickness (h) and to the drug diffusion coefficient (D) through that membrane by

$$t_1 = \frac{h^2}{6D}$$

$$(4.5)$$

The lag time may be found by extrapolation of the linear portion of the penetration profile (Fig. 4.6). This procedure allows the calculation of D, the drug diffusion coefficient through the tissue, by application of equation (4.5). The lag time is shortest for the transappendageal route, and longest for the transepidermal pathway. For percutaneous local anaesthesia, the lag time is effectively the time taken to establish a constant concentration gradient across the stratum corneum. Since transdermal systemic drug delivery systems require the establishment of this gradient across a much thicker section of skin, through to the upper regions of the dermis, the lag time phenomenon is much less significant with percutaneous anaesthesia. Nevertheless, short but measurable lag times have been observed during *in vitro* studies on the penetration characteristics of local anaesthetics through model polydimethylsiloxane (Silastic®) barrier membranes (McCafferty *et al.*, 1988).

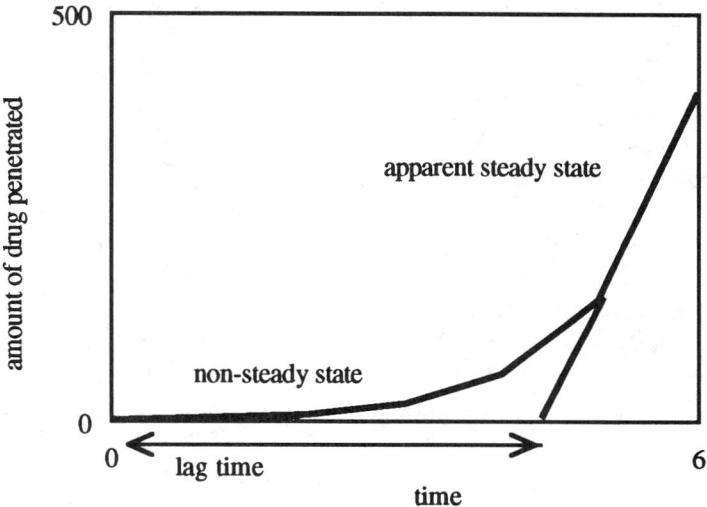

Fig. 4.6 — Percutaneous penetration profile showing estimation of the lag time by extrapolation of the linear portion of the curve

Overall, then, a complex picture is presented with regard to the penetration of drugs through the skin (Table 4.1). However, specifically for the percutaneous penetration of local anaesthetics, a simplified model of drug penetration can be adopted in which the stratum corneum barrier, and the drug partition coefficient between it and the vehicle, may be considered as the major factors.

4.3.2 Transport of local anaesthetics through the stratum corneum: the two-compartment model

The stratum corneum can best be considered as a two-compartment system in which the individual cells, the corneocytes, are surrounded by a continuous lamellar lipid phase. This model has been described by Elias (1988) as "bricks and mortar", in which the keratin-rich corneocytes are the bricks and the intercellular lipid is the mortar. Thus, a penetrant molecule may pass through the bricks (the intracellular route) and/or through the mortar (the intercellular route), as depicted in Fig. 4.7.

Corneocytes are surrounded by an envelope, which is lipoidal on the exterior and is in contact with the intercellular lipid. The interior is hydrophilic and is in contact with the cell contents (Wertz and Downing, 1989). The corneocytes, which are also covered with keratin filaments, occupy the largest volume of the stratum corneum. Their contribution to the barrier function resides in the water-insoluble protein fraction (Matoltsy *et al.*, 1968).

Table 4.1 — Some parameters of percutaneous penetration

	diffusion coefficient $cm^2 s^{-1}$
through stratum corneum	range 10^{-9} to 10^{-13}
water	$\approx 10^{-9}$
n-alkanols (hydrated tissue)	$\approx 10^{-9}$
n-alkanols (dry tissue)	$\approx 10^{-10}$
small nonelectrolytes	10^{-9} to 10^{-10}
progesterone	$\approx 10^{-11}$
cortisone	$\approx 10^{-12}$
hydrocortisone	$\approx 10^{-13}$
through follicular pore (sebum)	10^{-7} to 10^{-9}
through viable tissue	$\approx 10^{-6}$
	tissue thickness μm
dry stratum corneum(normal)	≈ 10
hydrated stratum corneum (occlusion)	20 to 30
pore (diffusional length)	60 (maximum)
viable tissue	150-2000
	route fractional area
transepidermal	≈ 1
transfollicular	$\approx 10^{-3}$
transeccrine	$< 10^{-5}$

Reprinted from Flynn (1979) by courtesy of the copyright holders, Marcel Dekker Inc., New York

It is now generally accepted that the main penetration route for a drug molecule traversing the stratum corneum is through the intercellular lipid matrix, and that very little drug penetration occurs via the intracellular corneocyte route (Loth, 1989; Wiechers, 1989). Much work has been done on elucidating the chemical architecture of this intracellular lipid matrix. Freeze-fracture studies on isolated stratum corneum membranes (Breathnach *et al.*, 1973) have clearly demonstrated that the intercellular lipid is organised in multiple, broad bilayers (Fig. 4.8).

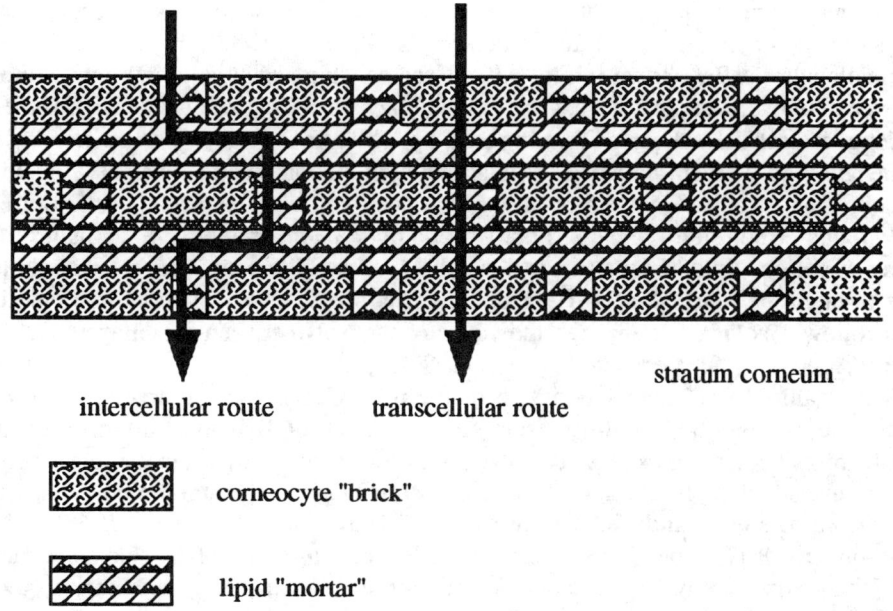

intercellular route   transcellular route   stratum corneum

corneocyte "brick"

lipid "mortar"

Fig. 4.7 — The "bricks and mortar" model of percutaneous penetration

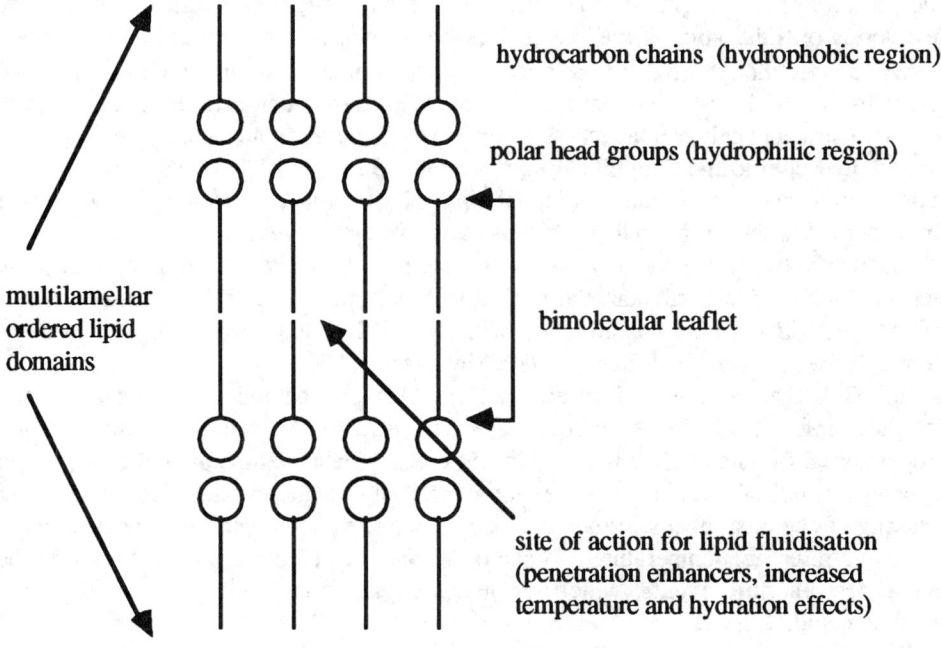

hydrocarbon chains (hydrophobic region)

polar head groups (hydrophilic region)

multilamellar
ordered lipid
domains

bimolecular leaflet

site of action for lipid fluidisation
(penetration enhancers, increased
temperature and hydration effects)

Fig. 4.8 — Organisation of the intercellular lipid of human stratum corneum

The lipid components present in the stratum corneum consist largely of ceramides, sterols (mainly cholesterol), and free fatty acids (Smith *et al.*, 1982). Each lipid bilayer, the bimolecular leaflet shown in Fig. 4.8, alternates with a relatively hydrophilic area formed by the hydrated polar head groups of the lipids, thus forming an aqueous channel. The long, saturated alkyl chains forming each lipid bilayer are tightly packed forming a unique and highly organised barrier with strong hydrophobic interactions. Hydrophilic interactions are stabilised by the presence of ceramides which have a predominance of free alkyl groups. Cholesterol imparts rigidity to the hydrophobic region and facilitates the mixing of various lipid components (Potts, 1989). Lipophilic penetrants are thought to move through the lipid bilayers (Nemanic and Elias, 1980) whereas more hydrophilic drugs follow a polar route through the aqueous channels between the bilayers (Loth, 1989; Wiechers, 1989; Wertz and Downing, 1989).

The organised, multilamellar nature of the intercellular lipid matrix is of prime importance in determining the barrier characteristics of human stratum corneum (Landmann, 1988), and thus represents the main obstacle to the percutaneous absorption of local anaesthetics. Extraction of the lipid components of the stratum corneum has been shown to significantly reduce the barrier function (Matoltsy *et al.,*, 1968). The barrier function is also notably reduced in clinical conditions such as fatty acid deficiency in which an abnormality has been demonstrated in the lamellar body secretory system responsible for the generation of the intercellular lipids (Prottey, 1977; Elias and Brown, 1978).

4.3.3　Percutaneous absorption of amethocaine: effect on stratum corneum lipids

The penetration of lipophilic molecules through the stratum corneum involves some disordering or fluidisation of the intercellular lipid domains. Penetration enhancers such as Azone® are thought to exert their activity by this mechanism in which the chemical inserts itself into the ordered bilayer structure. The consequent disruption to the tightly organised structure causes a reduction in barrier function and an increased ease of passage for both hydrophilic and lipophilic drug molecules (Barry, 1987). Similar effects on the hydrocarbon chains of stratum corneum lipid bilayers have been noted when either temperature or skin hydration have been increased (Knutson *et al.*, 1985).

The thermotropic behaviour of biological membranes may conveniently be studied by thermal analysis. In particular, the related techniques of differential thermal analysis (DTA) and differential scanning calorimetry (DSC) have been widely used in biomembrane research (McElhaney, 1982; Melchior, 1984).

In DTA the sample and reference crucibles are heated at a constant rate. Thermocouples attached to each crucible or embedded in their contents detect when a temperature difference occurs between the crucibles. Such a temperature difference can occur as a result of an endothermic event, which may be due to a melting transition or breaking of chemical bonds. When this occurs, the sample temperature lags behind the increasing reference temperature and can be recorded as either a peak or trough in the signal. Exothermic events, which are generally secondary processes, produce the opposite result.

DSC differs from DTA in allowing the energy involved in the thermal transition or process to be quantified. The detection of a temperature difference between the crucibles causes an auxiliary heater to supply power to either crucible in order to restore the original position. Thus, peak area integration gives a measure of the resulting enthalpy change. Changes in the heat capacity of the sample can also be quantified.

The thermotropic behaviour of human stratum corneum membranes has been studied by numerous workers. Van Duzee (1975) obtained four endothermic transitions with DSC. These occurred at 40, 75, 85 and 107°C, with the endotherms at the two lower temperatures attributed to lipid melting and those at higher temperatures being due to protein denaturation. The effect of lipid extraction on these endotherms was investigated by Golden *et al.* (1986). The higher temperature transition was found to occur in both intact and lipid-extracted stratum corneum but not in the lipid extracts. Furthermore, stratum corneum membranes lacking intracellular keratin failed to show this transition, suggesting that the highest temperature endotherm is due to an irreversible protein transition involving keratin.

The endotherms at around 40 and 75°C were attributed to lipid melting as lipid-extracted stratum corneum did not show these transitions. The transition at 40°C was generally small and its occurrence was reported to vary from sample to sample. It has been suggested that this transition is due to the melting of sebaceous lipids (Golden *et al.*, 1986) since it was reduced or abolished by hexane washing of stratum corneum samples. The transition at 75°C was attributed to intracellular lipid melting. However, there were conflicting interpretations of the endotherm occurring at about 85°C. This endotherm is not observed in thermal profiles of lipid-extracted stratum corneum. This endotherm has been shown to be partly reversible if the sample is heated to 95°C but becomes irreversible if the sample is heated to 140°C. Although initial suggestions (Golden *et al.*, 1986) were that this transition was due to a lipid-protein association, more recent evidence (Goodman and Barry, 1989) suggests that it is the result of complete disruption of the normal stratum corneum lipid structure.

The effect of percutaneously absorbed amethocaine has been studied by DSC (Woolfson *et al.*, 1991). DSC was performed on untreated samples (Fig. 4.9), samples treated with the gel vehicle alone (Fig. 4.10), and samples treated with amethocaine percutaneous gel for either 1 hour (Fig. 4.11) or 24 hours (Fig. 4.12). The thermal profiles obtained for untreated samples, and gel vehicle or amethocaine percutaneous gel (1 hour) treated samples, were similar. Endotherms at about 71 and 85°C , although not sharp, were consistently apparent. These peaks could no longer be identified in stratum corneum samples treated with amethocaine percutaneous anaesthetic for 24 hours. Samples treated for 24 hours with gel base, or untreated samples maintained at 37°C for this period, still gave the characteristic endotherms.

Abolition of endotherms at about 71 and 85°C is typical of thermal profiles obtained with stratum corneum samples treated with established penetration enhancers such as Azone® and oleic acid (Goodman and Barry, 1989). DSC studies with amethocaine suggest that this lipophilic base may also solubilise and fluidise, to some extent, lipid bilayers in a similar manner to certain known penetration enhancers. Most DSC studies with known penetration enhancers report at least a 24 hour pretreatment of stratum corneum prior to analysis. Lipid fluidisation appears to be both dose and time dependent.

Amethocaine, together with other local anaesthetics, has been shown (Racansky *et al.*, 1988) to lower the gel-to-liquid crystalline phase transition temperature of a model dipalmitoyl-phosphatidylcholine lipid membrane. In the case of stratum corneum, only a 24 hour treatment prior to DSC resulted in abolition of lipid-related endotherms

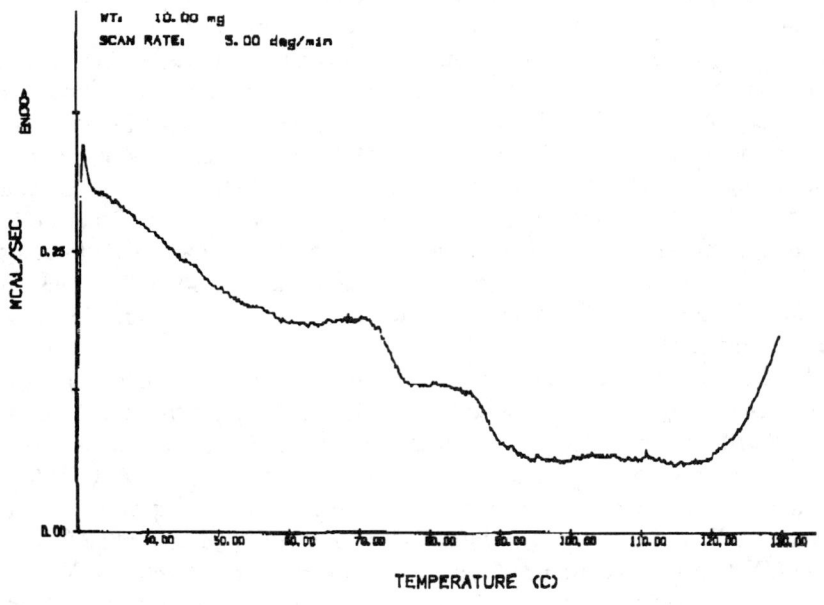

Fig. 4.9 — Differential scanning calorimetry of human stratum corneum following maintenance at 37°C for 24 hours

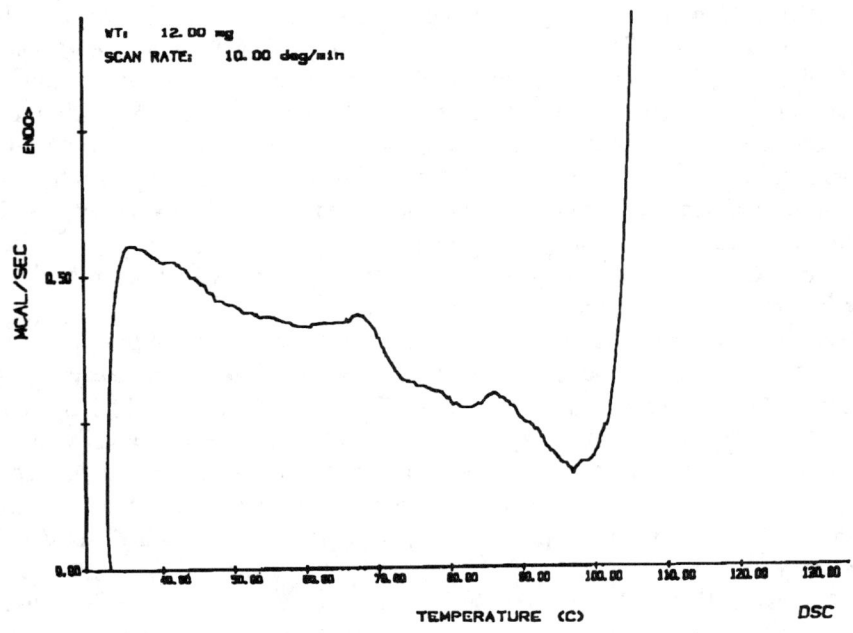

Fig. 4.10 — Differential scanning calorimetry of human stratum corneum following treatment with gel vehicle only at 37°C for 24 hours

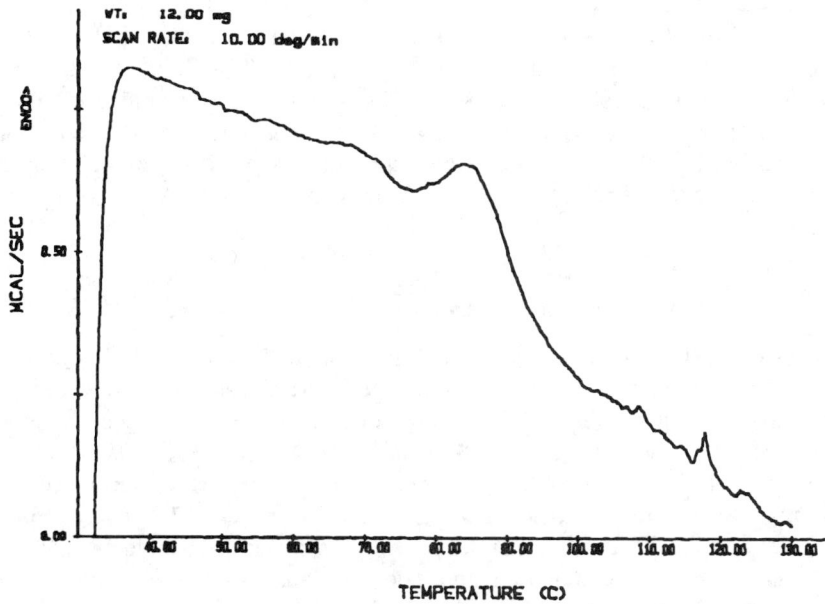

Fig. 4.11 — Differential scanning calorimetry of human stratum corneum following treatment with amethocaine percutaneous anaesthetic gel at 37°C for one hour

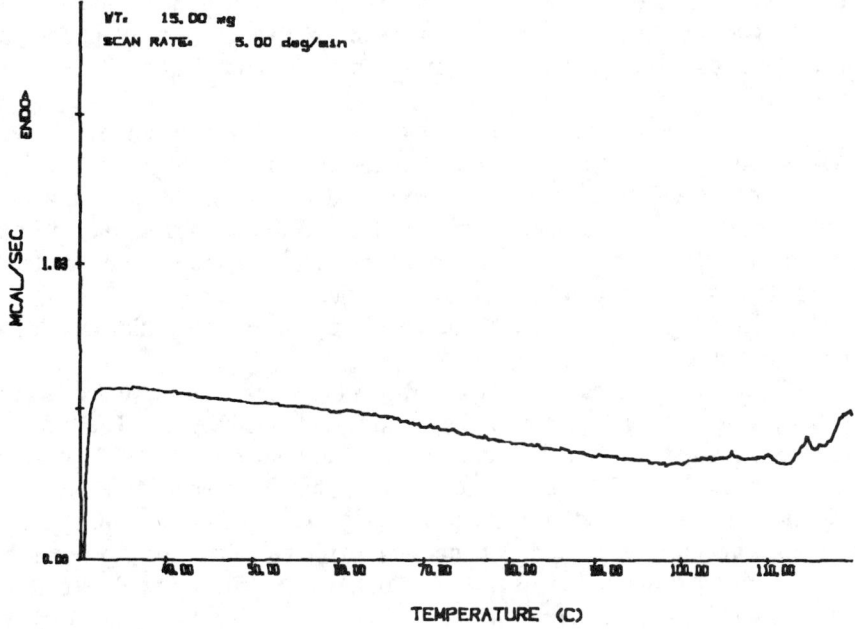

Fig. 4.12 — Differential scanning calorimetry of human stratum corneum following treatment with amethocaine percutaneous anaesthetic gel at 37°C for 24 hours

whereas a 1 hour treatment did not abolish these signals. From a clinical viewpoint amethocaine, when formulated as a percutaneous anaesthetic, acts rapidly following a skin application time of 30 minutes (Woolfson *et al.*, 1990a). Therefore, the extent of this fluidising effect on skin lipids is unlikely to produce any clinically significant adverse effects. Nevertheless, it does suggest that the drug may penetrate through the stratum corneum largely via the intercellular lipid route, and this has implications for the successful formulation of percutaneous local anaesthetic preparations.

4.4   CUTANEOUS METABOLISM OF LOCAL ANAESTHETICS

Traditionally, the skin has been regarded as a passive, inert structural barrier between the body and its environment. However, it is now clear that the skin also possesses enzyme systems capable of metabolising both endogenous substrates and exogenous chemicals (Pannatier *et al.*, 1978; Mukhtar and Bickers, 1981; Martin *et al.*, 1987). Cutaneous enzyme systems include simple, non-specific esterases. The action of skin in hydrolysing short-chain fatty acid esters has been demonstrated by several studies, as reviewed by Findlay (1955). In addition to hydrolysis, skin is capable of other phase 1 functionalisation reactions (oxidation and reduction) and phase 2 conjugation reactions such as glucuronide or glutathione formation (Pannatier *et al.*, 1978).

The possible extent of metabolism during the percutaneous absorption of exogenous chemicals has been considered by Bronaugh *et al.* (1989) using radiolabelled model compounds and rat skin. It was concluded that, for many compounds, metabolism during skin absorption will be small and, for many others, metabolic effects will be undetectable. Nevertheless, the importance of even a small amount of metabolism was emphasised with respect to either the activation or inactivation of a potent compound, and also with regard to the accurate determination of the skin pharmacokinetics of the absorption process.

With local anaesthetics, particularly the more potent drugs that are most suitable for percutaneous local anaesthesia, cutaneous drug metabolism, if significant, could affect both the onset time and duration of anaesthesia. Inactivation by cutaneous metabolism could also be advantageous in detoxification of the local anaesthetic, thereby further reducing the risk of systemic toxicity due to the drug reaching the general circulation in appreciable amounts. A potent local anaesthetic could then be regarded as a soft drug, that is, an active drug moiety inactivated by enzymic or other biotransformation reactions in the skin (Nacht *et al.*, 1981).

Metabolic studies on percutaneously absorbed local anaesthetics have been restricted to members of the ester group, notably benzocaine and amethocaine. These drugs are subject to enzymatic hydrolysis of the ester linkage. Nathan *et al.* (1990) studied the skin absorption and metabolism of benzoic acid, para-aminobenzoic acid and benzoic acid in the hairless guinea pig and also, for benzocaine itself, in human skin. This study used benzocaine only as a model compound, with the absorption process being maintained over 48 hours. This is quite unlike the true clinical situation for percutaneous local anaesthesia, in which the skin application period is generally from 30 minutes to 2 hours. However, during the prolonged absorption period used in this study, extensive metabolism of benzocaine was observed, largely by N-acetylation, to which the drug is particularly susceptible, rather than by hydrolysis. Absorption and metabolism of benzocaine were reduced when human, rather than guinea pig, skin was used.

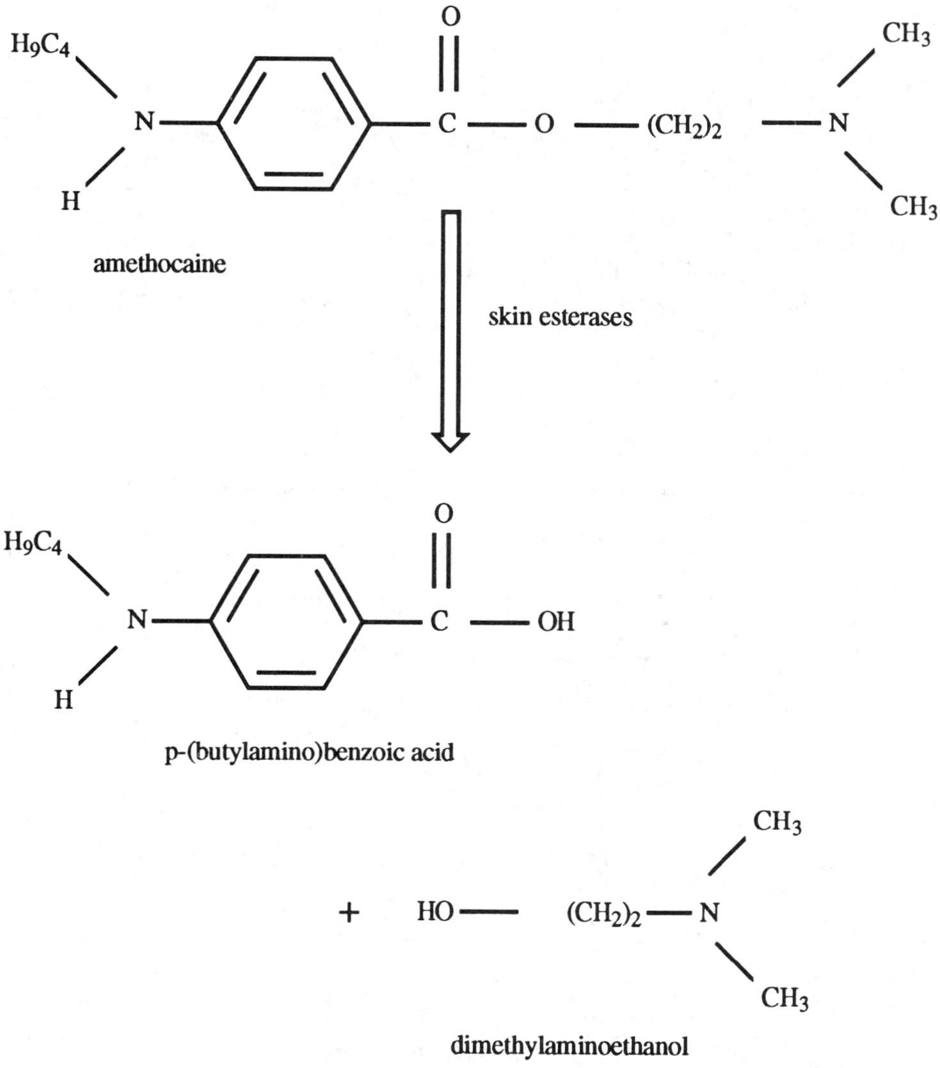

Fig. 4.13 — Cutaneous metabolic pathway of amethocaine

The metabolism of amethocaine by human and porcine skin homogenates has been investigated by Woolfson *et al.* (1990b). Skin homogenates were shown to possess enzymic activity with respect to non-specific esterases by incubation with a standard esterase substrate, p-nitrophenyl acetate, and subsequent spectrophotometry. The pattern of amethocaine skin metabolism was shown to be identical to that experienced when amethocaine was incubated in solution with the enzyme, pseudocholinesterase.

Metabolism by skin homogenates proceeded via simple hydrolysis of the ester sidechain, yielding p-(butylamino)benzoic acid and dimethylaminoethanol (Fig. 4.13). Unlike systemic metabolism, there was no evidence of further transformation to yield the allergen, p-aminobenzoic acid, as the final product.

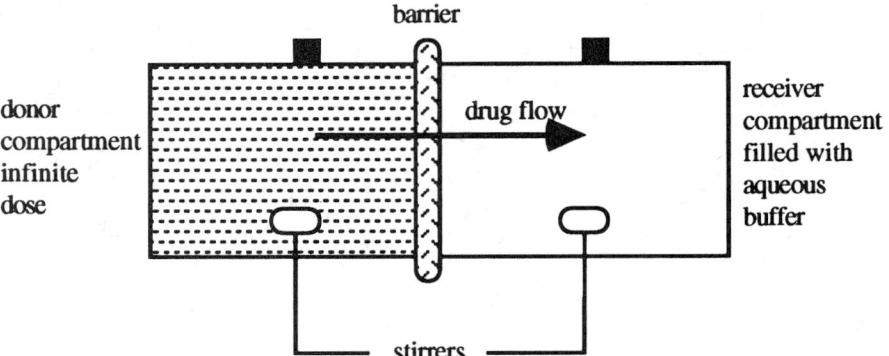

Fig. 4.14 — Infinite dose percutaneous penetration apparatus

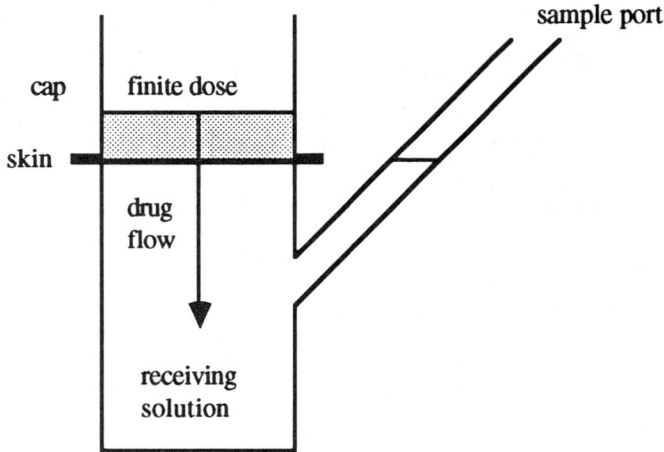

Fig. 4.15 — Finite dose percutaneous penetration apparatus

Metabolism of amethocaine with porcine and human whole skin extracts (Figs 4.14 and 4.15) demonstrated that a loss of drug substrate could only confidently be observed after a 24 hour incubation period. However, the reaction could be followed from the early stages by monitoring the appearance of the metabolite, p-(butylamino)benzoic acid. The data obtained in both cases showed a good fit to a simple linear model, enabling zero order rate constants (Table 4.2) to be calculated from the slopes of the regression lines. There was reasonable agreement between observed losses of amethocaine substrate and those predicted from the experimental data on human skin homogenates (Table 4.3).

Table 4.2 — Rate constants for the metabolism of amethocaine by human and porcine skin homogenates

sample no.	rate constant $(mol10 \ ml^{-1} \ min^{-1})$
human whole skin	
1	$7.647 \times 10^{-10} \pm 3.152 \times 10^{-11}$
2	$7.183 \times 10^{-10} \pm 6.033 \times 10^{-11}$
3	$5.729 \times 10^{-10} \pm 2.427 \times 10^{-11}$
porcine whole skin	
1	$2.854 \times 10^{-9} \pm 1.656 \times 10^{-10}$
2	$3.334 \times 10^{-9} \pm 1.606 \times 10^{-10}$
human epidermis	
1	$5.900 \times 10^{-10} \pm 2.086 \times 10^{-11}$
2	$4.453 \times 10^{-10} \pm 3.331 \times 10^{-11}$
3	$4.723 \times 10^{-10} \pm 2.947 \times 10^{-11}$

Reproduced from Woolfson *et al.* (1990b) with permission of the copyright holder, Elsevier, Amsterdam

Table 4.3 — Comparison of predicted and observed losses of amethocaine during incubation with human skin homogenates

sample no.	time (min)	observed loss of amethocaine (μg)	predicted loss of amethocaine (μg)
1	2880	546	582
2	1440	309	274
3	1320	253	199

Reproduced from Woolfson *et al.* (1990b) with permission of the copyright holder, Elsevier, Amsterdam

Although comparisons with control experiments have confirmed that the skin is capable of metabolising amethocaine, and by implication other ester local anaesthetics, the observed rate of drug loss was slow. It seems likely that a comparatively bulky molecule such as amethocaine has a low affinity for the non-specific esterases found in the skin. Certainly, in a realistic clinical situation the drug will be in contact with the skin for much less than the time required *in vitro* to achieve significant metabolic transformation.

Although the total enzyme yield of whole skin was considered (Woolfson *et al.*, 1990b), it must be remembered that any local anaesthetic drug molecule reaching the dermis will be rapidly cleared via the dermal capillaries. Thus, although the dermis may be up to 5000 μm in thickness, drug penetration is unlikely beyond about the upper 200 μm. Thus, it is unlikely that drug metabolism in the dermis is of any practical consequence (Martin *et al.*, 1987). The problems in relating *in vitro* skin metabolic studies to the *in vivo* situation have been considered in some detail by Potts *et al.* (1989).

4.5 *IN VITRO* METHODOLOGY FOR ASSESSMENT OF THE PERCUTANEOUS PENETRATION OF LOCAL ANAESTHETICS

Test systems for studying the percutaneous absorption of local anaesthetics, or other drug penetrants, may be based on either *in vivo* or *in vitro* methodologies. Clearly, results from *in vivo* studies are much preferable in terms of reliability and clinical relevance. *In vivo* experimentation may involve the use of radiolabelled penetrants or, in some cases, non-invasive techniques may be used to monitor drug absorption. Such methods are discussed in Chapter 5. However, when a formulation is still in the developmental stage, a certain amount of *in vitro* experimentation is necessary. This is partly dictated by practical considerations, including the availability of human volunteers, potential drug toxicity and expense. With percutaneous local anaesthesia, *in vivo* studies are comparatively straightforward, but laboratory studies can still provide much useful information and thereby substantially reduce product development time.

In vitro experimentation inevitably involves the use of a suitable barrier membrane (Franz, 1975). Human skin is ideal, but other animal models or synthetic barriers are often employed. The major objection to the use of excised human skin is that it may not completely duplicate the physiological role of the skin *in vivo*. However, the use of isolated human skin membranes in diffusion cells enables drug penetration rates to be obtained simply and with reasonable reproducibility (Marzulli *et al.*, 1969). Data obtained by this means can be useful in the formulation of an optimised drug delivery system. It can also be used to predict the likely amount of penetrant that may be absorbed through the skin, such information being of toxicological importance.

4.5.1 The infinite dose technique

The percutaneous absorption of drugs is commonly assessed *in vitro* using human skin, or other suitable barrier membrane, mounted in a diffusion chamber. The barrier membrane is positioned between two fluid-filled chambers which are synchronously stirred (Fig. 4.14). The candidate drug is in solution on one side of the barrier (the donor solution). Drug passing through the barrier is determined by sampling, at intervals, the receiver fluid on the other side. The amount of drug that penetrates the barrier during the experiment is generally small relative to the total amount of drug in the donor solution. Thus, there is no significant reduction in the amount of drug remaining in the donor solution as a result of drug crossing the barrier into the receiver solution during the course of the experiment. In practice, the available dose is infinite (Franz, 1978).

Studies on the percutaneous absorption of local anaesthetics are not well served by the infinite dose technique. No account is taken of the influence of formulation factors in promoting drug penetration since only aqueous solutions, with or without co-solvents, can be used. Water is not a suitable vehicle for topical formulations and the skin penetration characteristics of a given drug obtained from an aqueous solution will have little relevance when that drug is formulated in a semi-solid or other vehicle.

A further serious problem relates to the hydration state of the barrier, particularly when human or animal skin is used. Both sides of the skin barrier will be in contact with aqueous solution, and therefore both sides will be fully hydrated. This is certainly not realistic, since the outer surface of the skin is usually dry and hydration effects can dramatically alter the permeability of the stratum corneum (Barry, 1983b).

Lipophilic anaesthetic bases have very low solubility in water. Thus, the dose available for the establishment of a concentration gradient across the barrier will be low unless the donor solution is buffered to an acidic pH, in which event the available dose will be unrealistically large and the ionised local anaesthetic will be a poor penetrant. Thus, for all of these reasons, the infinite dose technique is of little practical value in the development of percutaneous local anaesthetic formulations. If the inherent penetration characteristics of local anaesthetic bases are to be determined on a comparative basis, it is better to formulate each in an identical semi-solid vehicle (McCafferty *et al.*, 1988).

4.5.2   The finite dose technique

The disadvantages inherent in the infinite dose technique are largely avoided with the finite dose model. Here, human skin, or other suitable barrier membrane, is mounted in specially constructed diffusion chambers (Franz, 1978). Such chambers are often referred to as Franz diffusion cells (Fig. 4.15). The membrane is clamped between the flanges of a lower receiving fluid chamber and an upper cell cap which is open to the atmosphere. The dermis, or lower surface of the barrier membrane, is bathed by pH 7.4 buffered saline acting as the receiving fluid. The solution temperature is maintained at 37°C by a thermostatically controlled water circulating system in conjunction with a water jacket surrounding each receiving chamber.

Several diffusion cells can be mounted on a single drive console which provides two manifolds for water circulation via an external pump. The drive console also permits synchronous stirring of the receptor fluid in all cells to ensure a homogeneous temperature distribution through the fluid. This is achieved by small magnetic stirring bars driven by an external magnet mounted on a timing motor in the drive console. The arrangement allows convenient replication of finite dose diffusion experiments (Franz, 1985).

In the finite dose technique the skin barrier membrane is held under conditions closely approximating the living state. Since the outer surface of the skin or the donor vehicle are exposed to the atmosphere, water and temperature gradients which exist under real conditions are maintained in the Franz model. Any type or amount of vehicle can be used, including creams, ointments, liquids, gels, polymeric films and transdermal patch systems. Thus, small finite doses typically associated with the clinical use of dermatological preparations can be used, as can the larger applications more usually associated with percutaneous anaesthetic systems. This contrasts favourably with the infinite dose technique in which the failure to approximate the amount of drug used *in vivo* produces results which have little resemblance to those found in man. The finite dose technique has produced results (Franz, 1978) which show good correlation with previously reported human volunteer studies using radiolabelled penetrants (Feldmann and Maibach, 1970).

4.5.3 Choice of barrier membrane for *in vitro* penetration studies on local anaesthetics

If meaningful results are to be obtained from *in vitro* penetration studies, the choice of barrier membrane to be used in the diffusion cell is of major importance. Although much argument has been expended on the topic, there is no doubt that human skin is the ideal barrier membrane for any *in vitro* percutaneous absorption study. However, a number of considerations apply even in this case. The source of the skin sample, whether cadaver or living skin, the skin racial type and age, the degree of hydration, and the body area from which the sample originates are all important variables which can affect the reliability of the data obtained. Appropriate storage conditions for the skin prior to use in the laboratory are also important. Despite these variables, a human skin barrier is certainly preferable to any alternative membrane, but there is often a practical difficulty in obtaining sufficient supplies of human skin for *in vitro* percutaneous absorption studies. Thus, many workers have considered alternative membranes. These can broadly be divided into animal skin of various species and those which are formed from artificial materials.

A wide range of animal species, as listed in Table 4.4, have been proposed as alternative barriers to human skin. Generally, the skin of common laboratory animals is more permeable to exogenous chemicals than human skin (Wester and Maibach, 1987). Each model has its own advantages and disadvantages, proponents and detractors.

Table 4.4 — List of species used to provide skin barrier membranes for *in vitro* percutaneous penetration studies

species
cat
chimpanzee
dog
goat
Guinea pig
hairless mouse
horse
monkey
rat
rabbit
pig
snake (shed squamate epidermis)
weanling pig

Hairless mouse skin has been particularly widely used as a model barrier membrane because of its availability and ease of preparation. Generally, a rectangle of skin from the abdomen is simply excised with scissors. Since the skin is not firmly attached to the viscera, it is easily lifted away from the animal. Adhering fat and other cellular debris can then be removed with tweezers. Hairless mouse skin, although having many anatomical features in common with human skin (Durrheim *et al.*, 1980), is significantly more permeable than its human counterpart (Hinz *et al.*, 1989). Rigg and Barry (1990) noted a 37-fold increase in water permeability of hairless mouse skin compared to human skin over an 8 day test period and concluded that hairless mouse skin was unsuitable for penetration studies in excess of 24 hours. Although the time periods involved with percutaneous anaesthetic studies are of much shorter duration, the tendency of hairless mouse skin to overestimate percutaneous penetration makes it an unsuitable model for this application.

Barry (1990) has pointed out that investigative problems should not be made more complex by selection of an animal tissue to represent human skin. This is undoubtedly sensible advice. If an animal model alternative to human skin is unavoidable, newborn porcine skin has been found to correlate well with human skin during percutaneous penetration studies on the local anaesthetic agent, amethocaine (Woolfson *et al.*, 1992). In general, porcine and monkey skin are probably the best models of human skin penetration characteristics (Wester and Maibach, 1987). However, the quality of such correlations certainly varies to some extent with the chemical properties of the penetrant, and no absolute conclusions as to the "best" animal model can confidently be made.

In any formulation development exercise it is often necessary to make comparisons as to the potential efficacy of the candidate formulations. In such a case, when it is desirable that biological variation within the study should be eliminated from the experimental design, there is some case to be made for the use of artificial membranes. Although such membranes differ radically from human or animal skin, they can, if carefully chosen, indicate important differences between formulations and thus contribute to the formulation optimisation process.

In common with the wide range of animal models investigated as alternative skin barrier membranes, many different artificial or semi-artificial membranes have been used for *in vitro* percutaneous absorption studies. The choice of membrane must, however, be related to the physicochemical characteristics of the penetrant. Thus, a polar penetrant cannot be studied using a lipophilic membrane. Transport of the penetrant through the artificial membrane, which is typically composed of a polymeric material, is generally dependent on the relative adsorption of the diffusing penetrant molecules to the face of the membrane and consequent solubility of those molecules in the membrane.

Artificial membranes used as barriers to drug diffusion in *in vitro* penetration studies have included polydimethylsiloxane, cellulose acetate, lyophilised porcine skin dressing sheets (Corethium[®]) and the Sartorius system comprising a double-layer membrane of a hydrated hydrophilic foil soaked in an oily liquid (McClelland, 1986). Polydimethylsiloxane, an isotropic polymer sold as preformed Silastic[®] sheets or as a kit comprising monomer, initiator and curing agent, is a lipophilic barrier which has been shown to provide a useful comparative basis for studying the percutaneous absorption of lipophilic local anaesthetic bases (McCafferty *et al.*, 1988). Silastic[®] has demonstrated reasonable agreement for lipophilic penetrants with Fick's laws of diffusion (Garrett and Chemburkar, 1968). The variation in performance of each of these barrier membranes is illustrated in Table 4.5 with respect to the average penetration fluxes of amethocaine, from an identical formulation batch, through each membrane.

Table 4.5 — Comparative fluxes of amethocaine through various barrier membranes

membrane	flux μmol cm^{-2} h^{-1} $\pm$ s.d.
Corethium$^{®}$ epidermis	12.55 $\pm$ 0.51
Corethium$^{®}$ epidermis plus dermis	1.45 $\pm$ 0.08
Corethium$^{®}$ dermis	2.23 $\pm$ 0.11
Sartorius system	0.18 $\pm$ 0.08
Silastic$^{®}$	0.28 $\pm$ 0.03

4.6 PERCUTANEOUS PENETRATION CHARACTERISTICS OF LOCAL ANAESTHETICS

A finite dose penetration study on eight local anaesthetic bases has been reported by McCafferty *et al.* (1988). Each anaesthetic base was formulated in an identical standard water-miscible cream vehicle in order to assess, on a comparative basis, the intrinsic suitability of the drugs as percutaneous penetrants. The local anaesthetics used in this study were chosen on the basis of their anaesthetic potency, lipophilicity, availability and clinical acceptability. The drugs were formulated on an equimolar rather than an equipotent basis since determination of the ability of the anaesthetics to reach the target site of action was the prime interest in this study. Furthermore, drug release from the formulation matrix and the consequent establishment of a concentration gradient across the barrier membrane are dependent upon drug concentration. Hence, the latter had to be constant for each formulation.

The modified Sartorius absorption system (McClelland, 1986) was used to determine the apparent steady state fluxes, lag times and permeability coefficients of the anaesthetic bases (Table 4.6). Since the study was performed on a comparative basis, a lipophilic Silastic$^{®}$ sheet was used as the barrier membrane, thus eliminating the variability inherent in the use of biological membranes.

All the local anaesthetics in Table 4.6 (except bupivacaine, which did not penetrate the barrier) exhibited a characteristic lag phase followed by apparent steady state penetration of the barrier membrane. Flux values for the various drugs appeared to decrease as the lag time increased, an observation previously reported in drug penetration studies using Silastic$^{®}$ as the barrier membrane (Flynn and Roseman, 1971). The lag period can be interpreted as the time required for the diffusion of drug molecules into and through the barrier before appearing in the receiving fluid.

In this general comparative study the highest apparent steady state flux values obtained were for amethocaine, lignocaine and the topically active local anaesthetic ether, fomocaine. However, a better comparison is that made on the basis of the permeability coefficients for the drugs, which takes into account the actual drug concentration present in each case. Using this criterion penetration decreased in the order lignocaine > amethocaine > fomocaine > benzocaine. The most lipophilic agent in the series, bupivacaine, failed to penetrate the barrier membrane, probably due to poor availability from a non-optimised formulation. Lignocaine and amethocaine showed similar penetration properties, notwithstanding the greater lipophilicity of the latter. The low apparent steady state flux of mepivacaine, however, might have been predicted from a knowledge of its relatively low lipophilicity (Covino, 1986).

Table 4.6 — Indices of *in vitro* penetration for local anaesthetics through a polydimethylsiloxane barrier membrane

local anaesthetic	flux mg cm^{-2} h^{-1}	lag time (min)	permeability coefficient cm^{-2} h^{-1} x 10^{-4}
amethocaine	0.95 ± 0.08	18	5.16
amylocaine	0.39 ± 0.06	22	2.34
benzocaine	0.33 ± 0.06	16	2.82
bupivacaine	-	-	-
cinchocaine	0.45 ± 0.09	22	1.87
fomocaine	0.71 ± 0.05	25	3.24
lignocaine	0.89 ± 0.10	19	5.40
mepivacaine	0.23 ± 0.03	31	1.34

Reproduced from McCafferty *et al.* (1988) with permission of the copyright holder

A reasonable conclusion from the data in Table 4.6 is that the affinity of the drug for the vehicle is a factor additional to drug lipophilicity in controlling the drug penetration of a lipophilic barrier membrane, and that amethocaine, taking into account its known anaesthetic potency, might be a particularly suitable drug for use as a percutaneous local anaesthetic.

4.6.1 Percutaneous penetration characteristics of benzocaine

Benzoic acid and its derivatives, including benzocaine, are often used as model compounds for *in vitro* percutaneous absorption studies. Although the local anaesthetic and physicochemical properties of benzocaine make it unsuitable as a percutaneous anaesthetic for intact skin, the drug is quite widely used in formulations for application to the mucosa. It may also be regarded as a model ester local anaesthetic, particularly with respect to the study of skin metabolic processes for these drugs.

The importance of drug availability from the vehicle was emphasised in a study on the percutaneous penetration of benzocaine from polyoxyethylene nonylphenol surfactant solutions through hairless mouse skin (Dalvi and Zatz, 1981). In this example, it was found that benzocaine penetration of the membrane was proportional only to the free drug in solution. The solubilised portion of the drug was not available for skin penetration.

Nathan *et al.* (1990) investigated the *in vitro* skin absorption and metabolism of benzoic acid, p-aminobenzoic acid and benzocaine through hairless guinea pig skin and, for benzocaine alone, through human skin. Both viable and non-viable skin were used by these workers. Skin was made non-viable by being bathed in distilled water alone from the receiver compartment rather than by isotonic buffered saline. Differences were noted in the percutaneous absorption of the two acidic compounds through viable and non-viable skin, and these were ascribed to pH changes occurring during degeneration of non-viable skin. Benzocaine absorption was similar in both viable and non-viable skin, the drug being applied in an ethanol vehicle at a dose of approximately 2 μg cm^{-2} over a 48 hour period. The percentages of the applied benzocaine doses that were absorbed were 76.6% (guinea pig) and 49.5% (human). These values are high, but the differences in application time for a percutaneous anaesthetic (typically less than 60 minutes) compared to a chronic dosing study of 48 hours should be remembered. This means that, in effect, minimal benzocaine would be absorbed through the stratum corneum in a true clinical scenario, and that the drug would be quite ineffective for anaesthetising intact skin.

4.6.2   Percutaneous penetration characteristics of lignocaine

Although lignocaine has been the subject of much effort to produce an effective percutaneous anaesthetic preparation (Monash, 1957; Lubens and Sanker, 1964; Lubens *et al.*, 1974) comparatively little work has been done *in vitro* on the cutaneous disposition of the drug.

The effect of pH changes on the percutaneous penetration of lignocaine hydrochloride through guinea pig skin was investigated by Menczel and Goldberg (1978). An infinite dose study design was used with the skin membrane separating a donor solution of buffered lignocaine hydrochloride from a receiving solution of isotonic phosphate buffer (pH 7.4). The donor solutions contained either 10 or 40 mg of lignocaine hydrochloride per 100 ml. In common with many percutaneous absorption studies, drug penetration was monitored over a 48 hour period. Not surprisingly, it was concluded that the percutaneous penetration of lignocaine hydrochloride was affected by pH. The amount of the drug accumulating on the dermal side of the diffusion cell in the buffered receiving fluid was directly proportional to the initial concentration of the applied drug at the two alkaline pH values studied, 7.42 and 7.9. When the donor solution was at pH 2 no percutaneous penetration of lignocaine was observed, again emphasising the importance of drug lipophilicity for the percutaneous absorption of local anaesthetics. After 48 hours, the maximum drug accumulation in the receiving fluid was approximately 550 μg.

The transfer of lignocaine from the skin into the isotonic, buffered, receiving solution occurred after a characteristic lag period during which the skin became quasi-saturated. Irrespective of drug concentration in the donor solution, the transfer rate from the skin into the receiving fluid fell as the donor solution pH was increased, although the partition coefficient of the drug between donor solution and skin increased with increasing pH (Table 4.7). It was suggested that concomitant absorption into the skin of the alkaline buffer from the donor solution resulted in better retention of the drug in the lipoidal skin.

Clearance of the drug from donor solution into epidermis, and subsequent transfer from the dermal region into the receiving solution, analogous to absorption *in vivo* into the dermal microcirculation, was concluded to be a two-stage process. It was suggested that, if the epidermal clearance rate could be maximised and the dermal clearance rate minimised, then the drug would remain largely localised in the epidermal region. This would both increase the duration of anaesthesia and reduce the possibility of systemic absorption of the local anaesthetic agent. Unfortunately, it is not practical to administer a percutaneous anaesthetic in an aqueous, buffered, liquid vehicle. Therefore, there is a minimum practical possibility of sufficient aqueous buffer being absorbed into the skin from a typical semi-solid vehicle such that the epidermal retention of the local anaesthetic would be significantly enhanced.

Table 4.7 — Effect of pH on the epidermal clearance constants of lignocaine hydrochloride solutions determined with guinea pig abdominal skin

	pH 2	pH 7.42	pH 7.9
percentage unionised	< 0.001	25	50
partition coefficient	0	7.2 - 7.3	13-14
epidermal clearance constant (days^{-1}) 10 mg%	0	0.38	0.52
epidermal clearance constant (days^{-1}) 40 mg%	0	0.40	0.54
dermal clearance constant (days^{-1}) 10 mg%	0	0.072	0.041
dermal clearance constant (days^{-1}) 40 mg%	0	0.082	0.037

Reproduced from Menczel and Goldberg (1978) with permission of the copyright holder, S. Karger AG, Basel

The possible enhancement by surfactants of lignocaine base through hairless mouse skin has been investigated by Sarpotdar and Zatz (1986). The enhancers were polyoxyethylene sorbitan monoesters in co-solvent formulations containing various propylene glycol concentrations. Both infinite and finite dose designs were used in the study. In both cases, the steady state flux of lignocaine through the skin barrier was enhanced by the presence of surfactant at high propylene glycol concentrations. However, the partitioning of the drug from solution into skin decreased with increasing co-solvent concentration in the donor solution. These conflicting trends are emphasised in the data in Table 4.8. Clearly, as the polarity of the donor solvent decreased the affinity of the solution for the lipophilic drug was increased, emphasising again the importance of formulation factors in promoting the percutaneous absorption of local anaesthetic bases.

Table 4.8 — Effect of non-ionic surfactants on the penetration of 1% lignocaine solutions through hairless mouse skin in the presence of various propylene glycol concentrations

	steady-state flux μg cm^{-2} h^{-1} $\pm$ s.d.		
surfactant	propylene glycol 40% w/w	propylene glycol 60% w/w	propylene glycol 80% w/w
1% polysorbate 20	51.4 ± 1.74	22.3 ± 3.53	24.8 ± 9.84
1% polysorbate 60	49.2 ± 3.47	27.7 ± 3.28	26.7 ± 6.14
3% polysorbate 60	23.0 ± 1.36	-	-
no surfactant	59.9 ± 8.08	18.6 ± 2.45	8.3 ± 0.19

Reproduced from Sarpotdar and Zatz (1986) with permission from the copyright owner, the American Pharmaceutical Association

4.6.3 Percutaneous penetration characteristics of amethocaine through various barrier membranes

Unlike many other local anaesthetics, amethocaine is known to produce effective percutaneous anaesthesia when formulated specifically for this purpose. Percutaneous anaesthesia with amethocaine is profound and is characterised by a short application period and prolonged activity (Woolfson *et al.*, 1990a). Thus, much valuable information can be gained by establishing the penetration characteristics of this drug through various skin strata, and by comparing these data with those obtained using alternative barrier membranes.

4.6.3.1 Amethocaine penetration characteristics through human and porcine whole skin and stratum corneum, and through human epidermis

A series of studies on amethocaine penetration of skin, or skin component strata, have been reported by Woolfson *et al.* (1992). In these penetration studies, amethocaine base was formulated as aqueous gels McCafferty and Woolfson (1988). The drug concentrations used ranged from 2 to 6% m/V. The study design involved a replicated finite dose technique using Franz diffusion cells with the gels applied as a thin film to the upper side of the barrier membrane. Phosphate-buffered saline at pH 7.4 and 37°C was used as the receiving fluid.

The percutaneous penetration characteristics of amethocaine are shown in Figs 4.16 - 4.18 for each of three different drug concentrations. Generally, as the concentration of amethocaine increased, the flux through each barrier membrane also increased. Given the

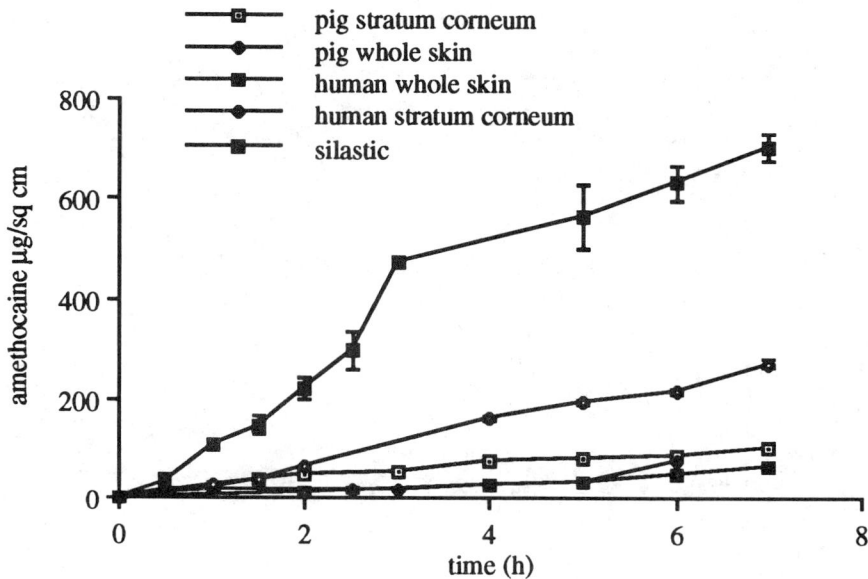

Fig. 4.16 — Comparison of amethocaine penetration characteristics from a 2% m/V gel formulation through various barrier membranes. Reproduced from Woolfson *et al.* (1992) with permission of the copyright holder, Elsevier, Amsterdam

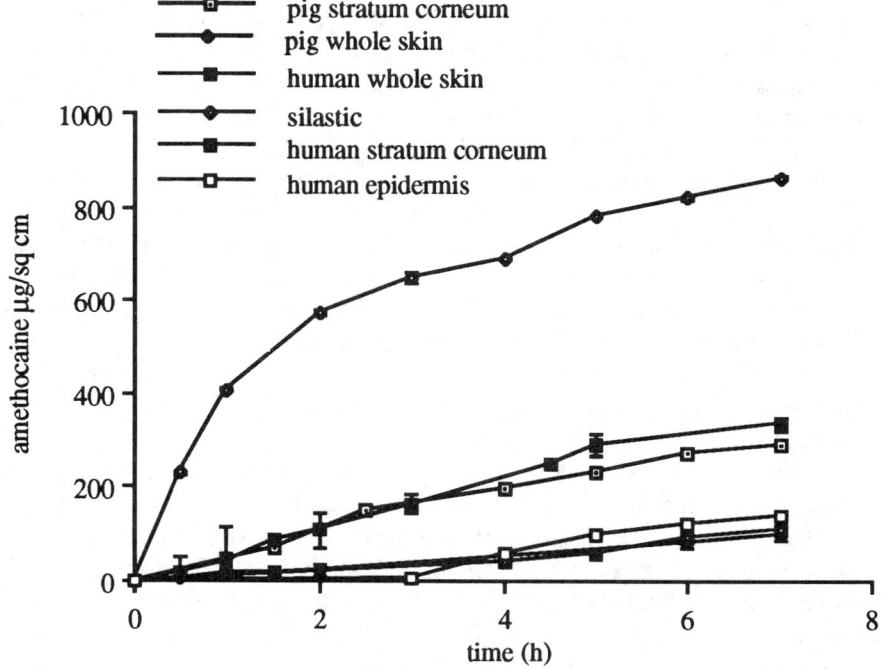

Fig 4.17 — Comparison of amethocaine penetration characteristics from a 4% m/V gel formulation through various barrier membranes. Reproduced from Woolfson *et al.* (1992) with permission of the copyright holder, Elsevier, Amsterdam

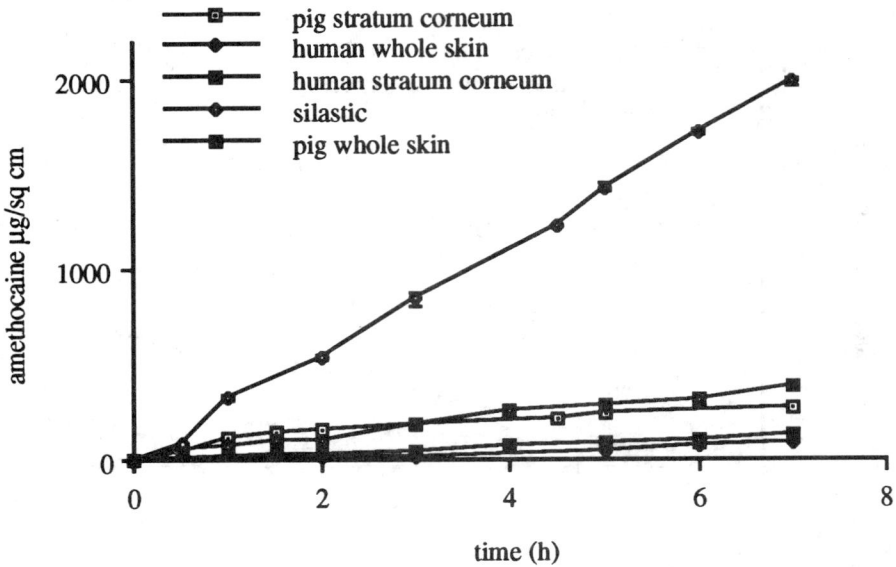

Fig 4.18 — Comparison of amethocaine penetration characteristics from a 6% m/V gel formulation through various barrier membranes

nature of the formulation, this is unlikely to be due to the conventional increase in concentration gradient resulting in an increased thermodynamic driving force for diffusion. Since these formulations are not suspensions but, in effect, viscous aqueous suspensions of an oily drug, the larger drug concentration results in a greater surface area of drug being in contact with the barrier and, hence, an increased flux. Thus, increasing the amethocaine concentration from 2 to 4% m/V produced a corresponding increase in flux through human stratum corneum from 39.58 to 52.07 $\mu g \ cm^{-2} \ h^{-1}$ (Table 4.9). However, a further increase to 6% m/V amethocaine in the gel did not produce such a large increase in flux, suggesting that surface area packing of the drug is nearing a maximum and that the penetration process is, in effect, saturable. Of course, tissue variation will affect flux values inter-experiment, although intra-experiment values were obtained using single-source membranes. This is inevitable given the size of skin samples usually obtainable, particularly of human skin, and the amount required for an extensive study.

Porcine skin is more readily obtainable than human skin and is therefore of interest as a possible realistic alternative barrier membrane. Porcine skin samples used in this study were from neonatal pigs that were either stillborn or died shortly after birth, in the latter case as a result of accidental crushing by the mother. Both human and porcine samples were treated identically after harvesting. Amethocaine fluxes from the various formulations through both porcine whole skin and stratum corneum were much closer to the values obtained with human skin than was observed in the case of Silastic®. Although the differences in fluxes between equivalent human and porcine skin barriers were significant (P < 0.05), as determined by a multiple range test (Newman-Keuls), the orders of magnitude were similar in each case. Comparison of the effect of drug

Table 4.9 — Amethocaine fluxes from an aqueous gel formulation through various barrier membranes

barrier membrane	amethocaine flux $\mu g\ cm^{-2}\ h^{-1}$	standard deviation
2% m/V amethocaine gel		
porcine stratum corneum	13.45	1.08
porcine whole skin	4.19	0.25
human stratum corneum	39.58	0.22
human whole skin	8.65	0.42
Silastic®	101.60	0.78
4% m/V amethocaine gel		
porcine stratum corneum	42.38	0.33
porcine whole skin	13.76	1.11
human stratum corneum	52.07	1.13
human whole skin	15.27	0.95
human epidermis	21.42	0.72
6% m/V amethocaine gel		
porcine stratum corneum	32.87	2.09
porcine whole skin	18.46	0.52
human stratum corneum	52.00	0.98
human whole skin	12.14	1.34

concentration on flux followed essentially the same pattern between human and porcine barriers (Table 4.10). Thus, amethocaine fluxes from a standard 4% m/V amethocaine gel were 13.76 $\mu g\ cm^{-2}\ h^{-1}$ (porcine whole skin) and 15.27 $\mu g\ cm^{-2}\ h^{-1}$ (human whole skin). For stratum corneum the flux values were 42.38 $\mu g\ cm^{-2}\ h^{-1}$ (porcine) and 52.07 $\mu g\ cm^{-2}\ h^{-1}$ (human). These results suggest that studies using porcine skin are a good model with respect to the percutaneous penetration of amethocaine.

Table 4.10 — Comparison of amethocaine fluxes from an aqueous gel through various barrier membranes (Newman-Keuls Multiple Range Test)

barrier membrane	comparison in terms of amethocaine gel conc. (% w/w)	significance of difference
porcine stratum corneum	2 vs. 4	$P < 0.05$
	2 vs. 6	$P < 0.05$
	4 vs. 6	$P < 0.05$
porcine whole skin	2 vs. 4	$P < 0.05$
	2 vs. 6	$P < 0.05$
	4 vs. 6	$P < 0.05$
human whole skin	2 vs. 4	$P < 0.05$
	2 vs. 6	$P < 0.05$
	4 vs. 6	$P < 0.05$
human stratum corneum	2 vs. 4	$P < 0.05$
	2 vs. 6	$P < 0.05$
	4 vs. 6	$P > 0.05$

Reproduced from Woolfson *et al.* (1992) with permission of the copyright owner, Elsevier, Amsterdam

A further barrier membrane investigated in the study was human epidermis, the outermost non-vascular region of the skin, which includes the stratum corneum as the external layer. The epidermis is approximately 200 μm in thickness. Beneath the epidermis, the dermis is some 10 to 20 times thicker and possesses a rich blood supply. The hair follicles and various glands, such as the apocrine glands, all originate in the dermis. Epidermal samples were prepared by heating the whole skin at 60°C for 2 minutes followed by careful dissection to remove the dermis. For this particular study only data obtained with the 4% m/V amethocaine gel were reported. The epidermal flux value for amethocaine through human epidermis (21.42 μg cm^{-2} h^{-1}) was found to be less than for human stratum corneum and greater than that for human whole skin, as might be expected. Comparing the fluxes through the various skin layers, it is clear that, although allowing the largest flux of amethocaine, the stratum corneum provides the main barrier to penetration of exogenous chemicals, given that it is only some 15 μm thick. The extended passage through the much thicker epidermis and dermis affords substantial opportunity for loss of drug due to biotransformation and/or protein binding (Woolfson *et al.*, 1990b). Hence, fluxes through the epidermis and dermis are lower but this reduction in amethocaine flux does not reflect the comparative thicknesses of these layers compared to stratum corneum, indicating that the epidermis (less stratum corneum) and dermis do not constitute a substantial barrier to amethocaine penetration. Since the target nociceptors for the drug lie at, or near, the dermo-epidermal junction, relatively close to the skin surface, the penetration characteristics of the drug established in this study correlated well with the clinical efficacy of an amethocaine percutaneous anaesthetic gel and with the *in vivo* concentration-response profile (Woolfson *et al.*, 1988).

4.6.3.2 Influence of application time on amethocaine skin penetration characteristics

The data in Figs. 4.16 - 4.18 were obtained using a continuous application of drug-loaded gel matrix to the barrier membrane. This is common practice in skin penetration studies. This type of experimental design yields fundamental information on the skin penetration characteristics of a given drug, together with data on drug absorption during chronic dosing. However, this situation does not relate directly to that normally pertaining with percutaneous local anaesthesia. Unlike the more typical transdermal designs, a much shorter exposure to the anaesthetic formulation is usually made. This may be as short as 30 minutes, and certainly no longer than 2 hours. McGowan (1990) investigated the penetration characteristics of amethocaine using a design in which the exposure to the formulation was restricted to a short period corresponding to its clinical application. The formulation was carefully removed from the barrier membrane, which was rinsed with phosphate-buffered saline at 37°C, after which the appearance of drug in the receiving fluid continued to be monitored until a constant concentration was achieved in the receiving fluid, a situation in which no further drug was released from the skin barrier membrane (porcine and human whole skin and stratum corneum). Application times of 30 minutes and 2 hours were used.

Flux values measured with this design will, of course, be lowered compared to a continuous drug application since there will be a gradual reduction in the amount of drug appearing in the receiving fluid as the barrier drug reservoir becomes exhausted. This compares with the continuous steady state observed when the formulation is left in contact with the skin throughout and is well illustrated by the data in Figs 4.19 and 4.20. Here, amethocaine penetration (4% m/V amethocaine gels) through human stratum corneum and human whole skin respectively are compared for continuous, 30 minute and 2 hour application periods. In the case of the 30 minute application to human stratum corneum (Fig. 4.19), the drug is delivered only for about 90 minutes after the formulation is removed, as shown by the constant drug concentration in the receiving fluid. With a 2 hour application there is about a further 2 hours of drug penetration before the membrane becomes exhausted of drug. These data show that there is comparatively little reservoir effect with amethocaine in the stratum corneum and, further, no possibility of a build-up of the drug in this layer during successive applications, for example, over several days. Fig. 4.21 shows the comparative properties of porcine skin compared to human skin in terms of a 30 minute application of the 4% m/V amethocaine gel. Similarly, Fig. 4.22 refers to a 2 hour application time. The picture is qualitatively similar to human skin in both cases, although the reservoir properties of porcine stratum corneum are even less pronounced with only a further 30 minutes of drug delivery following removal of the formulation after a 30 minute application.

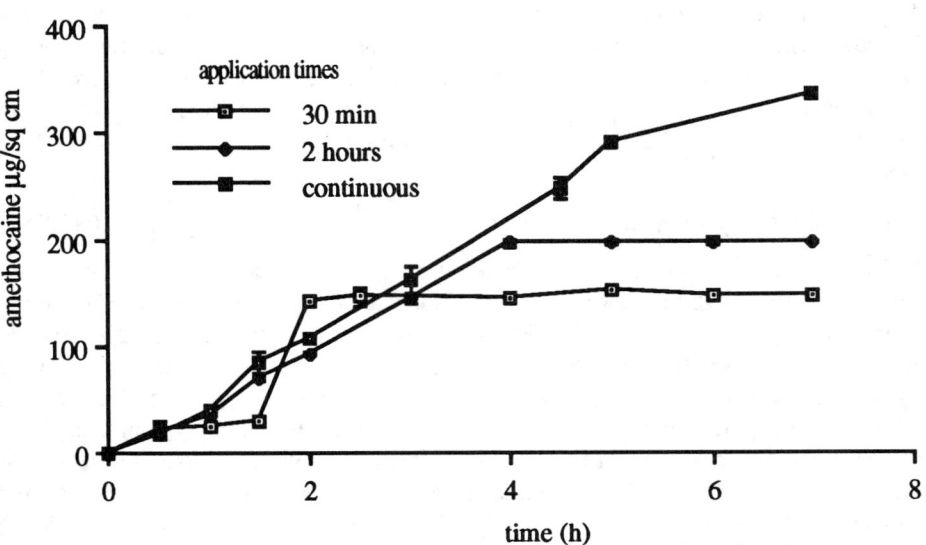

Fig. 4.19 — Influence of application time on amethocaine penetration (4% m/V gel)
through human stratum corneum

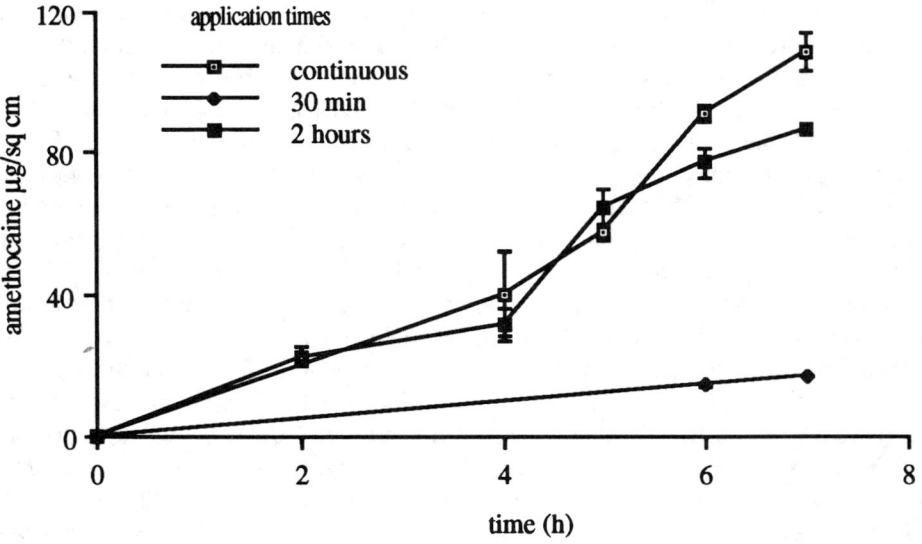

Fig. 4.20 — Influence of application time on amethocaine penetration (4% m/V gel)
through human whole skin

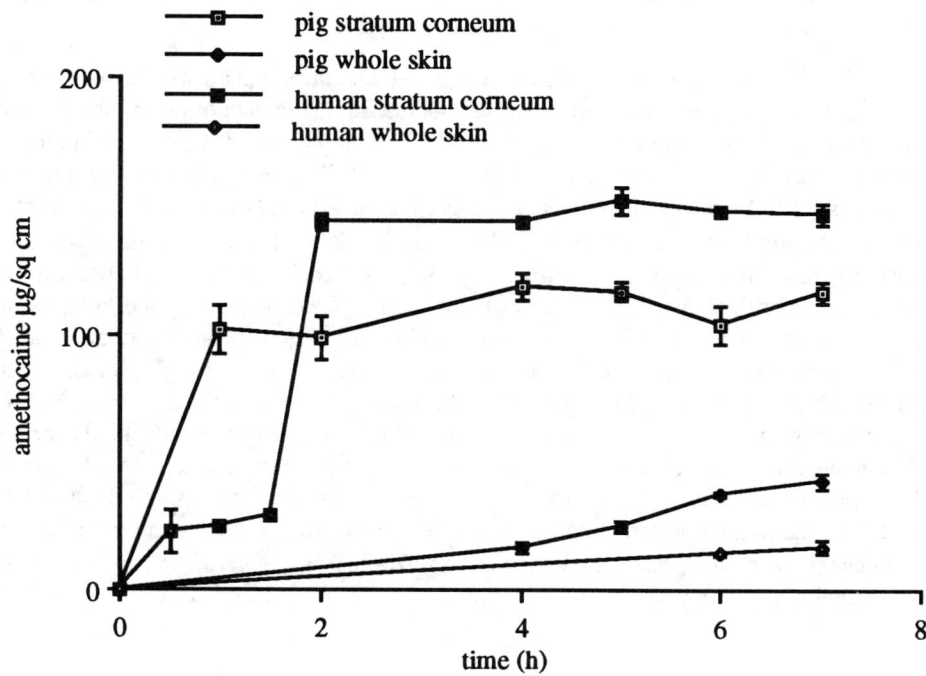

Fig. 4.21 — Comparison of amethocaine penetration (4% m/V gel) through various
barrier membranes using a 30 minute application time

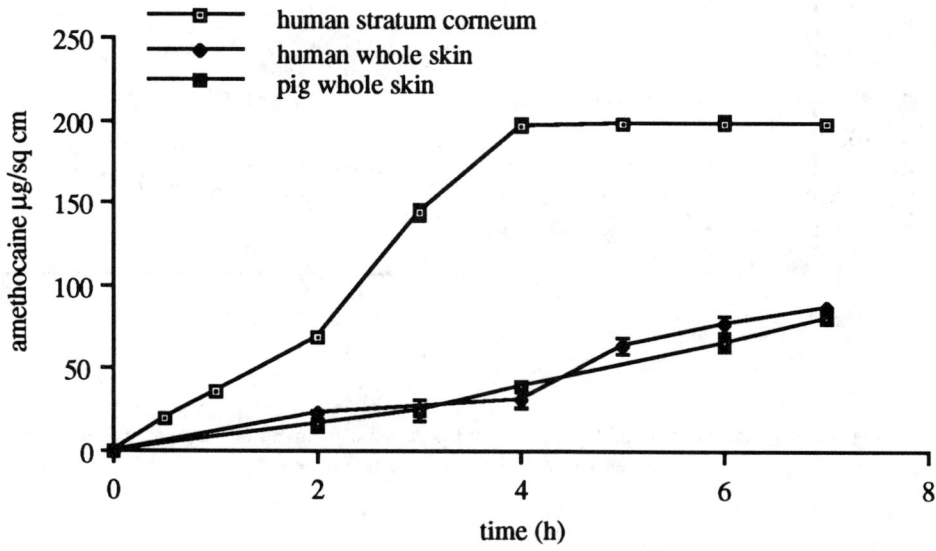

Fig. 4.22 — Comparison of amethocaine penetration (4% m/V gel) through various
barrier membranes using a 2 hour application time

4.6.3.3 Penetration characteristics of lignocaine and prilocaine bases from a eutectic mixture

EMLA® cream consists of a eutectic mixture of lignocaine and prilocaine bases forming the oil phase of an oil-in-water emulsion. Total anaesthetic concentration in the product is 5% w/w, each anaesthetic being 2.5% w/w. The preparation requires a minimum 1 hour application for venepuncture. McGowan (1990) investigated the penetration characteristics of both anaesthetic bases through human whole skin and stratum corneum using a continuous application of EMLA® onto the skin membrane. The penetration characteristics of both bases are shown in Fig. 4.23. Prilocaine penetrated better through both human whole skin and stratum corneum than lignocaine, though the latter is the more potent anaesthetic of the two. The flux of prilocaine through human stratum corneum was 33.86 μg cm^{-2} h^{-1}, some 2.5 times greater than through human whole skin (13.41 μg cm^{-2} h^{-1}). For lignocaine the flux was 21.00 μg cm^{-2} h^{-1}, 2.2 times greater than human whole skin (9.83 μg cm^{-2} h^{-1}). The corresponding fluxes for 4% m/V amethocaine were 52.07 μg cm^{-2} h^{-1} (human stratum corneum) and 15.27 μg cm^{-2} h^{-1} (human whole skin). Thus, amethocaine fluxes were greater through each barrier than either lignocaine or prilocaine individually. However, a more appropriate model was to consider the total anaesthetic penetration from EMLA® compared to that for the amethocaine formulation.

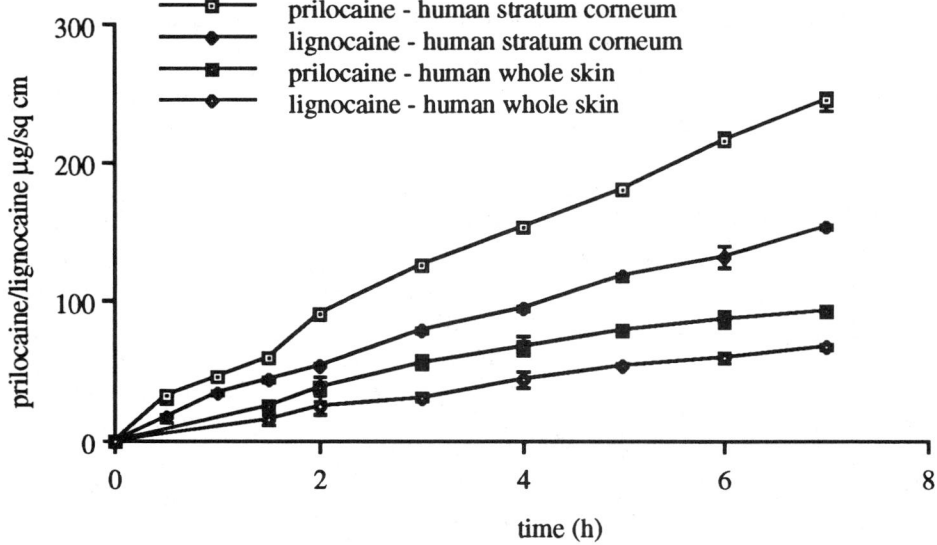

Fig. 4.23 — Penetration of lignocaine and prilocaine from Emla® cream through human stratum corneum and whole skin

A typical skin area used clinically for venepuncture is about 9 cm^2. Using the calculated flux values, a 30 minute application period in each case gives prilocaine absorption through human stratum corneum as 152.37 μg and through human whole skin as 60.35 μg. For lignocaine the corresponding values are 94.5 μg and 44.24 μg. Thus, the total anaesthetic penetration from EMLA® in this model was 246.87 μg (human stratum corneum) and 104.59 μg (whole skin). Since the clinical application time for EMLA® is 1 hour these values should really be doubled to 493.74 μg and 209.18 μg respectively. For 4% m/V amethocaine the corresponding amounts of anaesthetic penetrating in the clinically recommended 30 minute application period, as calculated from continuous application flux values, were 234.32 μg (human stratum corneum) and 68.72 μg (human whole skin). Thus, total anaesthetic delivery was similar from both preparations given the same application period but substantially greater anaesthetic penetration occurred with EMLA® when the clinically recommended application period was considered. Overall, the difference between the two preparations was not with respect to their relative efficacies at delivering the anaesthetic to the target nociceptors, since the amounts of anaesthetic penetrating human stratum corneum in a 30 minute application were similar. Rather, it was the greater potency of amethocaine, compared to either lignocaine or prilocaine, which produced cutaneous anaesthesia for relatively less drug at the target site of action. The combination of further delivery from the stratum corneum after the amethocaine preparation is removed, taken together with its inherent potency, probably explains the prolonged activity of amethocaine gel compared to EMLA®.

4.7   NON-INVASIVE MONITORING OF PERCUTANEOUS LOCAL ANAESTHESIA *IN VIVO*

In studying candidate percutaneous local anaesthetic formulations a particular difficulty encountered is the inevitably subjective nature of pain assessment, particularly in children. In order to determine the minimum concentration of anaesthetic required for effective dermal anaesthesia a non-invasive and non-subjective method of concentration-response analysis would clearly be advantageous. Laser-Doppler velocimetry (LDV) offers perhaps the best practical possibility of achieving this aim. LDV can be used to monitor blood perfusion through the cutaneous microcirculation (Holloway, 1983). Thus, its use has been reported in monitoring the percutaneous absorption of topically applied vasoactive compounds, notably potent vasodilators such as nicotinic acid esters (Guy *et al.*, 1983, 1986).

Vasodilatation and local anaesthesia are both due to a drug-receptor interaction. Many local anaesthetics are vasoactive (see 3.6.4) and their percutaneous absorption can therefore be monitored via LDV. The technique uses a low power laser light. When placed against the skin, this illuminating light undergoes partial reflection, and consequently a Doppler frequency shift, upon striking blood cells traversing the illuminated volume of skin. The actual quantity measured is blood cell flux, defined as the product of the number of red blood cells moving in the measured volume and the mean cell velocity. Thus, it is the velocity of cutaneous blood vessel perfusion that dictates the magnitude of the output signal obtained by LDV.

Amethocaine is a vasodilator and, although not as potent in this respect as the nicotinates, will therefore cause an increase in blood cell velocity. Woolfson *et al.* (1989) compared the percutaneous absorption of amethocaine, using three different concentrations in the amethocaine phase-change system, with a placebo. A standard protocol was used involving a 30 minute application time followed by removal of the preparation, attachment of the LDV probe to the treated site, and monitoring of the blood flow at 5 minute intervals for a period of 60 minutes.

Typical responses to each of the four test preparations by an individual subject are shown in Fig. 4.24. The perfusion curves demonstrated a marked increase in blood flow through the cutaneous microcirculation following treatment with each of the three amethocaine concentrations in the phase-change system. By contrast, the responses to placebo showed no significant increase during the monitoring period. The peak response increased with increasing drug concentration and in all cases occurred approximately 10 minutes after monitoring commenced, 40 minutes after the initial application of the preparation. This correlated well with the previously observed onset times for percutaneous anaesthesia in adults using the amethocaine phase-change system, which were typically about 40 minutes.

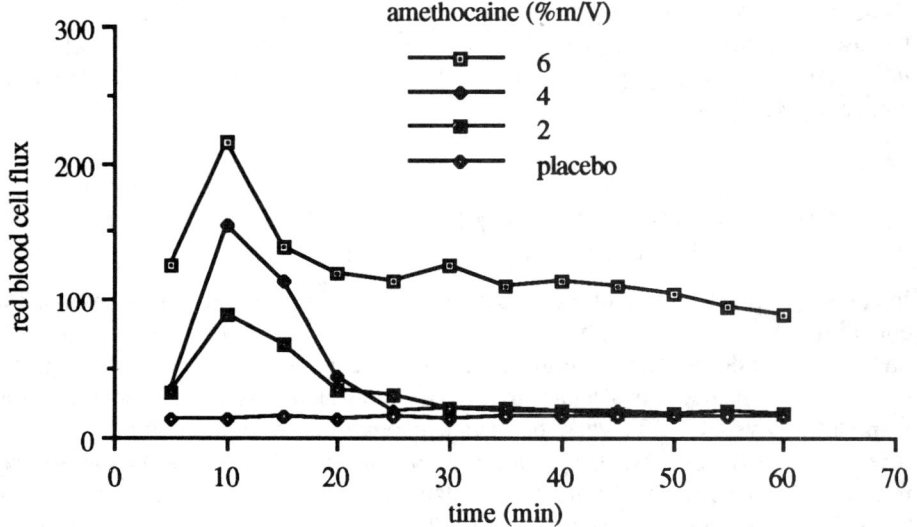

Fig 4.24 — Typical LDV perfusion curves following treatment of a subject with percutaneous anaesthetic formulations containing amethocaine. Reproduced from Woolfson *et al.* (1989) with permission of the copyright holder, Elsevier, Amsterdam

In addition to peak blood flow, results from an LDV experiment can also be evaluated with respect to the area under the perfusion curve (AUC). AUC data can be regarded as a measure of the duration of the effect, with peak response indicating its magnitude. Table 4.11 compares the peak and AUC data for each preparation in the study, analysed by a one-way analysis of variance with repeated measures. The formulations were significantly different in respect of both parameters and were further analysed by a multiple range test (Table 4.12). With peak flux data, all amethocaine concentrations were significantly different from placebo, and also from each other, with the peak flux increasing with increasing drug concentration. AUC data, however, gave a less well-defined result. Although the highest drug concentration was significantly different in its effect on cutaneous blood flow from all other concentrations, and from placebo, the other active preparations were not significantly different from each other, or from placebo.

Table 4.11 — Monitoring of percutaneous local anaesthesia by laser Doppler velocimetry following application of the amethocaine phase-change system to adult volunteers. Flux and AUC values are in arbitrary units

anaesthetic concentration (%m/V)	0	2	4	6	significance of difference
mean peak flux	16	59	92	132	$P < 0.01$
mean area under curve	833	1499	1692	3027	$P < 0.01$

Table 4.12 — Comparison of perfomances in the amethocaine phase-change system as determined by laser Doppler velocimetry. Peak red blood cell flux and area under the perfusion curve (AUC) were used as parameters of percutaneous anaesthetic penetration

comparison in terms of anaesthetic concentration (%m/V)	response	significance of difference
6 vs. 0	AUC	$P < 0.05$
6 vs. 2	AUC	$P < 0.05$
6 vs. 4	AUC	$P < 0.05$
4 vs. 0	AUC	$P > 0.05$
4 vs. 2	AUC	$P > 0.05$
2 vs. 0	AUC	$P > 0.05$
6 vs. 0	peak flux	$P < 0.05$
6 vs. 2	peak flux	$P < 0.05$
6 vs. 4	peak flux	$P < 0.05$
4 vs. 0	peak flux	$P < 0.05$
4 vs. 2	peak flux	$P < 0.05$
2 vs. 0	peak flux	$P < 0.05$

Since the peak flux value on the perfusion curve is a measure of the magnitude of the response to the vasodilatory effect of amethocaine, it is perhaps not surprising that this measure appears to follow the percutaneous absorption of the drug as determined subjectively (Woolfson *et al.*, 1988). However, at 90 minutes following the initial application of each preparation, the flux and, therefore, the AUC values were in decline, in many cases reaching basal levels again. This occurs even though all subjects treated with the two highest amethocaine concentrations still had complete cutaneous anaesthesia. Therefore, it was not surprising that the use of AUC as a parameter in this study failed to differentiate adequately between the preparations. Although AUC is a measure of the duration of the drug effect on the peripheral microcirculation, this latter factor is related only to the onset of anaesthesia and not its duration.

Considering that LDV is a saturable process and that the dose response curves may not be linear (Guy *et al.*, 1983, 1986), the results obtained by the use of LDV were nevertheless promising as a non-subjective method of monitoring the onset of percutaneous anaesthesia. However, the method does rely on evaluating a pharmacological response to a percutaneously administered drug rather than directly following drug penetration through the stratum corneum. A method of direct non-invasive monitoring of percutaneous drug absorption has been proposed by Mak *et al.* (1990a). This involves the use of attenuated total reflectance infrared spectroscopy (ATR-IR). This followed a study on the effects of the penetration enhancer, oleic acid, on the ordering of human stratum corneum lipids (Mak *et al.*, 1990b). In this study it proved possible to approximate the amount of the enhancer in the outer layers of the stratum corneum by following the infrared absorbance at 1710 cm^{-1}, the carbonyl stretching band of the carboxylic acid group in oleic acid. Similarly, ATR-IR could be used to monitor the concentration of any topically applied drug in the outer region of the stratum corneum, provided that the drug possesses a unique IR absorbance distinct from that of the stratum corneum itself. The regions available for monitoring drug absorption by this method are restricted to wavelengths between 1700 and 2500 cm^{-1}, and the near IR region. This method has not yet been applied to local anaesthetics, and its utility will obviously depend on the structure and consequent IR spectrum of the drug. Nevertheless, it is a method that may hold some future promise.

4.8 CLINICAL FACTORS AFFECTING THE PERCUTANEOUS ABSORPTION OF LOCAL ANAESTHETICS

Much useful information can be gained from *in vitro* modelling of percutaneous drug absorption. However, there are a number of clinically relevant factors that can significantly affect this process and are sometimes difficult to consider in the laboratory. The age of the the patient, and therefore the drug penetration characteristics of the skin, is certainly important in this respect. This is particularly so in percutaneous local anaesthesia, where many of the patients will be children. There may also be differences in percutaneous drug absorption characteristics shown by skin of different racial types. Finally, there is a likelihood that skin of different thicknesses, and from different parts of the body, will have different resistances to the penetration of exogenous chemical agents, including drugs.

Rasmussen (1979) commented that paediatricians and dermatologists have long believed that children's skin is more "sensitive" than adults to topically applied chemicals and that such skin is "thinner" and "more tender". This, in turn, has led to a general caution, or even reluctance, in the use of topical drug therapy on children, mostly in association with the application of corticosteroid treatment.

The major source for concern in the use of the percutaneous route of drug delivery in children is probably when newborn infants are involved. In this situation there are real hazards associated with topical drug therapy, involving agents for the treatment of nappy rash, topical antiseptics and dermatological preparations (Rutter, 1987). The newborn infant's skin is not a complete barrier to drug absorption, particularly if it is damaged, diseased or immature, with the latter being the most important factor. Very immature infants have a poorly developed epidermis, which is readily permeable to drugs. This presents a risk, but also offers the benefits of transdermal therapy, with drugs such as theophylline being delivered by this route. Evans and Rutter (1989) have summarised both the risks and potential benefits of topical drug therapy of the newborn infant.

In the specific case of percutaneous local anaesthesia it could be argued that a policy of non-use in infants and very young children would be the safest course of action. This is based on the attitude, still somewhat prevalent, that babies will cry irrespective of feeling pain. Therefore, alleviation of pain in babies is often given a low priority. This unfortunate viewpoint is confirmed in a recent survey of neonatal intensive care units in the UK and Ireland conducted by Tohill and McMorrow (1990). They found that policies of pain relief in such units were poorly defined and that analgesics in general were underprescribed by physicians and often underadministered by nurses (Table 4.13). They recommended the increased use of local anaesthetic creams and sprays, together with other forms of analgesia when warranted by post-operative or other painful conditions.

Caution should rightly be applied in the use of percutaneous local anaesthesia in the newborn or very young babies but the only category really at risk from the sensible use of this form of pain relief is probably the preterm infant. Certainly, it has been the authors' personal experiences that use of a percutaneous anaesthetic prior to routine vaccination of babies at three months and later is of major, even spectacular, benefit to all concerned in an otherwise often histrionic procedure.

For children, generally, there appears to be no real cause for anxiety in the use of percutaneous local anaesthesia. There is no firm evidence that a child's skin is thinner than that of an adult as a matter of anatomy. Rather, it is more likely that changes in an adult's skin, and, consequently, in resistance to percutaneous drug penetration, are the results of environmental factors. This would explain why percutaneous local anaesthetics act quicker in children than in adults. It is not that the child's skin is thinner but rather that the stratum corneum in adults may become thicker, notably as a result of exposure to the sun. Increased melanocyte formation may also retard the percutaneous penetration process. In any case, the authors have observed (admittedly on an empirical basis) over ten years of trials with percutaneous local anaesthesia using exposed skin areas such as the forearm, that those subjects who lead an outdoor lifestyle, such as those addicted to the royal and ancient game, are invariably the slowest to achieve onset of complete skin anaesthesia!

In addition to children, percutaneous drug absorption in the elderly requires some consideration. Roskos et al. (1989) compared the percutaneous penetration characteristics of several drugs in two groups of patients, a young group aged from 18 to 40 years and an older group where all patients were older than 65 years. The drugs

Table 4.13 — Neonatal intensive care unit questionnaire on analgesic practices

question	percentage of units answering yes
Do you accept babies feel pain?	100
Do you have a unit policy on analgesia?	71
Is this a written policy?	12
What criteria do you have to recognise pain?	
grimace	96
posturing	96
crying	100
tachycardia	85
high blood pressure	40
restlessness	60
Is analgesia routine in the following conditions?	
necrosing enterocolitis	25
neural tube defects and anencephaly	40
meningitis	18
Is analgesia sedation given before the following?	
endotracheal intubation	6
insertion of chest drain	71
lumbar puncture	6
heel stabs	4
venepuncture	0
removal of skin probes	0
Do you agree that:	
analgesia is commonly underprescribed by doctors	70
nalgesia is commonly underadministered by nurses	33

Reproduced from Tohill and McMorrow (1990) with permission of the copyright holder, The Lancet Ltd

investigated ranged from relatively hydrophilic substances, such as acetylsalicylic acid and caffeine, to lipophilic agents such as testosterone and oestradiol. There was a significant reduction in the percutaneous penetration of the more hydrophilic agents in the older age group compared to the younger group, whereas the penetration characteristics of the more lipophilic drugs was similar in both cases. It was postulated that the reduced lipid content of older skin will adversely affect the percutaneous penetration of those agents whose lipophilicity is relatively low to begin with, whereas highly lipophilic drugs will still be able to dissolve readily in the stratum corneum even when the available lipid content of this barrier layer is reduced. These effects may be further enhanced by the typically reduced hydration of the stratum corneum in older patients. With percutaneous local anaesthesia, the main application to older patients is in the harvesting of split skin grafts (see section 6.7), in which there appears to be no discernible difference between onset, duration and efficacy of skin anaesthesia in elderly patients compared to their younger counterparts (Small et al., 1988). This probably reflects the relatively high lipophilicity of the local anaesthetic free bases, which are, therefore, unaffected by any diminished stratum corneum lipid content in the elderly.

Most applications of percutaneous local anaesthetics involve venepuncture, either to the dorsum of the hand or the forearm, or the cutting of a split skin graft from the thigh. Although, to some extent, different skin thicknesses can be expected in these regions, such differences that do occur are not likely to be clinically significant, an observation supported by practical clinical experience, where effective percutaneous anaesthesia can now be routinely achieved at all these sites. Of greater significance may be the effect of using the technique on skin of different racial types. Gean et al. (1989), using methyl nicotinate as a model penetrant, compared by laser Doppler velocimetry the erythematous responses of black, oriental and Caucasian skin to this potent topical vasodilator. The results of this particular study were somewhat inconclusive and failed to demonstrate any significant overall difference between the behaviour of the three skin types, either on a visual basis or with respect to the objective LDV results. Of more relevance to percutaneous local anaesthetic absorption is the study by Hymes and Spraker (1986) which appeared to demonstrate a delay in the onset of action and a reduction in efficacy of percutaneous local anaesthesia with the lignocaine-prilocaine eutectic system (EMLA® cream). It was suggested that the increased density and more compact nature of the stratum corneum in black skin might slow the absorption of a topically applied agent. Thus, Hellgren et al. (1989) used a two hour application time with EMLA® in studying pain relief for venepuncture in a group of Tanzanian schoolchildren. The results were broadly similar to those achieved with a one hour application of the same preparation to Caucasian children. However, they did not actually study the effect of the shorter application period on the trial group so that the necessity of using a more prolonged application period on black compared to Caucasian skin has not been clearly established. This may reflect the fact that, at the time of writing, the technique of percutaneous local anaesthesia has largely been restricted, in terms of commercial availability, to Western Europe.

REFERENCES

Anderson, R.L. and Cassidy, J.M. (1973) Variations in physical dimensions and chemical composition of human stratum corneum. *J. Invest. Dermatol.* **61** 30-32.

Barry, B.W. (1983a) *Dermatological Formulations.* Marcel Dekker, New York, pp. 1-48.

Barry, B.W. (1983b) *Dermatological Formulations.* Marcel Dekker, New York, pp. 155-158.

Barry, B.W. (1990) Some problems in predicting human percutaneous absorption via *in vitro* animal models. In: Scott, R.C., Guy, R.H., and Hadgraft, J. (eds) *Prediction of percutaneous penetration*. IBC, London, pp. 204-212.

Barry, B.W. (1987) Penetration enhancers. In: Shroot, B. and Schaefer, H. (eds) *Skin Pharmacokinetics*. Karger, Basel, pp. 121-137.

Bissett, D.L. (1987) Anatomy and biochemistry of skin. In: Kydonieus, A.F. and Berner, B. (eds) *Transdermal delivery of drugs*, Vol. I, CRC Press, Boca Raton, Florida, pp. 29-42.

Blank, I.H. (1965) Cutaneous barriers. *J. Invest. Dermatol.* **45** 249-256.

Blank, I.H. and Scheuplein, R.J. (1969) Transport into and within the skin. *Brit. J. Derm.* **81** Suppl. 4. 4-10.

Breathnach, A.S., Goodman, T., Stolinski, C. and Gross, M. (1973) Freeze fracture replication of cells of stratum corneum of human epidermis. *J. Anat.* **114** 65-81.

Bronaugh, R.L., Stewart, R.F. and Storm, J.E. (1989) Extent of cutaneous metabolism during percutaneous absorption of xenobiotics. *Toxicol. Appl. Pharmacol.* **99** 534-543.

Brown, L. and Langer, R. (1988) Transdermal delivery of drugs. *Am. Rev. Med.* **39** 221-229.

Covino, B.G. (1986) Pharmacology of local anaesthetic agents. *Brit. J. Anaesth.* **58** 701-716.

Dalvi, U.M. and Zatz, J.L. (1981) Effect of non-ionic surfactants on penetration of dissolved benzocaine through hairless mouse skin. *J. Soc. Cosmet. Chem.* **32** 87-94.

Durrheim, H., Flynn, G.L., Higuchi, W.I. and Behl, C.R. (1980) Permeation of hairless mouse skin I: Experimental methods and comparison with human epidermal permeation by alkanols. *J. Pharm. Sci.* **69** 781-786.

Ebling, F.J.G. and Rook, A. (1979) Hair. In: Rook, A., Ebling, F.J.G. and Wilkinson, D.S. (eds) *Textbook of dermatology*, 3rd. edn., Vol. 2. Blackwell, Oxford, pp. 1733-1824.

Elias, P.M. and Brown, B.E. (1978) The mammalian cutaneous permeability barrier. Defective barrier function in essential fatty acid deficiency correlates with abnormal intercellular lipid deposition. *Lab. Invest.* **39** 574-583.

Elias, P.M. and Leventhal, M.E. (1980) Intercellular volume changes and cell surface area expansion during cornification. *Eur. J. Cell Biol.* **22** 439a.

Elias, P.M. (1981) Lipids and the epidermal permeability barrier. *Arch. Dermatol. Res.* **270** 95-117.

Elias, P.M. (1988) Structure and function of the stratum corneum permeability barrier. *Drug Dev. Res.* **13** 97-105.

Evans, N. and Rutter, N. (1989) Transdermal drug delivery to the newborn infant. In: Hadgraft, J. and Guy, R.H. (eds). *Transdermal Drug Delivery*. Marcel Dekker, New York, pp. 155-176.

Feldmann, R.J. and Maibach, H.I. (1970) Absorption of some organic compounds through the skin in man. *J. Invest. Dermatol.* **54** 399-404.

Findlay, G.H. (1955) The simple esterases of human skin. *Br. J. Dermatol.* **67** 83-91.

Flynn, G.L. and Roseman, T.J. (1971) Membrane absorption II: influence of physical absorption on molecular flux through heterogeneous dimethylpolysiloxane barriers. *J. Pharm. Sci.* **60** 1788-1796.

Flynn, G.L. (1979) Topical drug absorption and topical pharmaceutical systems. In: Banker, G.R. and Rhodes, G.L. (eds) *Modern pharmaceutics*. Marcel Dekker, New York, pp. 263-327.

Flynn, G.L., Yalkowsky, S.H. and Roseman, T.J. (1974) Mass transport phenomena and models: Theoretical concepts. *J. Pharm. Sci.*, **63** 479-510.

Franz, T.J. (1975) Percutaneous absorption. On the relevance of *in vitro* data. *J. Invest. Dermatol.* **64** 190-195.

Franz, T.J. (1978) The finite dose technique as a valid *in vitro* model for the study of percutaneous absorption in man. *Curr. Probl. Dermatol.* **7** 58-68.

Franz, T.J. (1985) Systems for the measurement of percutaneous absorption of pharmaceutical compounds, cosmetics and toxic substances. Catalog. No. Pa-1-85. Crown Glass Co., Somerville, New Jersey.

Garrett, E.R. and Chemburkar, R.B. (1968) Evaluation, control and prediction of drug diffusion through polymeric membranes. I. *J. Pharm. Sci.* **57** 944-948.

Gean, C.J., Tur, E., Maibach, H.I. and Guy, R.H. (1989) Cutaneous responses to topical methyl nicotinate in black, oriental and caucasian subjects. *Arch. Dermatol.* **281** 95-98.

Golden, G.M., Guzek, D.B., Harris, R.R., McKie, J.E. and Potts, R.O. (1986) Lipid thermotropic transitions in human stratum corneum. *J. Invest. Dermatol.*, **86** 255-259.

Goldschmidt, H. and Kligman, A.M. (1964) Quantitative estimation of keratin production by the epidermis. *Arch. Dermatol.* **88** 709-712.

Goodman, M. and Barry, B.W. (1989) Action of penetration enhancers on human stratum corneum as assessed by differential scanning calorimetry. In: Bronaugh, R.L. and Maibach, H.I. (eds) *Percutaneous Penetration*, 2nd edn. Marcel Dekker, New York, pp. 567-593.

Guy, R.H., Wester, R.C., Tur, E. and Maibach, H.I. (1983) Non-invasive assessment of the percutaneous absorption of methyl nicotinate in humans. *J. Pharm. Sci.* **72** 1077-1079.

Guy, R.H., Tur, E., Schall, L.M., Elamir, S. and Maibach, H.I. (1986) determination of vehicle effects on percutaneous absorption by laser Doppler velocimetry. *Arch. Dermatol. Res.* **278** 500-502.

Hellgren, U., Kihamia, C.M., Premji, Z. and Danielson, K. (1989) Local anaesthetic cream for the alleviation of pain during venepuncture in Tanzanian schoolchildren. *Br. J. Clin. Pharmacol.* **28** 205-206.

Hinz, R.S., Hodson, C.D., Lorence, C.R. and Guy, R.H. (1989) *In vitro* percutaneous penetration. Evaluation of the utility of hairless mouse skin. *J. Invest. Dermatol.* **93** 87-91.

Holloway, G.A. (1983) Laser Doppler measurement of cutaneus blood flow. In: Rolfe, P. (ed.) *Non-Invasive Physiological Measurements*, Vol. 2. Academic Press, London, pp. 219-247.

Homalle, A. (1853) Experiences physiologiques sur l'absorption par la tegument chez l'homme dans le main. *Union Med.* **7** 462-463.

Hymes, J. and Spraker, M. (1986) Racial differences in the effectiveness of a topically applied mixture of local anesthetics. *Re. Anest.* **11** 11-13.

Iggo, A. (1982) Cutaneous sensory mechanisms. In: Barlow, H.B. and Mollon, J.D. (eds) *The senses*. Cambridge University Press, Cambridge, pp. 369-406.

Jarrett, A. (1973) *The Physiology and pathophysiology of the skin*, Vol. 1: *The epidermis*. Academic Press, New York.

Knutson, K., Potts, R.O., Guzek, D.B., Golden, G.M., McKie, J.E., Lambert, W.J. and Higuchi, W.I. (1985) Macro and molecular physical-chemical considerations in understanding drug transport in the stratum corneum. *J. Contr. Rel.* **2** 67-87.

Landmann, L. (1988) The epidermal permeability barrier. *Anat. Embryol.* **178** 1-13.

Loth, H. (1989) Skin permeability. *Meth. Find. Exp. Clin. Pharmacol.* **11** 155-164.

Lubens, H.M. and Sanker, J.F. (1964) Anaesthetic skin patch. *Ann. Allergy* **22** 37-41.

Lubens, H.M., Ausdenmoore, R.W., Shafer, A.D. and Reece, R.M. (1974) Anesthetic patch for painful procedures such as minor operations. *Am. J. Dis. Child* **128** 192-194.

Mackenzie, I.C. and Linder, J.E. (1973) An examination of cellular organisation within the stratum corneum by a silver staining method. *J. Invest. Dermatol.* **61** 254-260.

Mak, V.H.W., Potts, R.O. and Guy, R.H. (1990a) Percutaneous penetration enhancement *in vivo* measured by attenuated total reflectance infrared spectroscopy. *Pharm. Res.* **7** 835-841.

Mak, V.H.W., Potts, R.O. and Guy, R.H. (1990b) Oleic acid concentration and effect in human stratum corneum: Non-invasive determination by total reflectance infrared spectroscopy. *J. Control. Rel.* **12** 67-75.

Martin, R.J., Denyer, S.P. and Hadgraft, J. (1987) Skin metabolism of topically applied compounds. *Int. J. Pharm.* **39** 23-32.

Marzulli, F.N., Brown, D.W.C., and Maibach, H.I. (1969) Techniques for studying skin penetration. *Toxicol. Appl. Pharmacol.* **46** Suppl. 3 76-83.

Matoltsy, A.G., Downes, A.M., and Sweeney, T.M. (1968) Studies of the epidermal water barrier. Part II. Investigation of the chemical nature of the water barrier. *J. Invest. Dermatol.* **50** 19-26.

Matoltsy, A.G. (1976) Keratinisation. *J. Invest. Dermatol.* **67** 20-25.

McCafferty, D.F. & Woolfson, A.D. (1988) Percutaneous local anaesthetic composition for topical application and associated method. U.K. Patent 2163956.

McCafferty, D.F., Woolfson, A.D., McClelland, K.H. and Boston, V. (1988) Comparative *in vivo* and *in vitro* assessment of the percutaneous absorption of local anaesthetics. *Br. J. Anaesth.* **60** 64-69.

McClelland, K.H. (1986) *Studies on percutaneous local anaesthesia*. Ph.D. thesis. The Queen's University of Belfast.

McElhaney, R.N. (1982) The use of differential scanning calorimetry and differential thermal analysis in studies of model and biological membranes. *Chem. Phys. Lip.* **30** 229-259.

McGowan, K.E. (1990) *Percutaneous local anaesthesia with amethocaine*. Ph.D. thesis. The Queen's University of Belfast.

Melchior, D.L. (1984) Some uses of differential scanning calorimetry in biomembrane research. *Anal. Calorimetry* **5** 307-324.

Menczel, E. and Goldberg, S. (1978) pH effect on the percutaneous penetration of lignocaine hydrochloride. *Dermatologica* **156** 8-14.

Miller, M.R. (1960) Cutaneous Innervation. In: Montagna,W. (ed) *Advances in biology of the skin, vol 1*. Pergamon Press, Oxford, p. 4.

Monash, S. (1957) Topical anesthesia of unbroken skin. *Arch. Dermatol.* **76** 752-756.

Mukhtar, H. and Bickers, D.R. (1981) Drug metabolism in skin. *Drug Metab. Dispos.*

9 311-314.

Nacht, S., Yeung, D., Beasley, Jr., J.N., Anjo, M.D. and Maibach, H.I. (1981) Benzoyl peroxide: percutaneous penetration and metabolic disposition. *J. Am. Acad. Dermatol.* **4** 31-37.

Nathan, D., Sakr, A., Lichtin, J.L. and Bronaugh, R.L. (1990) *In vitro* skin absorption of benzoic acid, p-aminobenzoic acid and benzocaine in the hairless guinea pig. *Pharm. Res.* **7** 1147-1151.

Nemanic, M.K. and Elias, P.M. (1980) *In situ* precipitation: A novel cytochemical technique for visualisation of permeability pathways in mammalian stratum corneum. *J. Histochem. Cytochem.* **28** 573-578.

Nimmo, W.S. (1990) The promise of transdermal drug delivery. *Brit. J. Anaesth.* **64** 7-10.

Osborne, D.W. (1986) Computational methods for predicting skin permeability. *Pharm. Manufacturing* **April/May**, 41-48.

Ostrenga, J., Steinmetz, C. and Poulsen, B. (1971) Significance of vehicle composition. I. Relationship between topical vehicle composition, skin permeability and clinical efficiency. *J. Pharm. Sci.* **60** 1175-1179.

Pannatier, A., Jenner, P., Testa, B. and Etter, J.C. (1978) The skin as a drug metabolising organ. *Drug Metab. Rev.* **8** 319-343.

Potts, R.O. (1989) Physical characterisation of the stratum corneum: The relationship of mechanical and barrier properties to lipid and protein structure. In: Hadgraft, J. and Guy, R.H. (eds) *Transdermal drug delivery.* Marcel Dekker, New York, pp. 23-57.

Potts, R.O., McNeill, S.C., Desbonnet, C.R. and Wakshull, E. (1989) Transdermal drug transport and metabolism. II. The role of competing kinetic events. *Pharm. Res.* **6** 119-124.

Prottey, C. (1977) Investigations of functions of essential fatty acids in the skin. *Br. J. Dermatol.* **97** 29-38.

Racansky, V., Bederova, E. and Piskova, L. (1988) The influence of local anesthetics on the gel-liquid crystal phase transition in model dipalmitoylphosphatidylcholine membranes. *Gen. Physiol. Biophys.* **7** 217-221.

Rasmussen, J.E. (1979) Percutaneous absorption in children. In: Dobson, R.L. (ed.) *The Year Book of Dermatology.* Year Book Medical Publishers Inc., Chicago, pp.15-38.

Reaven, E.P. and Cox, A.J. (1965) Histidine and keratinisation. *J. Invest. Dermatol.* **45** 422-431.

Rigg, P.C. and Barry, B.W. (1990) Shed snake skin and hairless mouse skin as model membranes for human skin during permeation studies. *J. Invest. Dermatol.* **94** 235-239.

Rosen, T., Lanning, M.B. and Hill, M.J. (1983) *The nurses atlas of dermatology.* Little, Brown and Co., Boston, pp. 2-5.

Roskos, K.V., Maibach, H.I. and gury, R.H. (1989) The effect of aging on percutaneous absorption in man. *J. Pharmacokinet. Biopharm.* **17** 617-630.

Rutter, N. (1987) Percutaneous drug absorption in the newborn: Hazards and uses. *Perinat. Pharmacol.* **14** 911-930.

Sarpotdar, P.P. and Zatz, J.L. (1986) Evaluation of penetration enhancement of lidocaine by non-ionic surfactants through hairless mouse skin *in vitro. J. Pharm. Sci.* **75** 176-181.

Scheuplein, R.J. (1967) Mechanism of percutaneous absorption . II. Transient diffusion and the relative importance of various routes of skin penetration. *J. Invest. Dermatol.* **48** 79-88.

Scheuplein, R.J. and Blank, I.H. (1971) Permeability of the skin. *Physiol. Rev.* **51** 702-747.

Scheuplein, R.J. (1972) Properties of the skin as a membrane. *Adv. Skin Biol.* **12** 125-152.

Scheuplein, R.J. (1976) Percutaneous absorption after twenty five years or "Old wine in new wineskins". *J. Invest. Dermatol.* **67** 31-38.

Schreiner, E. and Wolff, K. (1969) Die Permeabilitat des klein Molekulares Protein. *Arch. Klin. Exp. Dermatol.* **235** 78-88.

Small, J., Wallace, R.G., Millar, R., Woolfson, A.D. and McCafferty, D.F. (1988) Pain-free cutting of split skin grafts by application of a percutaneous anaesthetic cream. Brit. J. Plastic Surgery **41** 539-543.

Smith, W.P., Christensen, M.S., Nacht, S. and Gans, E.H. (1982) Effect of lipids on the aggregation and permeability of human stratum corneum. *J. Invest. Dermatol.* **78** 7-12.

Stoughton, R.B. (1972) Some bioassay methods for measuring skin absorption. *Adv. Biol. Skin* **12** 535-546.

Stuttgen, G. (1982) Drug absorption by intact and damaged skin. In: Brandau, R. and Lippold, B.H. (eds) *Dermal and transdermal absorption*, Wissenschaftliche Verlagsgesellschaft GmbH, Stuttgart, pp. 27-40.

Tohill, J. and McMorrow, O. (1990) Pain relief in neonatal intensive care. *Lancet* **336** 569.

Van Duzee, B.F. (1975) Thermal analysis of human stratum corneum. *J. Invest. Dermatol.* **65** 404-408.

Wertz, P.W. and Downing, D.T. (1989) Stratum corneum: Biological and chemical implications. In: Hadgraft, J. and Guy, R.H. (eds) *Transdermal drug delivery*. Marcel Dekker, New York, pp. 1-22.

Wester, R.C. and Maibach, H.I. (1987) Animal models for transdermal delivery. In: Kydonieus, A.F. and Berner, B. (eds) *Transdermal delivery of drugs*. Vol I. CRC Press, Boca Raton, Florida, pp. 61-70.

Wiechers, J.W. (1989) The barrier function of the skin in relation to percutaneous absorption of drugs. *Pharm. Weekbld. Sci. Ed.* **11** 185-98.

Wiechers, J.W. and De Zeeuw, R.A. (1990) Transdermal drug delivery: efficacy and potential applications of the penetration enhancer Azone®. *Drug Des. Del.* **6** 87-100.

Woodburne, R.T. (1965) *Essentials of human anatomy*. Oxford University Press, Oxford, p.6.

Woolfson, A.D., McCafferty, D.F., McClelland, K.H. and Boston, V. (1988) Concentration-response analysis of percutaneous local anaesthetic formulations. *Brit. J. Anaesth.*, **61** 589-592.

Woolfson, A.D. and McCafferty, D.F. (1989) Local anaesthesia of the skin. *J. Clin. Pharm. Ther.* **14** 103-109.

Woolfson, A.D., McCafferty, D.F., McGowan, K.E. and Boston, V. (1989). Non-invasive monitoring of percutaneous local anaesthesia using laser-Doppler velocimetry. *Int. J. Pharm.* **51** 183-187.

Woolfson, A.D., McCafferty, D.F. and Boston, V. (1990a) Clinical experiences with a novel percutaneous amethocaine preparation: prevention of pain due to venepuncture in children. *Brit. J. Clin. Pharmac.* **30** 273-279.

Woolfson, A.D., McCafferty, D.F. and McGowan, K.E. (1990b) The metabolism of amethocaine by porcine and human skin extracts: influence on percutaneous anaesthesia. *Int. J. Pharm.* **62** 9-14.

Woolfson, A.D., McCafferty, D.F. and McGowan, K.E. (1991) Differential scanning calorimetry of a novel amethocaine preparation and its effect on human stratum corneum. *Proc. 10th. Pharm. Tech. Conf.*, Bologna, Italy. pp. 405-423.

Woolfson, A.D., McCafferty, D.F. and McGowan, K.E. (1992) Percutaneous penetration characteristics of amethocaine through porcine and human skin. *Int. J. Pharm.* **78** 209-216.

5

Formulation of local anaesthetics for percutaneous delivery

Local anaesthetics do not readily penetrate intact skin (McCafferty *et al.*, 1988). Therefore, the formulation of an effective percutaneous anaesthetic presents a difficult challenge, which has been successfully met only in recent years. This point is well illustrated by the time interval between the first literature references to percutaneous anaesthesia and the first appearance of a commercial percutaneous anaesthetic product. In hindsight, it is possible to see that the delay has been caused, at least in part, by a combination of failure to move beyond the constraints of conventional dermatological systems and failure to select the optimum drug in the correct form. Since formulators, unfortunately, are not blessed with the gift of hindsight, it has been necessary to rely on the principles of topical formulation, perseverance and a little serendipidity!

A percutaneous anaesthetic is a topical formulation in that it is applied to an external, accessible body surface, the skin. It is arguable, perhaps, as to whether such formulations should be classed as dermatological products. Certainly, since they are specifically applied to intact, healthy skin, they are not therapeutic dermatological products. However, it does seem reasonable to regard them as prophylactic agents. The term prophylaxis generally refers to the prevention of disease. In the case of percutaneous anaesthetics, it is not disease but rather the pain due to unavoidable mechanical injury to the skin which is prevented. The injury to the skin is a consequence of a necessary clinical procedure such as venepuncture.

If a percutaneous anaesthetic formulation is regarded as a prophylactic dermatological preparation, it follows that the starting point for a successful formulation exercise must be a sound knowledge of the principles governing the formulation of dermatological vehicles. A further complication is that, uniquely in pharmacy, dermatological preparations are distinguished by an extraordinary variety of possible dosage forms. These can differ widely in their composition, physicochemical and aesthetic properties. Only certain formulation types will be appropriate as percutaneous anaesthetic vehicles although many different formulation types have been investigated for this purpose. In seeking to produce a clinically effective and acceptable percutaneous anaesthetic it is therefore essential to look at the complete range of available formulation options.

5.1 DERMATOLOGICAL VEHICLES FOR THE PERCUTANEOUS DELIVERY OF LOCAL ANAESTHETICS

Vehicles used for topical drug delivery may be broadly classified into four main groups: aerosols, liquids, solids, and semi-solids. All of these groups have been used at some time for the topical delivery of local anaesthetics, though the use of aerosols in this respect is almost exclusively confined to the delivery of fluorinated hydrocarbons as a freezing spray for sports injuries.

Liquid topical vehicles may be monophasic solutions, emulsions or suspensions. Solution vehicles may be aqueous, alcoholic, co-solvent or oil-based, and viscosity can be increased by the addition of a viscosity builder. Solubility requirements dictate that formulations of local anaesthetic bases cannot be simple aqueous solutions. Alcohol and co-solvent formulations are therefore of interest (Akerman, 1978). However, the fluidity of solutions makes them difficult to localise at the treatment site. Therefore, they must be used in the form of an absorbent pad soaked in the solution. A particular application of such fluid vehicles is in iontophoretic drug delivery (Banga and Chien, 1988). Fluid emulsions (lotions) and suspensions, although widely used as both topical drug delivery vehicles and cosmetics, offer few formulation possibilities or advantages with respect to percutaneous local anaesthesia and therefore merit no further consideration here.

Solid topical vehicles were originally restricted to powders, notably antibiotic dusting powders and abrasives used in acne treatment. More recently, polymeric film drug delivery systems have been developed. These may contain the active agent in solution or suspension, either as a coating or distributed throughout the polymer matrix. The use of composite films incorporating a rate-controlling membrane is now well-established. Such multilaminar patches are increasingly widely used in transdermal therapeutic systems (Dohner, 1987). Polymeric film delivery systems offer interesting possibilities for the percutaneous delivery of local anaesthetics (Woolfson and McCafferty, 1988).

Historically, the most important topical delivery systems are the semisolids (Fuhrer, 1982). From a rheological perspective a semi-solid is plastic until acted upon by an external deforming force, in which case the deformation remains permanent. Unlike fluid systems or powders, semi-solid formulations tend to adhere and conform to the treatment site. Thus, they are easily localised and contained, a property also shared by solid, flexible polymeric delivery systems. It is therefore not surprising that the formulation of local anaesthetics for percutaneous penetration has concentrated almost exclusively on this structurally unique group. However, the term semi-solid conceals a diverse range of physicochemical systems, many of which are unsuitable for the percutaneous delivery of local anaesthetics. In attempting to produce a formulation that satisfies pharmaceutical and clinical criteria, it is therefore necessary to be aware of all the available topical formulation options listed in Table 5.1, and in particular of the rheological properties and physicochemical nature of the semi-solids. Typical classes of constituents used in the formulation of semi-solids are listed in Table 5.2.

5.2   SEMI-SOLID VEHICLES

Semi-solids are not simply passive drug delivery devices. They can have a direct effect on the condition of the treated skin site, even in the absence of an active medicament. Since percutaneous anaesthesia is applicable only to intact, healthy skin, the main interest in vehicle effects on the skin concerns alterations in skin hydration, specifically

Table 5.1 — Formulation options for percutaneous local anaesthesia

fluids	semi-solids	solids
monophasic solutions - aqueous, alcoholic, co-solvents, oily	ointments - water-free, hydrophobic hydrocarbons	dusting powders
multiphasic solutions - o/w and w/o emulsions	ointments - water-free, hydrophobic silicones	patch transdermal therapeutic system - multilaminate technology
suspensions	ointments - absorption bases forming w/o emulsions	patch transdermal therapeutic system - "form-fill-seal" technology
fluid/absorbent pad system	ointments - emulsifying bases forming o/w emulsions	dried hydrogel - multilaminate film matrix system
	gels	
	creams - o/w emulsions	
	creams - w/o emulsions	
	creams - multiple emulsions	
	pastes	

Table 5.2 — Classification of constituents of semi-solid topical formulations

classification of constituents
hydrophobic vehicles
co-solvents/water-miscible vehicles
matrix formers
gel formers, viscosity builders
w/o emulsifiers
o/w emulsifiers
preservatives

with regard to the water content of the stratum corneum. This can lead to an alteration in the permeability to a topically applied drug (Bucks et al., 1989). It is therefore necessary to be aware of the nature and properties of each potential semi-solid percutaneous anaesthetic formulation, which may be summarised as follows:

(i)   how the preparation will behave in respect of drug bioavailability

(ii)   physicochemical stability of the whole system

(iii)   chemical stability of the active agent(s)

(iv)   aesthetic appearance and patient acceptability

(v)   direct vehicle effects on the skin, including those of any additional specific penetration enhancers included in the formulation

(vi)   rheological properties.

5.2.1   Ointment vehicles

Hydrocarbon-based, anhydrous semi-solids which may contain dissolved or suspended drugs are referred to as ointments. Essentially, an ointment base consists of a higher melting component, the matrix former, which is a solid at room temperature, and a component which is fluid at room temperature. The semi-solid character of an ointment base is imparted by this mixture. Typically, hydrocarbon ointment bases are mixtures of C_{30} - C_{50} hydrocarbons with lower melting C_{15} to C_{30} hydrocarbons. The base is generally prepared by fusion. The stiffness of the final product is determined by the nature of the matrix former, the relative proportions of the two components and the speed of cooling during preparation of the base. Slow cooling produces a larger crystalline structure in the matrix former. The matrix is therefore less coherent and the resulting base is more fluid. Ointments may also be formulated without the use of hydrocarbons. Silicone ointments may be prepared in which dimethylpolysiloxane is incorporated into a molten wax which acts as the matrix former. The base sets on cooling, and is an excellent emollient.

Ointment bases tend to be greasy, difficult to remove and aesthetically unsatisfactory. They are occlusive, drying on the skin to form an adhesive film with water retaining properties. Being very lipophilic, they are poor vehicles for water-soluble drugs, although blending the base with a polar co-solvent may improve drug bioavailability in such cases. Local anaesthetic bases, of course, are lipophilic to various degrees and theoretically compatible with ointment bases. However, the partitioning characteristics of a lipophilic local anaesthetic are such that it will preferentially remain in the lipophilic environment of the vehicle in such cases, rather than partitioning into the skin. Thus, $K_{sc/w}$ in equation (4.3) will be small. Such vehicles will therefore offer poor bioavailability of a dissolved local anaesthetic base. The only way to counteract this is to increase the value of ΔC in equation (4.3). In practice, this means substantially increasing the drug loading of the base. This is wasteful of material, since most of the drug will not be absorbed, and results in a formulation with an unacceptably high drug concentration. In essence, then, this is the dilemma facing the formulator of a percutaneous local anaesthetic preparation. How can a high bioavailability of local anaesthetic base be achieved in order to promote absorption through intact skin without using an unacceptably high drug loading in the vehicle?

Although ointments are anhydrous bases, it is possible to formulate an ointment that is compatible with an aqueous environment. Absorption bases are ointments that possess intrinsic emulsifying properties. They can thus absorb a considerable volume of water, forming in the process a water-in-oil (w/o) emulsion. A water-soluble drug may be incorporated into the anhydrous base as its emulsified solution. However, the aqueous internal phase must be saturated with the drug in order to ensure adequate bioavailability, in a sense similar to the problem of formulating a lipophilic agent in a lipophilic system but with the added problems of more complex drug partitioning in a multiphase system. Since the external phase of these bases is an oil, they behave similarly on the skin to a hydrocarbon ointment. Thus, they present no additional opportunities with respect to the topical delivery of a local anaesthetic base.

Self-emulsifying ointment bases, which are themselves anhydrous, may be prepared by incorporating surfactants into a hydrocarbon base. Examples of such emulsifying ointments using anionic, cationic or non-ionic surfactants are seen in most major pharmacopoeias. The overall effect of the mixture of surfactants used in each vehicle formulation is to produce a base which, in the presence of water, will form an oil-in-water emulsion. It is possible that the surfactants may enhance the absorption of certain drugs from such bases, but the effect is unlikely to be significant. However, they are water-washable and have a greater cosmetic acceptability than other ointment bases.

Water-soluble, hydrophilic, non-occlusive ointment bases may be prepared from mixtures of high and low molecular weight polyethylene glycols (macrogols). These bases are cosmetically excellent, non-staining, water-washable and miscible with skin exudates. Examples of such bases are found in various official compendia. Lidocaine ointment U.S.P., which is intended for topical application to broken skin or mucosa, is formulated in a macrogol vehicle. Interestingly, such vehicles appear to be completely unsuitable for the percutaneous delivery of local anaesthetics through intact skin. When formulated with a high drug loading of either lignocaine or amethocaine free bases, macrogol formulations were completely inactive, producing no anaesthesia to pin-prick challenge (Woolfson and McCafferty, unpublished observations). Macrogol vehicles are incompatible with many chemicals, but it is more likely that, in the case of the anaesthetic bases, the lack of activity was due to poor drug bioavailablity from the formulations, thus preventing a sufficient concentration gradient being established across intact skin. However, the difference between the conventional topical use of local anaesthetics and their effective percutaneous absorption through intact skin is well illustrated by this formulation example.

5.2.2   Cream vehicles

The term cream is something of a misnomer, since it has a rather broader meaning in pharmaceutical science than elsewhere. In pharmaceutical terms a cream is simply a semi-solid emulsion. The characteristic appearance of a pharmaceutical cream is due to reflection of light by the internal phase of the emulsion. Cream emulsions may be of the w/o or o/w types. The use of this shorthand nomenclature can also be confusing since the two immiscible phases forming the emulsion are more accurately described as polar and non-polar. The polar phase may be water or another polar liquid. The oil phase is not necessarily an oil, in the true physical sense of that term, but can consist of long-chain alcohols (cetyl, C_{16}, or stearyl, C_{18}), long-chain esters (myristates C_{14}, palmitates C_{16} or stearates C_{18}), long-chain acids (palmitic or stearic), various oils of vegetable and animal origin, and waxes. A further point of confusion can arise between creams and absorption ointment bases. An absorption base forms an o/w (cream) on addition of water. Oily Cream B.P. is an example of this type of emulsified product. It is a cream by virtue of its visual appearance, which is creamy rather than translucent as in an anhydrous ointment. Flynn (1979) has suggested, however, that the term cream should apply only to semi-solid o/w systems, thus using a physicochemical rather than a visual system for characterising semi-solid topical vehicles.

Most creams are prepared, as for conventional emulsions, at a temperature above the melting point of the waxy components. Sufficient emulsifier is present to exist in the micellar phase. On cooling, some of the waxy material is solubilised in the micelles. Once the solidification point of the lipophilic components has been reached, the emulsion droplets solidify and the micelles achieve a liquid crystalline character imparting the semi-solid character to the base. The greater the amount of waxy material solubilised, and the higher the melting point of these components, the stiffer the consistency of the resulting cream. The internal phase of the emulsion constitutes between 15 and 40% w/w of the vehicle. Alternatively, a large proportion of internal liquid oil phase can be emulsified. In this situation, close packing distorts the emulsified particles, thus imparting the semi-solid character to the vehicle. These creams are more difficult to prepare than those made by conventional heating and cooling. A homogeniser is required to produce a stable emulsion.

Oil-in-water creams are readily diluted with water and have the aesthetic advantages of being non-greasy and non-staining. In normal therapeutic or cosmetic applications, the cream is rubbed into the skin, leaving a thin, invisible film which may contain the active ingredients. This explains their description as vanishing creams. Any active medicament must be soluble in the deposited film, and a water-miscible co-solvent may be necessary in the formulation to prevent the drug from crystallising as the film is formed.

For maximum bioavailability the dried film should be just saturated with the drug. However, even under these ideal circumstances, there will be a relatively low drug concentration gradient across the skin. Certainly, the concentration gradient achieved by the conventional application of a cream vehicle, that is by rubbing in the preparation to form the dry film, is not a viable method of promoting the percutaneous absorption of a local anaesthetic. Therefore, use of a cream formulation requires the application of a substantial quantity of material to the site, and its maintenance at the site for prolonged periods, in order to achieve passive drug diffusion along a concentration gradient.

Typically, the site may be covered with several grams of the formulation for periods of one hour or even longer. Since o/w creams are non-occlusive, an occlusive dressing may also be required to promote drug absorption by increasing the degree of hydration of the stratum corneum.

A further problem concerning adequate bioavailability arises from the multiphase nature of a cream formulation. The external phase may typically be water, but a local anaesthetic base will have to be dissolved in the lipophilic phase prior to forming the emulsion. This leads to partitioning of the drug between internal and external phases of the emulsion, and between the external phase and the skin.

The overall effects of using a conventional cream formulation for the percutaneous delivery of a local anaesthetic base is that a high drug loading will be required. In many cases, the required drug loading will, in fact, be unacceptably high. However, notwithstanding this requirement, it is possible to formulate a percutaneous anaesthetic base as an o/w cream and achieve positive clinical results with the resulting preparation. Thus, Woolfson *et al.* (1988) formulated amethocaine base in a vehicle consisting of Emulsifying Wax B.P. (16% w/w), liquid paraffin (4% w/w) and water. The cream was prepared by conventional means. Anaesthetic concentrations used ranged from 8 to 14% w/w, notably high compared to typical drug concentrations used in conventional topical preparations. The preparation was assessed in a volunteer trial in 20 adults aged from 18 to 37 years. Assessment was by a standard pin-prick technique (Pettersson, 1978; Russo *et al.*, 1980). The test site, which was occluded, was the ventral surface of the left or right forearm at or near the anterior cubital fossa. A 7 day washout period was used, with each formulation being applied for a 30 minute period, followed by removal and washing of the site. Each volunteer received all formulations, including a placebo. The results of this study (Table 5.3) indicated that effective percutaneous anaesthesia could be obtained with such a formulation approach, but that the drug concentration required to reliably anaesthetise 95% of the volunteers was 12% w/w. The mean onset of anaesthesia occurred after about 40 minutes, of which 30 minutes constituted the initial application period, and the duration of anaesthesia was about 3 hours. Apart from the high drug concentration required, these parameters were certainly acceptable clinically. However, this type of vehicle contained approximately 20% of lipid phase, excluding the

Table 5.3 — Concentration-response trial of a percutaneous anaesthetic preparation containing amethocaine base and formulated as an o/w cream

amethocaine (% w/w)	volunteers anaesthetised (%)	onset time (min) ± standard deviation	duration of anaesthesia (h) ± standard deviation
0 (placebo)	0	-	-
8	30	55.8 ± 6.6	1.6 ± 0.4
10	90	51.8 ± 5.8	1.9 ± 0.4
12	95	42.9 ± 5.8	2.7 ± 0.3
14	95	42.8 ± 5.8	3.0 ± 0.5

drug, and the preferential retention of drug in this phase resulted in the necessity for a high drug loading. The physical state of the drug in the formulation was also uncertain. At such a high concentration, it seemed that, although some drug was solubilised in the internal lipid phase, some was also present as suspended solid material. A conventional approach to formulating a percutaneous anaesthetic, such as the use of an o/w cream, therefore tends not to produce the optimum delivery system compatible with an acceptable drug loading and an effective, safe clinical response.

5.2.3   Gel vehicles

A gel is formed when a polar liquid, usually water, is constrained by entrapment and immobilisation within a solid, three-dimensional network formed by a polymeric component. Thus, gels are two-component systems with a high ratio of solvent to gel former. The polymeric network, which can have a variety of structures at the microscopic level (Pena, 1990), imparts the semi-solid nature to the vehicle, giving it viscoelastic properties.

Natural polymers that form gels include polysaccharides such as agar, tragacanth and gelatin. Ideally, gels should be clear and sparkling. However, pharmaceutical gel vehicles may be opaque due to suspended rather than dissolved gelling agent, or to the presence of suspended solid or oily medicament. Synthetic gel-forming polymers are generally easier to work with, have well-defined physicochemical properties, and are chemically stable. Perhaps most importantly, synthetic gel-formers are commercially available in a range of molecular weights, yielding solutions and gels of varying viscosities. Pharmaceutical gel-forming polymers are highly purified compared to chemically similar agents used for other industrial purposes. A master file usually exists on each polymer so that their presence in a topical formulation is immediately acceptable to the regulatory authorities.

As a system for promoting the percutaneous delivery of a local anaesthetic base, aqueous gels have an advantage over conventional creams and ointments in that they do not contain any lipophilic phase. Thus, there is no tendency by the vehicle to "hold" the drug rather than make it available for partitioning into the stratum corneum. This property can also be a problem, unfortunately, since lipophilic local anaesthetic bases have a negligible solubility in an aqueous vehicle. Formulation of the drug as a solid suspension in the gel will result in poor drug bioavailablity to the skin. If this problem could be overcome, then both $K_{sc/w}$ and ΔC in equation (4.3) would be increased and drug penetration effectively enhanced. Reconciliation of these two apparently conflicting observations is necessary for the successful percutaneous delivery of local anaesthetic bases.

5.2.3.1 Cellulose ethers

Cellulose is a polysaccharide composed of anhydroglucose rings linked by β-glycoside bonds. The degree of polymerisation of the polysaccharide is defined by the number of anhydroglucose rings in the polymer chain. Each ring carries three free hydroxyl groups. Cellulose ethers are formed by substituting one or more of these groups. The distribution of the substituents introduced into the polymer chain is largely determined by the relative reactivity of these three hydroxyl groups. The cellulose ethers produce aqueous solutions of various viscosities rather than true gels. In this sense they are really viscosity builders rather than gel formers but the more viscous solutions possess typical semi-solid properties very similar to a true gel vehicle.

A wide range of non-ionic cellulose ethers is commercially available. Methyl-cellulose, methylhydroxyethylcellulose, methylhydroxypropylcellulose and carboxy-methylmethylcellulose are all sold under the trade names Benecel™ and Culminal™. These ethers are all soluble in cold water. Hot water can be used as a dispersing non-solvent. The solubility will vary with the specific ether used, and also with the nature of any incorporated drug. Although low salt concentrations are tolerated, higher concentrations can result in salting out of the ether. Solutions tend to behave like non-Newtonian liquids. All are pseudoplastic, and some show limited thixotropic behaviour, that is, they regain their original viscosity on removal of an applied shear force. Generally, methylcellulose derivatives are difficult to process, and better alternatives are available for the formulation of a topical gel as a percutaneous drug delivery system. Nevertheless, they are widely used in the cosmetics industry and in tablet formulations.

Hydroxyethylcellulose (Natrosol™) is a cellulose ether which offers enhanced ease of processing as a gel former compared to methylcellulose and its derivatives. Activation of the three hydroxyl groups on the cellulose anhydroglucose ring followed by reaction with ethylene oxide yields the hydroxyethylether of cellulose. Further ethylene oxide moieties can become attached by reaction at a substituted hydroxyl and subsequent polymerisation to form a side chain. A range of hydroxyethylcelluloses of pharmaceutical purity are commercially available. These vary in molecular weights and solution viscosities according to the degree of substitution of each ring with ethylene oxide moieties. The main advantage of the hydroxyethylcelluloses are their ease of solubility in both cold and hot water. Additionally, water-soluble films can be knife-cast from aqueous solutions. Hydroxyethylcellulose films can be cured by heating for 5 minutes at 150°C.

Hydroxypropylcellulose (Klucel™) is another cellulose ether which produces clear, viscous, gel-like solutions which can be made semi-solid in character when a suitable drug is incorporated into the vehicle. Hydroxypropylcellulose must first be wetted and dispersed in a non-solvent and is therefore not as convenient to use as hydroxyethylcellulose. However, dispersal in hot water between 55 and 60°C, followed by addition of ice-cold water, yields clear solutions. A 3% w/w solution is suitable for incorporation of the drug and also produces excellent films on casting. Unfortunately, hydroxypropylcellulose films cannot be heat cured since the solution turns opaque at higher temperatures due to precipitation of the polymer. This limits the practical application of hydroxypropylcellulose films as drug delivery systems since air drying is time-consuming and not practical in a manufacturing situation.

5.2.3.2 Carbomers

Carbopol® water-soluble resins are widely used as semi-solid gel vehicles, and for many other formulation purposes, in the pharmaceutical and cosmetic industries. Chemically, these resins are derived from polyacrylic acid by cross-linking with allyl sucrose. Carbopol® resins are officially referred to as carbomers. Five different viscosity grades of Carbopol® are commercially available (Table 5.4).

The most commonly used Carbopol® grade for pharmaceutical applications is 934P, for which a master file has been established with the U.S. Food and Drug Administration. Formation of a gel with this resin, as with all Carbopol® grades,

Table 5.4 — Types of Carbopol® resins

grade	approx. molecular weight	properties	uses
907	450,000	high water solubility, low viscosity, good lubricity.	applications requiring high carboxylic acid content
910	750,000	good salt tolerance, long rheology, effective at low concentrations	dip-coating applications, modifying rheology of higher molecular weight resins
941	1,250,000	good tolerance in ionic systems	emulsion and suspension stabiliser at moderate viscosities, produces thin, clear gels
934	3,000,000	excellent stability at high viscosity	produces thick formulations such as heavy gels, emulsions and suspensions
934P	3,000,000	highly purified form of 934	all pharmaceutical applications
940	4,000,000	excellent thickening efficiency at high viscosities	forms sparkling, clear gels in aqueous or aqueous alcoholic systems, cosmetic applications, screen printing and spray applications

Modified from Technical Manual GC67, *Carbopol Water-Soluble Resins*, B.F.Goodrich Chemical Co., Cleveland, Ohio

requires the neutralisation of the carboxylic acid moieties to form a water-soluble salt. As the pH of the opalescent dispersion increases, viscosity and clarity also increase with optimum performance being achieved in the pH range 6 - 7. At the molecular level, there is a change from a flexible, random coil arrangement of the polymer chains to a more rigid, inflexible and uncoiled form. Neutralisation beyond the optimum range causes a reduction in viscosity. There is also a limited tolerance to the presence of ions. Even at low total ionic strengths there is a tendency for the polymer to be salted out of solution.

Carbopol® gels form excellent semi-solid topical vehicles with optimum rheological properties. The inherent pseudoplastic flow of these gels permits immediate recovery of viscosity when the shearing force is terminated. The high yield value and quick break allow convenient dispensing from automatic filling machines during industrial processing (Pena, 1990). However, incorporation of a local anaesthetic base into an acidic system is a source of obvious incompatibility in respect of any drug in the solution state. In such a situation, the Carbopol® salt of the local anaesthetic is formed and this has negligible skin penetration properties. Therefore, a Carbopol® gel vehicle for percutaneous anaesthetic delivery must be carefully neutralised before attempting to incorporate the base. Usually, a stirred dispersion of the resin is neutralised by the slow addition of a base such as sodium hydroxide, although other bases, including organic amines, may be used. This *in situ* neutralisation requires careful control to produce an identical gel without excess inorganic base being present, thus yielding a vehicle whose final pH may be unacceptably high. A more convenient method is to synthesise the Carbopol® salt, such as sodium Carbopol, which can be precipitated as a granular solid from methanolic solution (Lee and Nobles, 1959). This acts as an instant gelling agent, dissolving rapidly in aqueous solution to form a suitable semi-solid vehicle at concentrations in the range 2 - 5% w/w. Sodium Carbopol® has excellent storage properties under dry conditions. Incorporation of a local anaesthetic base yields a gel with a pH value of about 8. However, the same problem regarding the incorporation of a lipophilic drug in an aqueous system applies to the Carbopol® gels as to gels formed using cellulose derivatives, and this must be solved if a Carbopol® gel vehicle is to be used.

5.3 FORMULATION OF LIPOPHILIC ANAESTHETIC BASES IN AQUEOUS SYSTEMS

Lipophilic anaesthetic bases have negligible aqueous solubility. However, use of an oily vehicle retards their partitioning into the stratum corneum. To achieve a high concentration gradient across the skin, an aqueous system is required in which the drug is in a bioavailable form. The available options are to solubilise the drug in the aqueous vehicle, or to suspend it in solid form. However, a suspension of a poorly water-soluble drug will yield a low drug concentration gradient across the barrier membrane. Fortunately, it is possible to solve these difficulties, but it will be seen that the solutions available to date are drug specific, thus restricting the choice of local anaesthetic base which can be used as a percutaneous anaesthetic.

5.3.1   Eutectic mixture of local anaesthetics

A percutaneous local anaesthetic preparation containing a eutectic mixture of lignocaine and prilocaine bases, developed by Broberg and Evers (1981), is commercially available as EMLA® cream (Astra Pharmaceuticals). Eutectic mixtures are of considerable interest in pharmaceutical formulation. Their formation may be advantageous, or may constitute an incompatibility, as in powder technology when eutectic formation results in increased adhesion between components of the blend. However, studies on the formation of a eutectic mixture between two drugs, rather than between drug and excipient, are unusual (El-Banna *et al.*, 1978). The lignocaine-prilocaine system can, therefore, be regarded as both a unique and unconventional solution to the problem of the percutaneous delivery of local anaesthetics.

A simple, condensed, two-component system may be represented by a temperature-composition plot such as Fig. 5.1. It is assumed in this case that the two solid components, X and Y, do not interact chemically or form solid solutions. On addition of one solid component to the other there is a mutual lowering of the melting points as shown in the liquid-solid equilibrium curves which intersect at a triple point (E). This point represents the lowest temperature at which the liquid phase is stable and is known as the eutectic point. If the temperature is cooled below the eutectic point, the liquid phase is lost and a mixture of the two solid components is present.

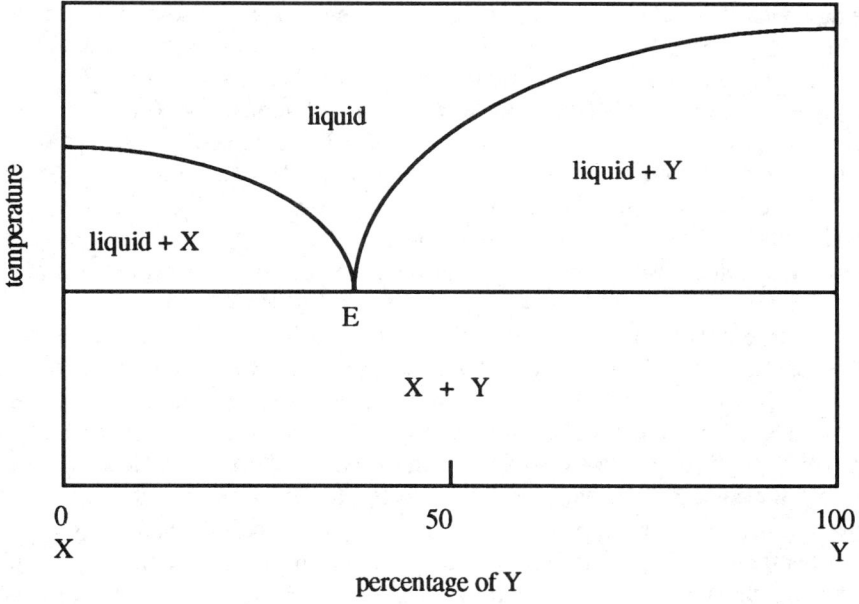

Fig. 5.1 — Phase diagram for a simple condensed system containing two solid components, X and Y, which are mutually soluble in the liquid state, and which do not form solid solutions or interact chemically

The phase behaviour of the lignocaine-prilocaine binary system has been extensively studied by Brodin *et al.* (1984) using differential thermal analysis, hot stage microscopy, infra-red spectrometry and X-ray diffraction. This study investigated whether the binary system was a true eutectic mixture, or whether there was any evidence for the presence of a solid solution. In a true solid solution one component is located in the interstitial spaces within the crystal lattice of the other component. A further possibility is a substitutional solid solution, non-crystalline in this case, in which one component replaces molecules of the second component in its crystal lattice. Infra-red and X-ray diffraction studies established that no solid solution was formed between lignocaine and prilocaine, and that there was no chemical interaction between the bases. Differential thermal analysis on non-equilibrated mixtures showed a single endotherm at about 35°C, the mixed melting point entity, with a second endotherm at about 20°C appearing when equilibrated samples were analysed. This latter peak corresponded approximately to the triple point on the lignocaine-prilocaine phase diagram obtained for an equilibrated system by hot-stage microscopy. The shape of the lignocaine-prilocaine phase diagram is broadly similar to that for the simple binary system shown in Fig. 5.1. However, the eutectic point is not sharp, possibly due to complex aqueous interactions between the bases and the slow establishment of equilibrium between solid and liquid phases. Nevertheless, the eutectic temperature was accurately established as 18±1°C.

Further studies by Brodin *et al.* (1984) on the aqueous solubility of the individual bases and their eutectic mixture showed that the heat of solution for lignocaine in the eutectic mixture was different from that of the pure base, whereas that for prilocaine remained unchanged. Overall, the eutectic mixture had a lowered solubility compared to the pure bases themselves but the differences were not considered significant. It was established that the lignocaine-prilocaine binary system was a simple eutectic containing no intermediate compounds and with a eutectic ratio of almost 1:1. From a formulation viewpoint, the most significant observation was that the eutectic mixture was an oily liquid at room temperature. For such a system, the oily eutectic may be directly emulsified to form an oil-in-water cream. The liquid state of the diffusible eutectic mixture allows enhanced topical bioavailability of the anaesthetic bases compared to a conventional solubilised system or an emulsion prepared with an inert internal oil phase as carrier.

When an emulsion is formed directly from an oily eutectic mixture, a complex system results in which the local anaesthetic bases may be present in three distinct phases. These are the freely dissolved state in the aqueous external phase, a surfactant solubilised state and an emulsified internal phase. The distribution of the drugs between these various physical states obviously has important implications in respect of achieving the maximum bioavailability from the formulation, and thus the optimum situation in which sufficient percutaneous penetration can be achieved within the limits of an acceptable total drug concentration. To obtain this information, the three phases constituting the formulation must be separated. An analysis of these phases was reported by Nyqvist-Mayer *et al.* (1985) following phase separation by membrane and gel filtration techniques, and ultracentrifugation.

Emulsification of the disperse phase of a lignocaine-prilocaine eutectic mixture can be achieved by the use of a suitable non-ionic surfactant. Nyqvist-Mayer *et al.* (1985) formed a 1:1 eutectic mixture from lignocaine and prilocaine bases. An emulsion concentrate was then formed using a surfactant consisting of polyoxyethylene fatty acid esters derived from hydrogenated castor oil, commercially available as Arlatone 289. The total anaesthetics to surfactant ratio was 2:0.76. Dilution with water produced emulsions of various anaesthetic concentrations.

The total concentration of lignocaine and prilocaine in the external aqueous phase was determined by Nyqvist-Mayer *et al.* (1985) using both ultracentrifugation and membrane filtration methods. Ultracentrifugation of the emulsified eutectic mixture (5%) yielded a clear aqueous phase consisting of 0.25% lignocaine, 0.40% prilocaine and 0.95% surfactant. Membrane filtration of the o/w emulsion gave a clear filtrate with a lignocaine to prilocaine ratio of 4.5:5.5. Emulsions with eutectic concentrations greater than 2.5% could not be filtered due to concentration polarisation of the membrane filter, but drug concentrations in the aqueous phases of these emulsions could be estimated by extrapolation of the data in Fig. 5.2. This shows the equilibrium concentrations of each local anaesthetic, and their combined (eutectic) concentration, in the aqueous phase as a function of the total drug concentration of the emulsion. Fig 5.2 also shows, for comparison, a plot of the equilibrium surfactant concentration in the aqueous phase against the total drug concentration of the emulsion. The positive slope of the local anaesthetic plots was considered to reflect surfactant solubilisation of the drugs in the aqueous phase of a system saturated in respect of freely dissolved drug. Extrapolation of the combined drug concentration to a zero emulsion concentration yields a value close to the aqueous solubility (0.52%) of the eutectic at 32°C, the normal skin temperature. Emulsion droplets with a size of approximately 200 nm were all dissolved, even at room temperature, when the emulsion was diluted below 0.7 - 0.8% lignocaine-prilocaine eutectic concentration. Below this level, although there was still some drug solubilised in the aqueous phase, the system was no longer saturated. Approximately 60% of the total surfactant was present in the external aqueous phase, with the remainder presumably located inside the emulsion droplets or at the oil-water interface.

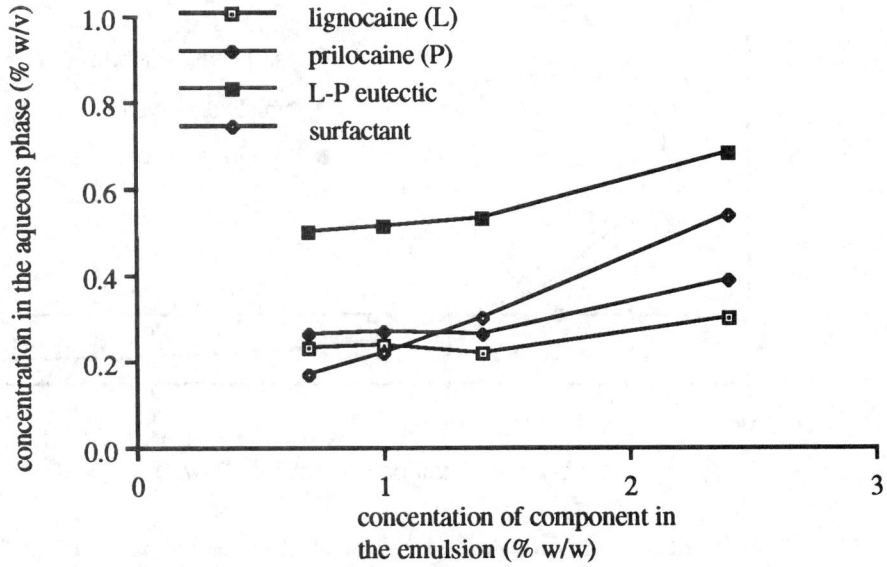

Fig. 5.2 — Equilibrium conditions in the aqueous phase of lignocaine-prilocaine emulsions at 32°C determined by filtration through polycarbonate membrane filters. Reproduced from Nyqvist-Mayer *et al.* (1985) with permission of the copyright owner, the American Pharmaceutical Association

The freely dissolved fraction of lignocaine-prilocaine present in the aqueous phase was estimated by gel filtration on a Sephadex G-200 column. The results indicated that each emulsion above about 0.75% lignocaine-prilocaine has a saturated external aqueous phase with a freely dissolved drug concentration of approximately 0.5%. With increasing surfactant concentration there is a corresponding increase in the amount of drug in the solubilised state, as in Fig. 5.2. However, when the total drug concentration in the emulsion was increased, and the drug to surfactant ratio held constant, there was a decrease in the freely dissolved fraction of drug and an increase in the emulsified fraction. The ratio of emulsified to solubilised drug remained constant (Fig. 5.3). This is interesting since, at a total drug concentration of 5% in the emulsion, the freely solubilised form approaches a minimum and the emulsified droplet form of the internal phase of the emulsion approaches a maximum (Fig. 5.3). Significantly, a percutaneous anaesthetic cream based on the lignocaine-prilocaine eutectic uses a total drug concentration of 5% (Ehrenstrom-Reiz and Reiz, 1982).

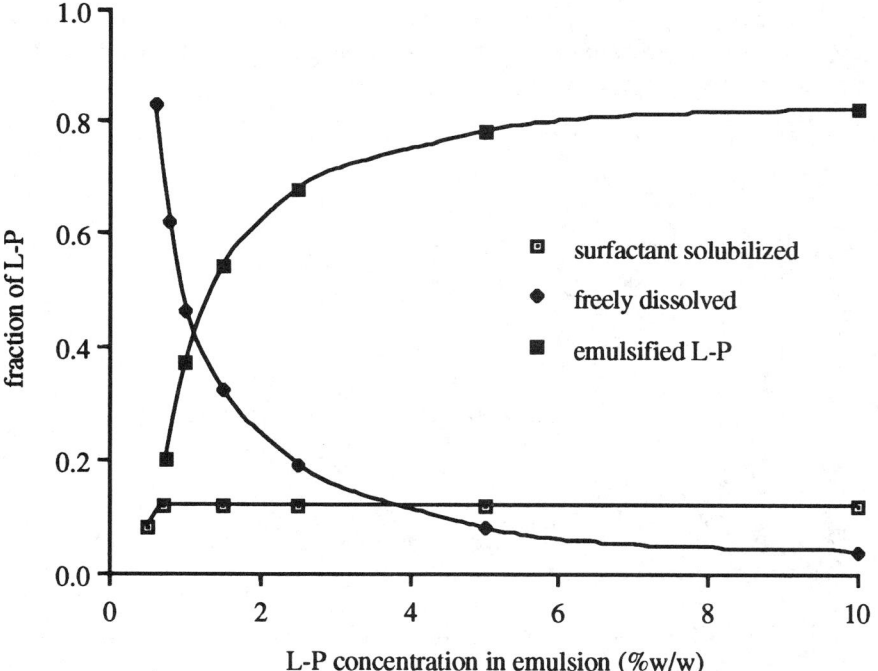

Fig. 5.3 — Distribution of lignocaine-prilocaine (L-P) between the phases of the emulsion system at a lignocaine/prilocaine/ surfactant ratio of 1:1:0.76. Reproduced from Nyqvist-Mayer *et al.* (1985) with permission of the copyright owner, the American Pharmaceutical Association

The direct emulsification of lignocaine-prilocaine eutectic as the dispersed phase without the addition of an inert oil phase yields a unique and unusual system classified by Nyqvist-Mayer *et al.* (1985) as a solid-liquid dispersion. Clearly, drug release characteristics from such a system, with drug present in three possible phases, will be complex. A detailed study of the drug release characteristics of the lignocaine-prilocaine eutectic system was reported by Nyqvist-Mayer *et al.* (1986). A polydimethylsiloxane (Silastic®) membrane was used to simulate a lipophilic barrier such as the stratum corneum. Partition coefficients and drug solubilities in the membrane were determined. Lignocaine, due to its greater lipophilicity, was more soluble in the membrane than prilocaine. The membrane solubilities of the lignocaine-prilocaine eutectic mixture were lower than their individual membrane solubilities, a similar situation to that pertaining with aqueous solubilities. Diffusion coefficients for both drugs in water were essentially the same, in line with their similar chemical structure. There was observed solution interaction between the drugs such that their diffusion properties through an aqueous medium would be affected. In a diffusion experiment using a polydimethylsiloxane barrier membrane, maximum drug flux was observed with a lignocaine-prilocaine eutectic mixture since, in the absence of any solvent, the drugs were able to permeate

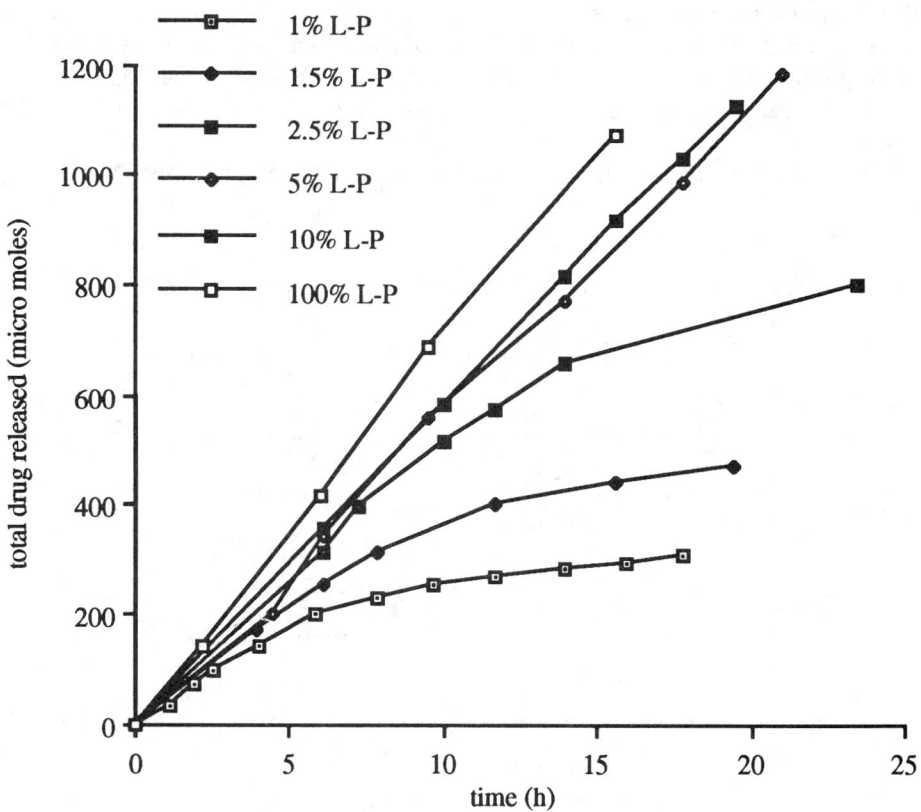

Fig. 5.4 — Drug release profiles for lignocaine-prilocaine (L-P) emulsions of different concentrations at 32°C and for the pure L-P eutectic mixture. Reproduced from Nyqvist-Mayer *et al.* (1986) with permission of the copyright owner, the American Pharmaceutical Association

directly into the membrane without their diffusional flux being reduced by the presence of an aqueous diffusion layer. Lignocaine, due to its greater lipophilicity and solubility in the membrane, had a higher steady-state flux than prilocaine.

Drug release characteristics from the lignocaine-prilocaine emulsion system were also investigated. Total drug release was initially linear with respect to time (Fig. 5.4), allowing calculation of the drug release rate from this initial steady-state portion (Fig. 5.5). When both donor and receptor compartments were stirred, there was no significant difference in the initial drug release rates with varying lignocaine-prilocaine concentrations in the emulsion. It would appear that the effective drug concentration in the emulsions, which is the diffusible drug available for penetration, was the same in each emulsion irrespective of total drug present. This concentration was calculated to be about 0.55%, similar to the concentration of freely dissolved drug at 32°C (Nyqvist-Mayer et al., 1985). When the donor phase was unstirred the plot of release rate versus drug concentration in the emulsion rose steeply before approaching the plot for the stirred emulsion at higher emulsion concentrations. It was suggested that this difference may have been due to the presence of a thicker aqueous diffusion layer on the unstirred donor side of the membrane. The decrease in the difference in release rates between stirred and unstirred emulsions at higher drug concentrations suggested the involvement of the micellar phase in addition to the emulsified droplets. This is in agreement with the proposal of Amidon et al. (1982) that, in saturated surfactant solutions, micelles can act as drug carriers across the aqueous diffusion layer, thus reducing diffusion layer resistance.

The drug release characteristics from the lignocaine-prilocaine emusified system can

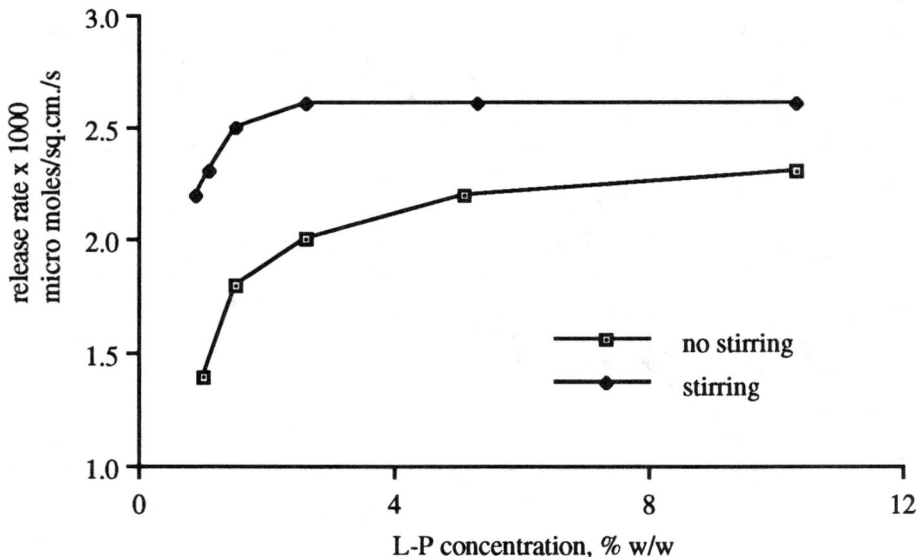

Fig. 5.5 — Drug release rate at 32°C as a function of lignocaine-prilocaine (L-P) concentration in the emulsion, with and without stirring in the donor phase. Reproduced from Nyqvist-Mayer *et al.* (1986) with permission of the copyright owner, the American Pharmaceutical Association

best be represented as a dynamic equilibrium between the three drug phases, that is, freely dissolved, surfactant solubilised and emusified droplets.   At higher drug concentrations, when the aqueous phase is saturated with drug, transfer of local anaesthetics across the barrier membrane proceeds from the saturated aqueous layer via penetration of freely dissolved drug.   The emulsified droplets then act as a reservoir, restoring drug saturation in the aqueous layer by rapid dissolution as the amount of freely dissolved drug is, in turn, diminished by transfer across the membrane.   This situation, which may be likened to a zero order release pattern in rate-controlled systems, results in the maintenance of a constant concentration gradient of dissolved lignocaine-prilocaine across the diffusion layer.   This concentration gradient can be maintained for several hours.   As the droplets are gradually diminished, the surfactant to drug ratio is increased since the surfactant does not penetrate the polydimethylsiloxane membrane.   Thus, the amount of drug in the solubilised phase gradually increases.   However, this effect only becomes significant after delivery times well in excess of anything seen in the clinical use of the eutectic emulsion system and can be disregarded.

In the emulsified eutectic system there is an increased thermodynamic activity of the local anaesthetics since they are not partitioned into an inert oil phase as in a conventional emulsion.   Thus, the system resembles a suspension rather than an emulsion.   Unlike a solid drug reservoir in a suspension, the fluid droplet reservoir in the emulsified eutectic system has a fast dissolution rate, promoting replenishment of the saturated aqueous phase.

The lignocaine-prilocaine emulsified system is too fluid for clinical use.   It is thus thickened with a viscosity builder, Carbopol 934P neutralised with sodium hydroxide. This yields a preparation referred to as a cream, but which is really an oil-in-water emulsion trapped within a gel matrix.   The pH of this formulation, 9.4, ensures that both drugs are present almost entirely in their uncharged forms.   Further drug release studies on this gelled emulsified eutectic (Nyqvist-Mayer et al., 1986) showed that the aqueous drug diffusivities were not decreased in this higher viscosity system.   However, at longer application times the release rate from the gel fell substantially compared to the low viscosity system due to formation of a depletion layer at the gel-barrier interface.   At this point the release process became vehicle-controlled rather than controlled by the barrier membrane and the aqueous diffusion layer.   However, for typical clinical application times of about one hour, this observation is not significant.   It does, however, suggest the diminishing returns that may be expected from the use of longer application times with this system.

The use of the eutectic local anaesthetic mixture, its direct emulsification and subsequent addition of the viscosity builder represents an elegant solution to the problem of achieving a high drug concentration gradient across the skin barrier, and at the same time having an acceptably low drug concentration in the formulation.   Direct emulsification solves the problem of the incompatibility of the anaesthetic bases with an aqueous environment.   The major advantages of the formulation as a percutaneous local anaesthetic delivery have been summarised by Nyqvist-Mayer et al. (1986). These are

   (i)   the drugs are present in their lipophilic uncharged forms in order to promote skin penetration;

   (ii)   the use of water, a poor solvent, as the vehicle, provides a saturated system at low total drug concentration;

   (iii)   the absence of inert lipophilic solvent in the dispersed phase increases the thermodynamic activity of the anaesthetic bases since their distribution coefficients between the skin and the formulation would otherwise be decreased;

(iv)   the droplets consist of dissolvable drug and act as reservoirs to obtain steady-state release;

(v)   the fluid state of the excess drug provides a higher dissolution rate than from the solid state.

The disadvantages seen with this system, long application times and short durations of clinical effect, are due to the pharmacological properties of the drugs used rather than to their formulation.

5.3.2   The amethocaine phase-change system

Amethocaine has many of the characteristics of an ideal percutaneous anaesthetic agent. These include high lipophilicity and, consequently, good anaesthetic potency and extended duration of activity. However, conventional topical delivery systems fail to produce significant anaesthesia of the skin unless high drug concentrations are used. For percutaneous drug absorption to occur the local anaesthetic base must be presented to the skin in a mobile, diffusible form. This will be the case if the drug is in solution. However, amethocaine is approximately 20% ionised at pH 7 (Table 3.5). Although an aqueous solution can be prepared from the base, the amount of drug in the uncharged, lipophilic form is reduced. It is this form which is required for significant percutaneous absorption to take place. If the solid base is formulated as a solution in an inert oil, or if this oily solution is emulsified as the internal phase of an o/w emulsion, the thermodynamic activity of the drug will be substantially reduced, since it will be partitioned between the inert oil and skin phases. This again leads to the use of unacceptably high drug concentrations in order to achieve the desired level of clinical response.

Amethocaine base is a poorly defined crystalline compound, a fact supported by its melting point range of 40-42°C. A crystal structure of this type, with a low heat of fusion and a low melting point, is bound together by weak forces and readily lends itself to eutectic formation with solids that have similar properties. Such solids need not necessarily be local anaesthetics themselves. However, in the case of amethocaine, a novel formulation strategy is possible which does not require the formation of a eutectic mixture. This is based on the chance observation that amethocaine base, in the presence of moisture, undergoes a depression of its melting point. Depression of the melting point in the presence of an impurity, in this case water, is, of course, well recognised. Amethocaine base, however, undergoes an unusually large change in melting point in the moist state. In fact, the melting range is lowered to 30-32°C, a significant occurrence since the moist drug melts at or below skin temperature, representing a melting point depression of approximately 10°C.

Confirmation of the melting characteristics of moist amethocaine base has been confirmed by differential scanning calorimetry (DSC) of the drug in the dry and wet states (Woolfson et al., 1991). DSC of a sample of the base dried over silica in a vacuum dessicator gave a peak onset temperature of 41.01°C and an endothermic peak temperature of 42.12°C (Fig. 5.6). When one drop of water was added to the dry solid in the sample pan the onset temperature fell to 28.69°C and the endothermic peak temperature was reduced to 30.24°C (Fig. 5.7). Interestingly, these values gradually return to those corresponding to the dry state when DSC scans are obtained as the moist

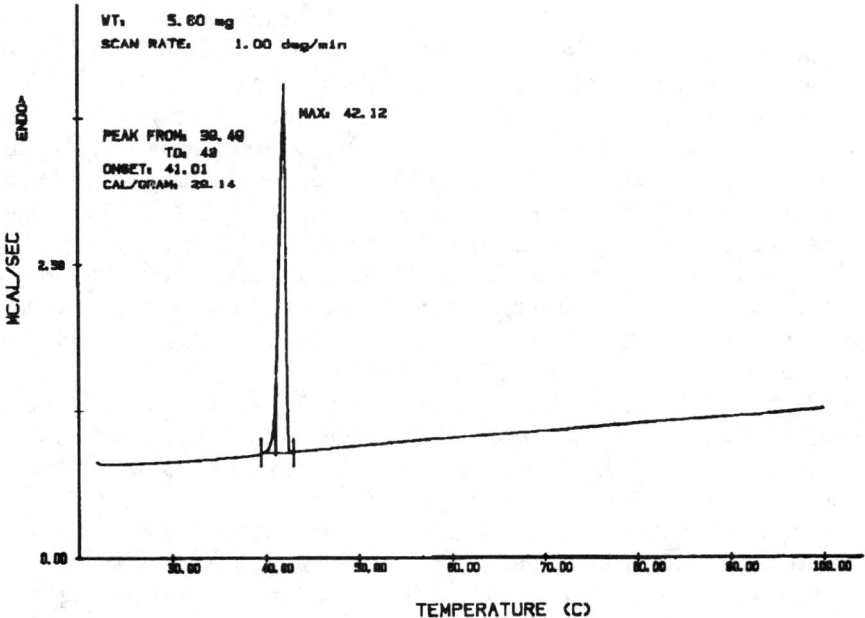

Fig. 5.6 — Differential scanning calorimetry of amethocaine in the dry state

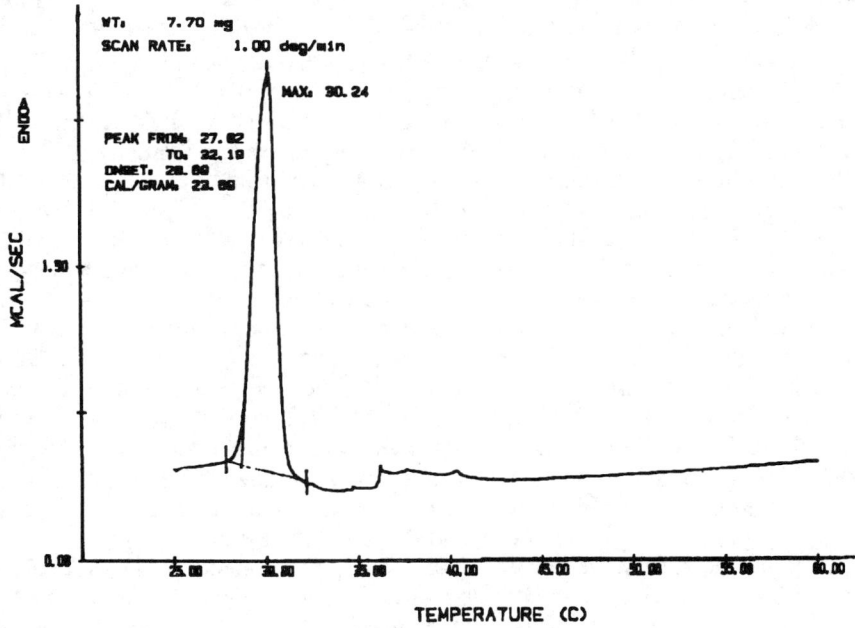

Fig. 5.7 — Differential scanning calorimetry of amethocaine in the wet state

sample gradually dries out. Adulteration of the dry base with a very small amount of water appears to yield a metastable hydrate. A true hydrate is not formed since the original DSC characteristics of the dry base are gradually restored.

Lowering of the melting point of amethocaine base results in a phase change from a crystalline solid to an oily liquid. This observation can readily be made using heated stage microscopy (McClelland, 1986). Thus, at skin temperature the drug undergoes a solid to liquid phase change which is the basis of its formulation as a percutaneous anaesthetic agent (McCafferty and Woolfson, 1988). Essentially, the drug may be formulated as an aqueous solid suspension. A viscosity builder is added to produce a preparation with semi-solid characteristics that allow the preparation to be located at the required skin site. In contact with the skin there is a rapid phase change, resulting in the formation of an aqueous suspension of fine oil droplets.

Amethocaine base is substantially more lipophilic than either lignocaine or prilocaine. Consequently, its aqueous solubility is much less. Solubility characteristics of amethocaine are complicated by the phase change occurring around 30°C. Thus, there is a sharp, non-linear increase in aqueous solubility between 25 and 32°C (McCafferty and Woolfson, unpublished data). At 32°C a saturated aqueous solution of amethocaine base contains only 240 μg ml^{-1} of the drug. This means that less than 1% of the total drug is present in the freely solubilised form in an amethocaine gel containing 4% w/w of total drug, the clinically effective concentration.

The nature of the amethocaine phase-change system is of importance in determining the clinical efficacy of amethocaine percutaneous local anaesthetic preparations. In a typical 4% w/w gel formulation there will be a large reservoir of undissolved drug present, in addition to the small fraction of dissolved drug in the aqueous phase. At temperatures in excess of 30°C, the undissolved drug reservoir will be in the fluid state as particles suspended in the aqueous gel. Fig 5.8 shows the drug penetration properties, through Silastic®, of gelled, saturated, aqueous amethocaine solutions at 25 and 37°C, these temperatures being, respectively, below and above the phase change in the system. Under these conditions there is no drug reservoir to replenish the aqueous diffusion layer at the barrier membrane interface. The resultant drug fluxes are, therefore, much lower than those resulting from a similar study using a 4% w/w amethocaine gel in which the drug reservoir is present. Indeed, the initial time period in Fig. 5.8 shows a higher, linear flux, which falls off rapidly in the absence of any excess drug to replenish the diffusion layer. The drug flux across the barrier membrane is higher, and the depletion effect more rapid, at the higher temperature. These effects may be contrasted with Fig. 5.9 in which the gelled saturated amethocaine solution was replaced by a 4% w/w amethocaine gel with, of course, a large drug reservoir available. Here, the drug penetration profile remains linear throughout at both temperatures due to constant replenishment of the aqueous diffusion layer by the excess available drug in suspension. Consequently, the drug fluxes in this situation are much higher than for gelled, saturated aqueous solutions. Furthermore, the drug flux at 37°C is much higher than that at 25°C, an increase greater than would be accounted for by the increased rate of drug diffusion at the higher temperature. This effect is due to the phase change in the system above 30°C, at which point the undissolved drug is in the fluid, more rapidly dissolvable oil state. This may be compared to the situation at 25°C, in which the drug is present as suspended solid particles. The phase change therefore produces a more efficient system with respect to rapid replenishment of the aqueous diffusion layer. This is important, given the much lower aqueous solubility of amethocaine compared to either lignocaine or prilocaine bases, resulting in a lower concentration gradient across the barrier

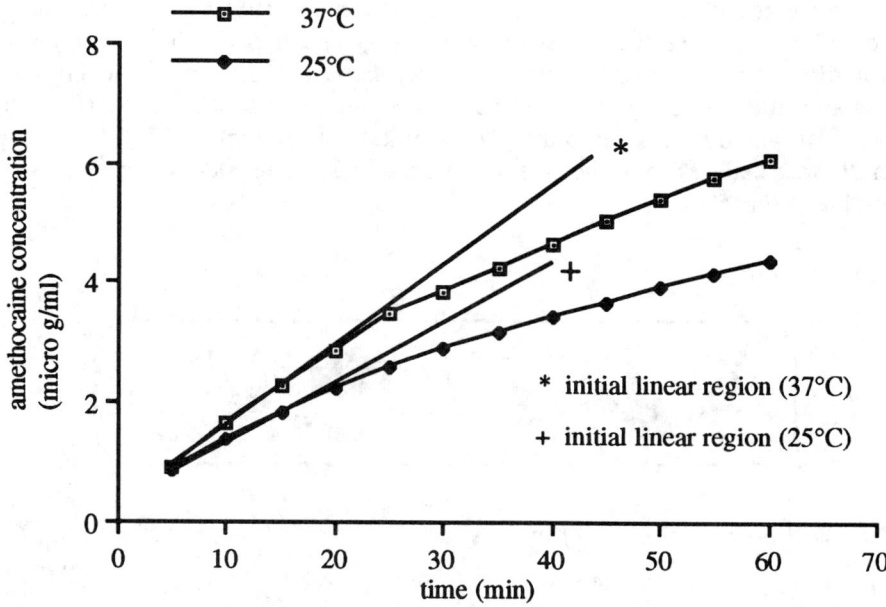

Fig. 5.8 — Penetration of amethocaine from gelled, saturated aqueous solutions of the drug through Silastic® membranes, at 25 and 37°C

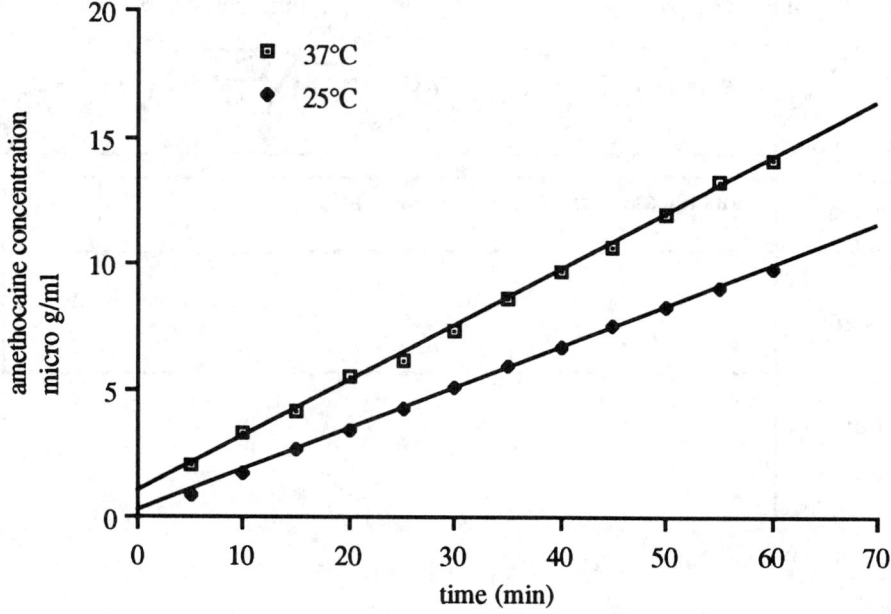

Fig. 5.9 — Penetration of amethocaine from 4% w/w amethocaine aqueous gels through Silastic® membranes, at 25 and 37°C

membrane. Despite this, the amethocaine phase-change system requires a shorter application time and has a longer duration of effect compared to the lignocaine-prilocaine eutectic mixture. Essentially, this is due to the greater lipophilicity of amethocaine, which results in substantially increased anaesthetic potency and, probably, better diffusion characteristics through the stratum corneum, though the latter effect will be offset somewhat by the reduced drug concentration in solution in the diffusion layer. Overall, drug delivery from the amethocaine phase-change system can be represented according to Fig. 5.10.

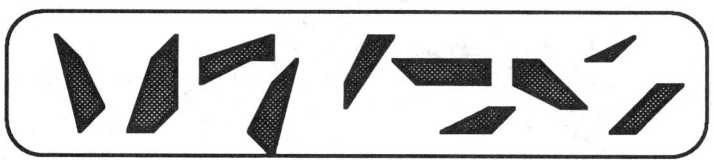

Product Matrix - below 32°C

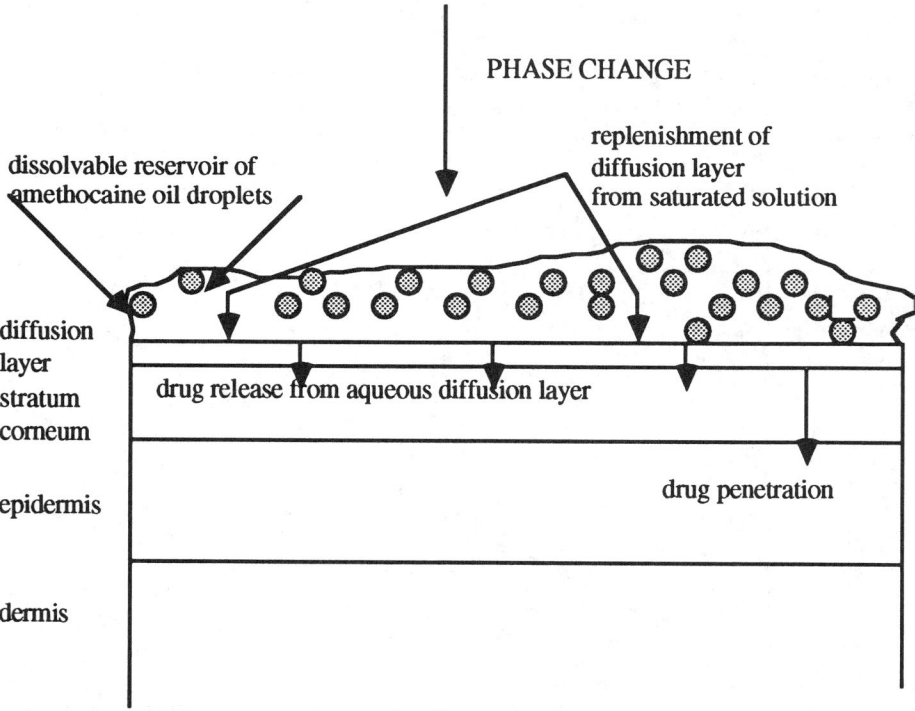

Product Matrix - above 32°C

Fig. 5.10 — Representation of the drug release characteristics of the amethocaine phase change system

5.3.3   Liposomal percutaneous anaesthetic systems

Liposomes are microscopic vesicles formed from amphipathic lipids arranged in one or more concentric bilayers. Their potential role as drug carriers for topical drug delivery has been recognised in several studies, notably those by Mezei and Gulasekharam (1980; 1982), and Schaeffer and Krohn (1982). Liposomes, which are lamellar in character, form spontaneously when lipid is added to an aqueous phase. Some of the aqueous phase is entrapped within the liposomes and is thus separated from the continuous, external aqueous phase by the bilayered lamellae, which are approximately 4 nm in thickness (Uster, 1990).

Liposomes may be classified according to the number of concentric lamellae enclosing the aqueous core. Multilammelar vesicles generally have greater than five concentric lamellar bilayers, yielding a milky aqueous dispersion. Small unilamellar vesicles, produced by sonicating a multilammelar vesicle preparation, yield a transparent dispersion. Large unilamellar vesicles can also be produced. Aqueous drugs can be entrapped in the liposomal core by first incorporating them in the aqueous buffer used to hydrate the lipid component. Lipophilic drugs must be incorporated in the lipid component before hydration. After liposome formation, such drugs will be located in the lipid bilayers (Fig. 5.11), or possibly at the aqueous-lipid bilayer interface. Multilamellar vesicles are most suitable where a lipophilic drug is to be encapsulated (Uster, 1990).

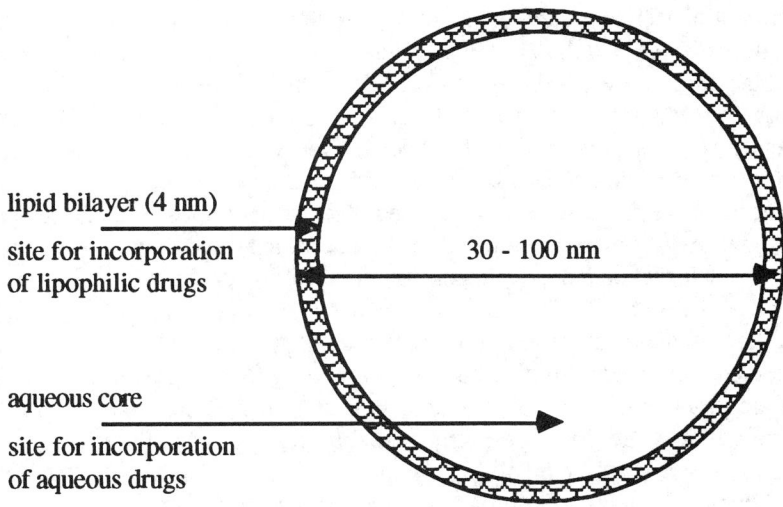

lipid bilayer (4 nm)

site for incorporation
of lipophilic drugs

30 - 100 nm

aqueous core

site for incorporation
of aqueous drugs

Fig. 5.11 — Possible sites for drug incorporation into liposomes

The mechanisms by which a liposomally entrapped drug can penetrate intact skin have been studied by Ganesan *et al.* (1984) using three model drugs (glucose, hydrocortisone and progesterone) and dipalmitoylphosphatidylcholine liposomes. *In vitro* diffusion experiments through hairless mouse skin were made with radiolabelled phospholipid in blank and drug-loaded liposomes. No radioactivity was found in any of the receiver compartments. Clearly, there is no evidence to support the view that liposomes themselves are capable of penetrating the intact skin barrier. This is not surprising, given that the size of even a small unilamellar vesicle is still as large as 30 nm.

Ganesan *et al.* (1984) proposed various mechanisms by which liposomally entrapped drugs can become available for skin penetration. For a water-soluble substance such as glucose the solute must first be released from the liposome into the aqueous external phase from which penetration can then occur. Thus, the process is controlled by the release rate of the solute from the liposome. Such solutes are found distributed in the aqueous core of the liposomes, which in this case were of the multilamellar vesicle type.

For hydrophobic drugs, two possible transfer mechanisms exist. Liposome entrapped solute may be release into the external phase, as with a more hydrophilic solute. Skin permeation of the free solute can, however, be coupled with direct liposome/skin solute transfer. Alternatively, direct hydrophobic solute/skin transfer may be the only participating mechanism. In either case, for hydrophobic drugs the direct transfer of solute from liposome to skin is the rate controlling step. Hydrophobic drugs, unlike their more polar counterparts, are found intercalated in the lipid bilayers of the vesicles. Their presence tends to either fluidise or solidify the lipid bilayers and this perturbation can readily be observed with differential scanning calorimetry (Jain and Wu, 1977).

Recent evidence from Egbaria and Weiner (1990) has suggested that liposomes formulated using lipid mixtures similar to those found in skin may have the ability to penetrate directly into the stratum corneum. Labelled model drug (14C-inulin) and lipid (3H-cholesterol) gave the same ratio of radioactivity in hairless mouse skin layers as in the formulation itself. A molecular mixing of liposomal bilayers with those of the stratum corneum was postulated, an effect which would be expected to occur most easily if liposomal lipids were similar to those of the skin. However, the limiting effect of liposomal size was not discussed and, since lipid vesicles are most frequently and conveniently prepared from phospholipid derivatives, which are not found in the stratum corneum, this penetration mechanism may be of small significance.

Enhancement of percutaneous drug penetration through liposomal entrapment of the penetrant appears to proceed in most cases by increasing the capacity of the vehicle for the drug. For hydrophobic drugs, this means that the drug loading of an aqueous external phase can be substantially increased compared to a simple aqueous solution. The concentration gradient for the penetrant molecule between vehicle and skin is therefore also increased, with a consequent improvement in drug flux. Gesztes and Mezei (1988) reported the formulation of a liposomal percutaneous anaesthetic preparation containing amethocaine base. The drug was encapsulated in the liposomes by a patented method (Mezei and Nugent, 1984) involving the preparation of multilamellar vesicles with phosphatidylcholine and cholesterol. The local anaesthetic base was present in a final concentration of 0.5% w/w. The preparation, which had a gel-like consistency, was tested in adult volunteers against a commercially available local anaesthetic cream (Pontocaine Cream) containing amethocaine hydrochloride equivalent to 1% w/w amethocaine base. Application times of both 30 and 60 minutes were used and the duration of anaesthesia was monitored over a 4 hour period following removal of the preparation (Table 5.5). Testing for anaesthetic effect was carried out by the pin-prick method using a set of 10 challenges over a 10 cm^2 site. Volunteers reported the number of pin-prick challenges to which there was total anaesthesia, thus giving a mean pain score with a maximum value of 10.

Table 5.5 — Comparison of the percutaneous local anaesthetic efficiencies of liposomal amethocaine free base and a commercial amethocaine hydrochloride topical formulation (Pontocaine)

application time (minutes)	monitoring time (minutes after removal of preparation)	mean pain score ± s.d. for liposomal amethocaine	mean pain score ± s.d. for Pontocaine
30	0	2.75 ± 3.25	0.25 ± 1.73
30	30	5.50 ± 3.94	1.08 ± 1.98
30	60	6.75 ± 3.28	1.08 ± 1.68
30	120	8.25 ± 2.45	1.08 ± 1.31
30	240	8.33 ± 2.31	0.25 ± 0.62
60	0	6.25 ±3.65	0.08 ± 0.29
60	30	8.08 ± 2.27	0.41 ± 0.99
60	60	8.83 ± 1.47	0.25 ± 0.62
60	120	9.50 ± 0.67	0.33 ± 1.15
60	240	8.75 ± 1.48	0.16 ± 0.57

Gesztes and Mezei (1988). Reprinted with permission from the International Anaesthesia Research Society (*Anaesthesia and Analgesia*)

The use of amethocaine for liposomal delivery is appropriate owing to its large hydrophobic moiety which anchors the molecule in the phospholipid bilayers. Liposomal amethocaine produced effective percutaneous anaesthesia reflected in the pain scores in Table 5.5, and this activity was significantly different from Pontocaine, in which the drug was present in charged form. However, a 30 minute application time did not produce a reasonably effective mean pain score of 8 out of 10 until 2 hours after removal of the preparation. This can be compared to a 1 hour application which produced a maximum pain score of 9.50 out of 10 some 2 hours after removal of the preparation, but also yielded higher scores throughout the monitoring period with a reasonable value at 1 hour after removal (a total waiting time of 2 hours). Although duration of anaesthesia was prolonged, and similar to that for the amethocaine phase change system, it seems that onset times are significantly longer than with the phase change system in which > 90% of adults are anaesthetised within 15 minutes of removing the preparation following a 30 minute application time. This delay in onset of anaesthesia appears to be similar to that experienced with the lignocaine-prilocaine emulsion system. The prolonged onset time seen with liposomally entrapped amethocaine probably reflects the additional time required for drug release from the vesicles prior to skin penetration, assuming that the transfer mechanism is primarily via a direct liposomal drug/skin partitioning. Further evidence for this mechanism comes from the low overall drug concentration in the formulation but comparatively high drug loading in the lipid bilayers. This will give a high drug concentration gradient between vesicles and skin, thus promoting drug flux across the skin barrier. Since the vesicles were of the multilamellar type, they would certainly be too large to act as direct drug carriers into the stratum corneum.

The encapsulation efficiency and physicochemical stability of liposomally entrapped amethocaine has been further studied by Foldvari *et al.* (1990) who reported an encapsulation efficiency of between 60 and 90%. Encapsulation efficiency was enhanced by increasing drug concentration and pH, and including negatively charged stearic acid or unsaturated lipids in the formula. Physicochemical stability of the liposomal anaesthetic system was followed over eight months, and was reported to be high, though no details were given. It can be presumed that the degradation of the drug, which proceeds by hydrolysis of the ester group, is significantly retarded if the majority of the drug is present in the lipid bilayers. The long-term stability of the system is likely to depend on the extent to which drug is transferred into the aqueous phase, where it will be subject to hydrolytic degradation. If this happens to a significant extent, a zero order degradation, in which the liposomally entrapped drug acts as a reservoir, may occur, and stability would be compromised.

5.3.4   Solution systems

Formulation of a percutaneous anaesthetic as a solution presents a number of problems, including drug stability and difficulties of administration and localisation of the formulation at the required skin site. Homogeneous solutions also generally require higher drug concentrations to promote skin penetration. A solution system for percutaneous anaesthesia that illustrates these difficulties was developed by the Swedish pharmaceutical company Astra Lakemedel AB, and variously reported by Ponten and Ohlsen (1977), Akerman (1978), Pettersson and Strombeck (1978) and Ohlsen and Englesson (1980). The local anaesthetic used was the highly lipophilic agent ketocaine (Appiani and Laveneziana, 1966).

Ketocaine base was formulated as a solution with a final drug concentration of 0.10 g ml^{-1}. The other solution components were isopropanol (0.45 g ml^{-1}), glycerol (0.12 g ml^{-1}) and water (0.25 g ml^{-1}). Acetic acid (0.001 g ml^{-1}) was added as a stabiliser. This sterile solution, of approximately 10% w/w ketocaine, was added to a compressed cotton wool/viscous cellulose pad. The pad, 8 x 10 cm and containing 840 mg of ketocaine, was kept moist by packaging in a plastic-coated aluminium foil. The formulation was given the trade name Ane-Pad®, the soaked pad concept being necessary in order to conveniently present a non-viscous solution to the skin site. Ane-Pad® was successfully applied in trials involving the harvesting of split skin grafts and the planing of human skin for therapeutic purposes (dermabrasion). The application time was 60 minutes with up to 2.5 g of drug being used per patient depending on the size of the site to be anaesthetised. Although the literature reports are favourable in respect of adverse reactions, further in-house assessments apparently demonstrated quite severe topical reactions. The product was therefore discontinued shortly before the marketing stage. It may be speculated as to whether the adverse reactions were entirely due to the particular drug used, or whether its presentation, as a saturated solution in an aprotic solvent mixture, may have been partly or even wholly responsible for the problems encountered.

More recently, Miller *et al.* (1991a) have proposed a solution formulation based on amethocaine in which a mixture of free base and salt forms of the drug are used in combination with co-solvent systems consisting of propylene glycol and saline. A co-solvent system consisting of 40:60 propylene glycol/normal saline containing 10% w/v of amethocaine hydrochloride and amethocaine free base in a 4:6 ratio was reported to produce an amethocaine flux of 200 μg cm^{-2} h^{-1}. The experimental model was hairless mouse skin as the barrier membrane in an *in vitro* diffusion experiment. Pure saline or propylene glycol solutions produced only half of this flux value. The mixed solvent/mixed drug system was claimed to control the partitioning behaviour and solubility of the drug mixture, with the salt form of the drug apparently enhancing the solubility of the free base and the free base form enhancing the diffusional properties of the salt in respect of the skin barrier. There was an optimum concentration of propylene glycol in the co-solvent mixture corresponding to the maximum drug flux, with higher non-polar solvent ratios retarding drug diffusion although enhancing free base solubility.

It is difficult to see the advantages of a mixed free base/salt local anaesthetic formulation although, once again, amethocaine proved to be the drug of choice as a percutaneous local anaesthetic. The free base solubility in the propylene glycol/saline system was 4.5 g l^{-1} rising to beyond 100 g l^{-1} in the presence of the salt. Since the solution was unbuffered such a dramatic increase in drug solubility suggests a pH effect. In any case, the stability of the free base in solution may well be compromised even though some improvement may be expected due to the presence of the less polar propylene glycol co-solvent.

Miller *et al.* (1991b) have also recently proposed a quasi-steady-state, one dimensional Fickian diffusion model for the percutaneous absorption of local anaesthetics. The model takes into account the non-linear diffusion characteristics of local anaesthetics from percutaneous formulations. Non-linear diffusion occurs as a result of the short application periods used in percutaneous local anaesthesia compared to conventional transdermal drug delivery. The model gave a good fit to *in vitro* diffusion data for amethocaine from propylene glycol-saline solutions using hairless mouse skin as the barrier membrane. The effect of skin swelling on predictions made with the proposed model was also considered. However, this has little real clinical significance given the short application times used in percutaneous local anaesthesia.

5.4   IONTOPHORESIS

The formulation of local anaesthetics for percutaneous delivery requires in all cases the use of the penetrable, lipophilic free base form of the drug. For almost all other clinical indications for local anaesthesia, however, the drugs are administered as their water-soluble salts. In this form the drugs are more stable, simpler to formulate and more readily available in pharmacopoeial quality than the free bases. However, local anaesthetic penetration through intact skin by passive diffusion along a concentration gradient will not occur to any significant extent when the charged form of the drug is used. Local anaesthetic salts can only penetrate intact skin if some other active mechanism is applied. The migration of ions or charged drug molecules under the influence of an electrical potential gradient offers one such possibility for the percutaneous delivery of local anaesthetic salts, a process referred to as iontophoresis.

Iontophoresis may be defined as the transport of a charged drug into tissue by the application of a direct electrical current through an electrolyte solution containing the charged drug species, using an appropriate electrode polarity (Bellantone *et al.*, 1986). Positively charged drugs, such as the salts of weak organic bases, are driven into the tissue (in this case intact skin) at the positive electrode or anode whereas negatively charged drugs, such as the salts of organic acids, are delivered from the negative electrode or cathode (Fig. 5.12). Iontophoresis should not be confused with two associated electrokinetic phenomena, electrophoresis and electroosmosis. Electrophoresis involves the movement of a dispersed phase, in this case a colloid, under an electrical potential gradient and electroosmosis is a process in which the dispersion medium itself is the moving phase (Banga and Chien, 1988).

The mechanisms applying to iontophoretic drug delivery through intact skin are still the subject of some debate. The stratum corneum has a relatively high electrical resistance but the underside of this layer is in contact with a conducting extracellular fluid. Thus, the applied voltage in iontophoresis results in a potential difference across the stratum corneum which provides the driving force under which a charged drug can penetrate the skin. The route by which this occurs does, however, present some further difficulties. Kligman and Papa (1966), Burnette and Marrero (1986) and Burnette and Ongpipattanakul (1988) have all produced evidence from dye penetration experiments that the primary route of iontophoretic drug transfer across the skin is via the shunt route comprising mainly the various skin appendages together with pores which may exist as a result of skin imperfections. This is not surprising since the intercellular lipid path generally favoured for the passive diffusion of uncharged drugs is poorly conductive. However, this may alter if the stratum corneum is substantially hydrated, allowing at least some direct iontophoretic drug transfer via the intercellular route.

Rosendal (1942) established that the isoelectric point of skin is between pH 3 and 4. At pH values greater than 4 the skin has a net negative charge, which is the case at physiological pH. This overall negative charge results from the carboxylic acid moieties of skin proteins and means that, for iontophoretic delivery, positively charged drugs (weak organic bases) can traverse the skin barrier via the shunt route more readily than negatively charged molecules, which must overcome an electrostatic repulsion barrier (Burnette and Marrero, 1986).

5.4.1   Chemical factors influencing iontophoretic drug transport

Drug charge and inherent conductivity of the charged species are the prime factors for effective iontophoretic drug transport through the skin. The drug is presented to the skin as an aqueous solution and the composition of this solution may effect the efficacy of iontophoretic transfer. In particular, the presence of buffer salts can have a retarding effect on the iontophoresis of drugs with good inherent conducting properties, since these extraneous ions compete with charged drug molecules for the electric current (Banga and Chien, 1988). The use of buffers in the delivery solution is therefore best avoided, or the buffer solution should be diluted to the minimum possible ionic strength compatible with ensuring that the drug is charged in solution. Ideally, greater than one half of the total conductivity of the delivery solution should reside in the charged drug molecules (Gangarosa *et al.*, 1978).

5.4.2   Electrical factors influencing iontophoretic drug transport

The total quantity of charged particles (ions or molecules) transported iontophoretically

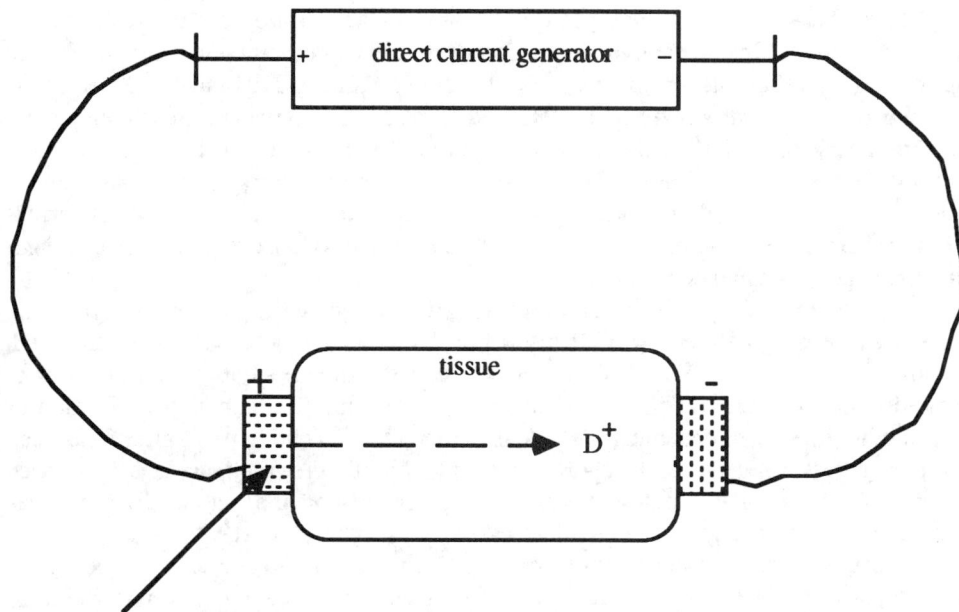

anode containing aqueous drug solution (DA)

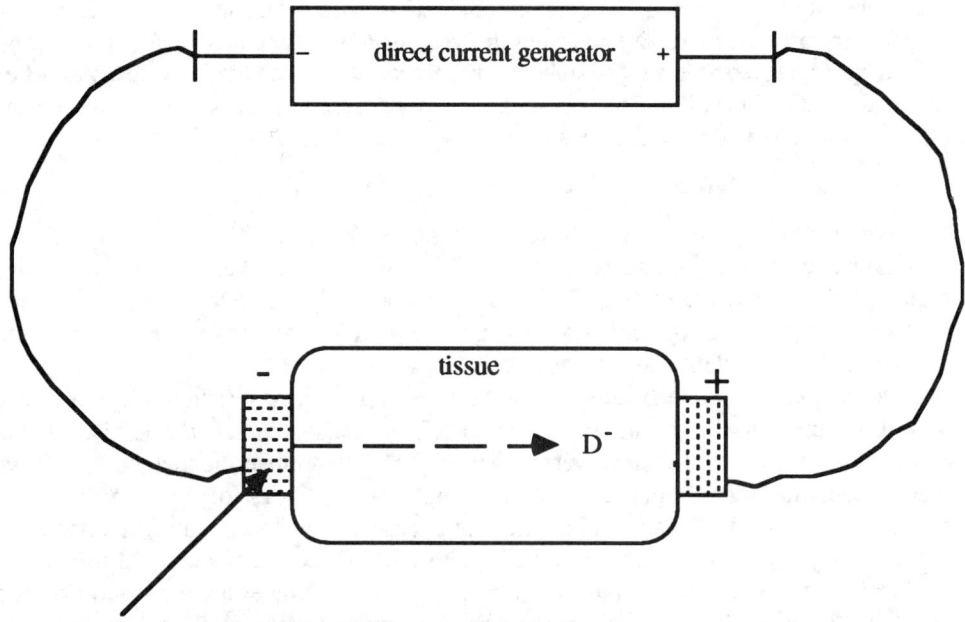

cathode containing aqueous drug solution (HD)

Fig. 5.12 — The principle of iontophoretic drug delivery

will be determined by Faraday's law according to the duration and intensity of the electrical current. In conventional iontophoretic delivery a constant direct current is often used. The current is slowly increased to its required value and maintained there for the desired period before slowly being returned to zero. Continuous current application, unfortunately, results in a charge build-up on the skin, which can lead to irritation and burning (Chien *et al.*, 1988). This limits the application period of constant current iontophoresis. A pulsed or depolarising current, which allows the skin short rest periods of zero current application, is preferable in this respect (Okabe *et al.*, 1986). Longer treatment periods can then be used.

In selecting the appropriate current and voltage settings for iontophoretic percutaneous drug delivery, it is clearly necessary to achieve a balance between a high enough current to provide the desired delivery rate and the necessity to prevent burning or irritation of the skin. It follows, of course, that the drug in a conducting solution or medium must be electrochemically stable under the chosen conditions. Currents between 40 µA and 10 mA have been reported for iontophoretic drug delivery and have been claimed to be painless in use, though much depends on the actual circumstances including the sensitivity of an individual's skin (Rapperport *et al.*, 1965).

A further consideration in iontophoretic drug delivery to the skin concerns the delivery and return electrodes. In the case of percutaneous local anaesthesia, where the location of the site to be treated can vary widely, it is particularly important that the electrode is both flexible and conformable in design. The drug reservoir delivery electrode can be of a simple type such as a moist gauze pad soaked in the drug solution, with a metal backing plate delivering the current. The return or dispersive electrode is generally larger than the delivery electrode and is placed on the body surface some distance from it. A more sophisticated delivery system can be designed using a drug-loaded hydrogel electrode with bioadhesive properties, which can then be directly attached to the skin site. This allows the possibility of combining the necessary electronics and electrodes in a miniaturised delivery system (Groning, 1987).

5.4.3   Percutaneous local anaesthesia by iontophoresis

Local anaesthetics have been shown to possess the necessary characteristics for iontophoretic delivery (Gangarosa *et al.*, 1978). In particular, local anaesthetics have high specific conductivities (Fig. 5.13). These conductivities tend to decrease as the pH is increased through the alkaline region, so that the drugs are best delivered iontophoretically as their water-soluble salts.

Iontophoretic local anaesthesia has long been reported for a range of applications, including anaesthesia of the tympanic membrane (Comeau *et al.*, 1973) and the conjunctiva (Sisler, 1978). However, Russo *et al.* (1980) applied the method to achieve local anaesthesia of intact skin by iontophoretic delivery of lignocaine as its hydrochloride. Both efficacy and duration of anaesthesia were separately assessed in a volunteer trial. A comparison was made with the effects of conventional lignocaine infiltration, and simply swabbing the test site with the drug solution. Iontophoretic delivery was achieved with a direct current which was slowly increased from zero to 2 mA over the first minute, and to 4 mA during the second minute. It was maintained at this level for a further 5 minutes, before being slowly reduced back to zero. The delivery electrode was therefore in contact with a topical 4% lignocaine hydrochloride solution for a total of 7 minutes.

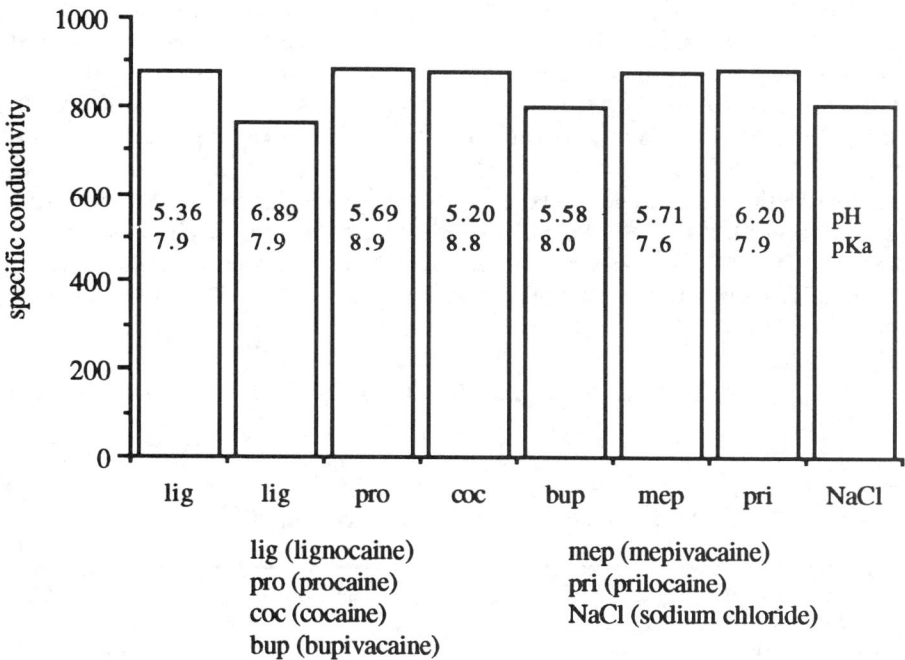

Fig. 5.13 — Specific conductivities of several local anaesthetic solutions (10 mM). Solution pH values are indicated on each bar. Reproduced from Gangarosa *et al.* (1978) with permission of the copyright owner, the American Pharmaceutical Association

A total of 27 subjects received iontophoretic lignocaine delivery. Of these, 10 experienced some degree of side effects requiring an alteration in the iontophoresis conditions, either in respect of the magnitude of the applied voltage, the duration of iontophoresis, or both. Side effects during iontophoresis included localised warmth, burning or cold, together with stinging and an isolated incidence of dizziness. Iontophoresis of lignocaine gave a mean duration of anaesthesia of 14.5 minutes, significantly better than a placebo or swabbing. However, the duration of anaesthesia was also significantly shorter than with lignocaine infiltration.

An important consideration pointed out by the authors is that, given the nature of the drug being delivered iontophoretically, there is a potential hazard in the resulting inability of the patient to detect a burn caused by the iontophoresis process. Clearly, however, local anaesthetics can be delivered percutaneously as their water-soluble salts by iontophoresis, although in the case of the study by Russo *et al.* (1980) the period of the effect was unrealistically short due, probably, to the limited application period which could be safely used.

A detailed volunteer study on the iontophoretic delivery of lignocaine hydrochloride through intact skin was reported by Gangarosa (1981). Solutions containing lignocaine hydrochloride with, or without, adrenaline were used to anaesthetise the skin by iontophoresis for 10 minutes at a constant current of 1 mA. The test mixtures were applied to the volar surface of the forearm as 0.3 ml of solution soaked onto a paper pad in contact with the anode. The return electrode was of a similar design but used sodium nitrate solution as the conducting medium. Anaesthesia was assessed in terms of a pin prick method. The effect was graded with respect to a nearby non-treated site from 0 (no pain) up to 5. Anaesthesia was further tested in respect of a needle penetration challenge, the depth of insertion being measured to the point at which discomfort was felt. Vasoconstriction was graded according to skin colour from -1 (blanched, due to vasoconstriction) through 0 (normal) to +1 (erythema, due to vasodilation). Statistical interpretation was made by sequential analysis with an experimental design involving a paired comparison on the same subject in each case. The main results reported are summarised in Table 5.6, with the mean durations of anaesthesia achieved in each case given in Table 5.7.

Overall, it was concluded that a practical solution for local anaesthesia of the skin by

Table 5.6 — Comparisons of local anaesthetic solutions for iontophoresis in respect of anaesthetic efficacy and vasoconstriction

drug pairs A vs. B		sequential analysis			
A	B	no. of trials	grade of effect	depth of effect	length of effect	vasocon-striction
2%L/Aw anodal	2%L anodal	9	A > B	A > B	A > B	A > B
2%L/Aw anodal	Aw anodal	7	A > B	A > B	A > B	A = B
2%L/Aw anodal	2%L/Aw no current	7	A > B	A > B	A > B	A > B
2%L/Aw anodal	5%L topical ointment	8	A > B	A > B	A > B	A > B
2%L/Aw anodal	4%L/Aw anodal	6	A = B	A = B	A = B	A = B
4%L/Aw anodal	4%L/As anodal	7	A = B	A = B	A = B	A = B

Key: L = lignocaine hydrochloride; Aw = weak adrenaline (1/50,000); As = strong adrenaline (1/10,000)

Table 5.7 — Comparisons of local anaesthetic solutions for iontophoresis in respect of mean durations of anaesthesia achieved

drug pairs A vs. B		no. of trials	mean duration ± s.e. A vs. B		P
A	B		A	vs. B	
2%L/Aw anodal	2%L anodal	9	65.6±5.4	33.3±3.3	< 0.001
2%L/Aw anodal	Aw anodal	8	53.6±8.4	25.8±1.0	< 0.02
2%L/Aw anodal	2%L/Aw no current	8	60.0±4.2	15.0±3.3	< 0.001
2%L/Aw anodal	5%L topical ointment	8	53.0±4.5	6.9±0.9	< 0.001
2%L/Aw anodal	4%L/Aw anodal	6	83.0±9.3	83.0±9.3	n.s.
4%L/Aw anodal	4%L/As anodal	7	76.0±8.9	76.0±8.9	n.s.

Key: L = lignocaine hydrochloride; Aw = weak adrenaline (1/50,000); As = strong adrenaline (1/10,000); s.e. = standard error

Reproduced from Gangarosa (1981) with permission of the copyright holders, J.R. Prous S.A.

iontophoresis should contain 2 to 4% lignocaine with between 1/50,000 to 1/10,000 adrenaline as a vasoconstrictor to maintain the drug at the nociceptors and thus increase the duration of anaesthesia. Although no details were given, lignocaine was considered superior, as an iontophoretic skin anaesthetic, to procaine, amethocaine, mepivacaine and bupivacaine. In this study the durations of anaesthesia achieved (up to 83 minutes) were impressive considering the short application time (10 minutes) used. However, no details of adverse effects were given, or, indeed, if any such effects occurred.

A clinical trial of lignocaine iontophoresis for painless venepuncture in adult blood donors was carried out by Arvidsson *et al.* (1984). The anodal delivery electrode consisted of multiple leaves of thin paper moistened with the anaesthetic solution of lignocaine hydrochloride, which was not described in detail. Electrical connection was made to the positive pole of a direct current source through a metal silver/silver chloride strip embedded in the paper. The current was slowly increased until the constant value was between 1.5 - 2.0 mA. This was maintained for 10 minutes.

The study design involved a randomised double-blind protocol in which the placebo solution was sodium chloride. Of the 47 volunteers who participated in the trial, 21 classified the subsequent venepuncture as painless, 14 perceived some pain and 3 experienced pain or discomfort at a level equivalent to their previous blood donation experiences. Thus, 89% of volunteers received complete or partial pain prophylaxis as a result of the procedure. Of the placebo group, 5 volunteers had some anaesthetic effect, with the rest reporting the normal level of pain associated with the procedure. There were some reported adverse effects in respect of reddening of the site and, in one case, a burning sensation at the treated site.

In order to overcome the adverse reactions and practical limitations associated with iontophoretic local anaesthesia of the skin, Petelenz *et al.* (1984) designed a so-called mini-set for topical analgesia. This device, which weighed only 400 g including batteries, was intended for home use by the patient. It consisted of a current generator of regulated current efficiency, together with a power supply system, current meter and battery container encased in a plastic container. The current range was from 0.5 - 5 mA with a maximum output voltage of 18 V. The set was equipped with an electrode assembly (cathode and anode) secured to the site by adhesive tape.

Table 5.8 — Numerical analysis of the effects on pain intensity of mini-set iontophoresis of lignocaine or placebo prior to intramuscular (i.m.) or intravenous (i.v.) injections

category	lignocaine		placebo	
	i.m.	i.v.	i.m.	i.v.
total no. of trials	29		24	
no. per category	12	17	11	13
painless	22		3	
no. per category	8	14	1	2
painful	7		21	
no. per category	4	3	10	11
pain category (intensity)				
light	n = 3		n = 8	
no. per pain category	1	2	3	5
medium	n = 4		n = 10	
no. per category	3	1	6	4
intense	n = 0		n = 3	
no. per category	0	0	1	2

Modified from Petelenz *et al.* (1984) with permission of the copyright owner

Lignocaine hydrochloride was delivered anodally via a gauze pad placed under the electrode and soaked in a 25% solution of the drug. In a double-blind clinical trial of the technique, the placebo solution was normal saline. The iontophoresis period was 10 minutes, in common with other studies, with a current of between 1 and 1.25 mA. Patients receiving either intravenous or intramuscular injections were employed in the trial, with the efficacy of the procedure for pain protection being self-assessed by means of a questionnaire. In total, 53 injections were made following iontophoresis of lignocaine hydrochloride or placebo, 29 being made following administration of the drug and 24 following iontophoresis of the placebo.

Table 5.8 summarises the results achieved in this particular study. Of those patients receiving the local anaesthetic, 76% (22 patients) felt no pain on subsequent injection whereas 87% of the placebo group (21 patients) experienced considerable or intense pain. This difference was statistically significant when the results were treated by a chi-square test. No adverse effects were apparent from the procedure. Interestingly, patients receiving intramuscular injection reported significant relief from post-procedure pain with prior lignocaine iontophoresis. The authors suggest that the anaesthetic may therefore have penetrated deeply into the tissue, but it seems more likely that the relief experienced was from surface referred pain.

In an attempt to quantify the percutaneous penetration of lignocaine hydrochloride through human skin, Siddiqui *et al.* (1985) used an *in vitro* diffusion cell in which the donor compartment contained a 0.1% drug solution at each of six various pH values and the receiver compartment contained normal saline. The two compartments were

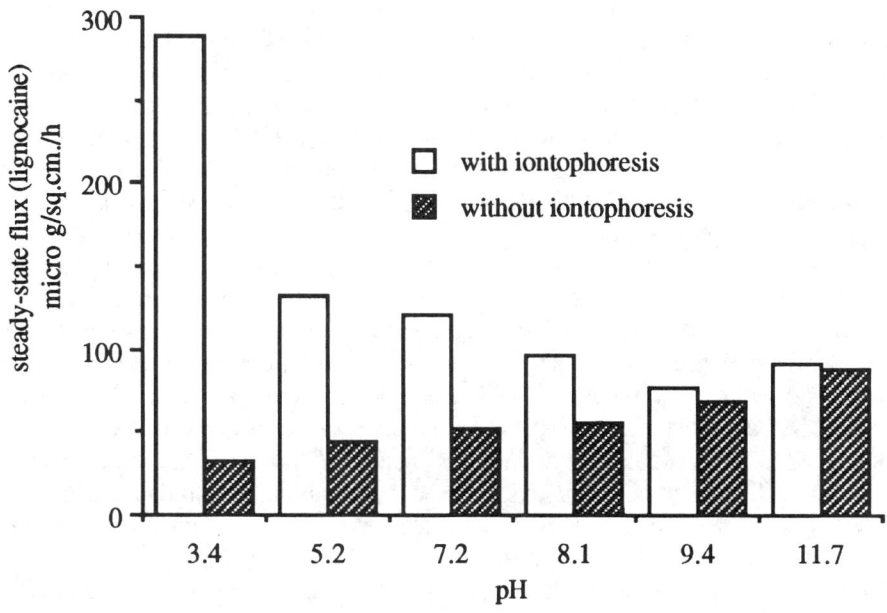

Fig. 5.14 — Steady-state penetration flux of lignocaine hydrochloride (0.1%) across human stratum corneum with and without iontophoresis. Reproduced from Siddiqui *et al.* 1985) with permission of the copyright owner

separated by a human stratum corneum barrier membrane. The donor solution was maintained at a positive potential relative to the receiver solution by means of an applied voltage across a platinum anode (donor) and platinum cathode (receiver). Iontophoresis at a constant current of 1 mA was applied for 3 minutes every hour starting at 10 minutes into the experiment, and the steady-state drug fluxes at various pH values determined, with and without iontophoresis, from the linear portion of the cumulative amount penetrated versus time plots (Fig. 5.14).

Iontophoretic delivery of lignocaine was found to be most efficient at a low pH value of 3.4, with the flux increasing by 8.5 times compared to penetration in the absence of iontophoresis. As the pH rises, iontophoretic delivery is decreased until it is almost identical to that without iontophoresis. This obviously represents the change from almost 100% of drug in the charged form at a low pH to almost all of the drug being present in the uncharged free base form at higher alkaline pH values. The change in pH values did not alter the permeability of the stratum corneum as shown by experiments in which the penetrant was tritiated water. In practice, a solution pH between 5 and 7 would be required in order to ensure compatibility with the skin but iontophoresis still showed significant penetration enhancement in respect of lignocaine.

Clearly, from the available experimental evidence there is little doubt that iontophoresis can achieve effective percutaneous local anaesthesia by promoting the absorption of local anaesthetic salts. Presently, all studies have related specifically to lignocaine hydrochloride. The duration of anaesthesia achieved by iontophoresis compares favourably with the lignocaine-prilocaine eutectic mixture but is much shorter than that possible with the amethocaine phase change system, or with liposomal amethocaine. This difference may reflect the choice of drug, but may also occur as a result of the comparatively short delivery times used in iontophoresis. The use of a constant current effectively limits the application period so a useful further step would be the iontophoretic delivery of local anaesthetics via a pulsed current, thus extending the delivery time and increasing the amount of drug penetrating the stratum corneum. However, this would negate to some extent the main advantage of iontophoretic delivery of local anaesthetics through the skin, which is that anaesthesia can be achieved with a much shorter application period than is presently possible with topical systems.

Although iontophoresis of local anaesthetics has been shown to work, at least to some extent, it is not, as yet, in routine clinical use for this purpose. A number of practical disadvantages remain to be overcome. These include the lack of a convenient, commercially available, small and, not least, inexpensive iontophoresis unit, together with the inconvenience of using pads soaked in drug solutions or saline as part of the delivery and return electrodes. This latter problem could be solved, perhaps, by incorporating the drug in a bioadhesive hydrogel delivery electrode. However, the further problem of adverse reactions, mainly the danger of burning the skin, remains, particularly if the patient is unable to detect the initial pain of a burn due to anaesthesia of the skin. With the availability of effective topical systems, the inevitable compromise necessary between minimum application time, effective and prolonged anaesthesia, and lack of serious adverse effects may well favour the topical approach to the exclusion of further development of iontophoresis for this particular application.

5.5   PHONOPHORESIS OF LOCAL ANAESTHETICS

The use of ultrasound to enhance the percutaneous absorption of drugs is known as phonophoresis, a technique first reported by Fellinger and Schmid (1954). Enhancement is thought to occur via the direct transfer of ultrasonic energy through a topical preparation located at the skin treatment site. It follows from this that a vehicle to be used as part of a phonophoresis drug delivery system must be formulated so as to efficiently transmit ultrasonic energy.

A number of reports have been made on the use of phonophoresis to promote the percutaneous absorption of local anaesthetics (Novak, 1964; Cameroy, 1966; Moll, 1979). However, phonophoresis involves massaging the drug-loaded vehicle against the treatment site. Careful controls are therefore required since rubbing in (inunction) can itself significantly promote percutaneous drug absorption. Such controls are, unfortunately, largely absent from most anecdotal reports relating to phonophoresis of local anaesthetics through intact skin.

A carefully controlled evaluation of the phonophoresis of an o/w cream containing 25% lignocaine base was made by McElnay *et al.* (1985). An experimental protocol was adopted which incorporated a standardised ultrasound intensity (2 W cm^{-2}), an initial cream application period (6 minutes followed by removal of the covering dressing), and a constant rubbing in period with the ultrasound probe (5 minutes with or without power). The study, which used 10 adult volunteers with a 7 day period between each treatment, was performed using a double-blind crossover design. It was concluded that there was no statistically significant difference in respect of the onset time for anaesthesia achieved, with and without, ultrasound. No assessment was made with regard to the duration of anaesthesia. Assessment was by a pin prick test.

The failure to achieve clinically significant anaesthesia with phonophoresis can be ascribed to a number of potential causes. The initial contact time was designed to saturate the stratum corneum with drug prior to the application of ultrasound. This is very unlikely to have been achieved. In addition, the choice of drug may have been unsuitable, the testing method too insensitive to detect any minor influence due to ultrasound, or the formulation may not have transmitted ultrasound energy in an effective manner. In any case, it is clear that ultrasound is unlikely to offer scope for the development of more effective percutaneous local anaesthetic preparations.

5.6   ENHANCEMENT OF THE PERCUTANEOUS PENETRATION OF LOCAL ANAESTHETICS BY CHEMICAL AGENTS

Penetration enhancers, sometimes also referred to as accelerants or sorption promoters, are chemical agents which have the ability to penetrate into the skin and reversibly decrease its resistance to the diffusion of topically applied drugs. The ideal properties required from a penetration-enhancing chemical have been summarised by Barry (1983).

(i)   The enhancer should be pharmacologically inert and possess no action of itself at receptor sites in the skin or the body generally.

(ii)   The material should be non-toxic, non-irritant and non-allergenic.

(iii)   The onset of action should be immediate, and the duration of the effect should be predictable and suitable.

(iv)   When the material is removed from the skin, the tissue should immediately and fully recover its normal barrier properties.

(v)   The barrier function of the skin should reduce in one direction only so as to promote penetration into the skin. Body fluids, electrolytes and other endogenous substances should not be lost to the atmosphere.

(vi)   The enhancer should be chemically and physically compatible with a wide range of drugs and pharmaceutical adjuvants.

(vii)   The enhancer should be an excellent solvent for drugs.

(viii)   The material should spread well on the skin and possess a suitable "skin feel".

(ix)   The enhancer should be capable of formulation into lotions, suspensions, ointments, creams, gels, aerosols and pressure-sensitive adhesives. To this list can now also be added transdermal therapeutic patch systems.

(x)   The enhancer should be odourless, tasteless, and colourless in order to be cosmetically acceptable.

It is true to say that, as with most things in life, the ideal situation rarely exists. Thus, no penetration-enhancing chemical can truly be considered ideal in the light of such demanding requirements. The literature on transdermal drug delivery and percutaneous drug absorption is prolific, and penetration enhancers now constitute a defined and separate area of study. A detailed treatment of this vast subject is outside the scope of the present text, and there are many excellent treatments of the subject available elsewhere. Nevertheless, in the quest for faster acting percutaneous anaesthetic preparations, it is worth considering the basic properties of available enhancers in the context of any possible benefits offered by their use.

5.6.1 Penetration enhancers

Hori *et al.* (1989) used a conceptual approach to classify penetration enhancers into three distinct groups based on an assessment of their so-called organic and inorganic characteristics. Classical penetration enhancers were assigned to group I. These were essentially liquids with good solvent properties such as dimethylsulphoxide, propylene glycol and 2-pyrrolidone. Group II enhancers included oleic acid and newer specifically designed enhancers such as Azone®. Group II agents were generally more effective at enhancing the percutaneous penetration of hydrophilic substances. Group III agents were those with a mainly "organic" character and were thus primarily enhancers for lipophilic penetrants. The chemical structures of several common penetration enhancers are shown in Fig. 5.15.

Penetration enhancers may promote percutaneous drug penetration either by interaction with the skin, or by increasing drug release from the vehicle, or possibly by a combination of both these effects. Pharmaceutical co-solvents such as propylene glycol appear to have no significant effect on the stratum corneum. Rather, they act by maximising the thermodynamic activity of the drug in the vehicle so that there is greater release of the agent from the vehicle and hence increased skin penetration (Woodford and Barry, 1986).

The most widely used penetration enhancers in the past have tended to be aprotic solvents, notably sulphoxides (dimethylsulphoxide and decylmethylsulphoxide) and amides (dimethylacetamide and dimethylformamide). These compounds, however, are irritant to the skin in high concentrations. In the case of dimethylsulphoxide (DMSO) a major problem in its topical application is the resultant unpleasant odour from the breath

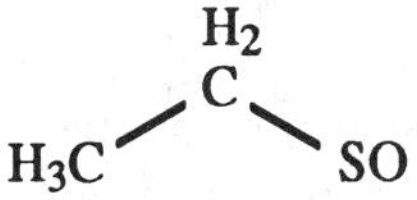

dimethylsulphoxide

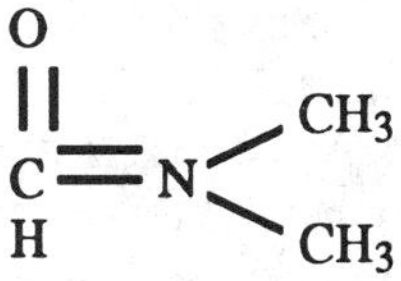

dimethylformamide

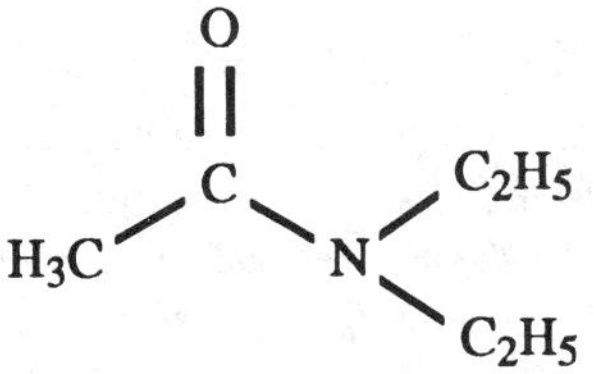

diethylacetamide

$CH_3. (CH_2)_7. CH = CH. (CH_2)_7. COOH$

oleic acid

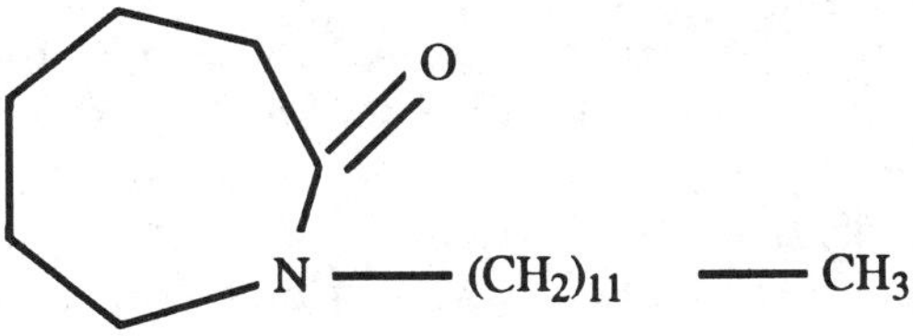

1-dodecylazacycloheptan-2-one (Azone, laurocapram)

Fig. 5.15 — Chemical structures of some enhancers of percutaneous drug penetration

and a bad taste in the mouth due to metabolic formation of dimethylsulphide. Kligman (1965) has summarised the topical pharmacology and toxicology of DMSO. Although the mode of action of DMSO is still not completely certain, it appears to act in part by its ability to replace water molecules associated with cellular structures and thus alter the conformational state of protein molecules in the stratum corneum. For many compounds the enhancement effect of DMSO is only evident at high enhancer concentrations. In this situation the enhancement mechanism may be due to the high osmotic pressure of the DMSO solution producing physical damage to the stratum corneum structure. Together with dimethylacetamide and dimethylformamide, which are thought to act similarly, the use of DMSO is certainly unwarranted for a non-therapeutic application such as percutaneous anaesthesia.

Pyrrolidones, particularly 2-pyrrolidone and N-methylpyrrolidone, are thought to have percutaneous penetration enhancing properties (Southwell and Barry, 1983: Sasaki et al., 1988). Their action may be related to an ability to enhance the moisture-retaining properties of the skin since they are chemically related to constituents of the natural moisturising factor (NMF) found in skin. NMF consists mainly of free fatty acids, urea, pyrrolidone carboxylic acid and its sodium salt, the latter apparently being the principal humectant responsible for increasing the water-binding properties of the stratum corneum. The pyrrolidones appear to be most effective on compounds penetrating via the polar route. Increased hydration of the skin is probably responsible for their activity since it is well known that, for many compounds, increased hydration results in a reduction of the stratum corneum barrier function (Wurster and Kramer, 1961). The pyrrolidones may therefore hold little promise for the enhancement of the percutaneous penetration of lipophilic local anaesthetic bases.

Free fatty acids, such as oleic acid and other *cis*-unsaturated fatty acids, have been shown to be effective penetration enhancers for quite a wide variety of penetrants (Aungst *et al.*, 1986; Green *et al.*, 1988). These compounds undoubtedly act on the intercellular lipid bilayers of the stratum corneum (Francoeur *et al.*, 1990). Increased lipid bilayer fluidisation, resulting in increased skin permeability to lipophilic penetrants, has been demonstrated by differential scanning calorimetry. Formulating a percutaneous local anaesthetic using this class of enhancer is problematical, however, since any beneficial enhancement of drug penetration may be negated by the presence of an exogenous oil phase. Local anaesthetic free base will tend to partition between the oily enhancer phase and the stratum corneum, thereby reducing the escaping tendency of the active component from the formulation. This is a problem which is not restricted solely to fatty acid penetration enhancers. In addition, fatty acids may be incompatible with the formulation of basic drugs.

In addition to aprotic solvents and fatty acids, other compounds and chemical groups have penetration enhancing properties. These include simple alcohols and all three major classes of surfactants (non-ionic, anionic and cationic (Walters, 1989)). However, perhaps the most interesting enhancer is a chemical agent specifically developed for this purpose, 1-dodecylazacycloheptan-2-one. The compound is generally referred to as Azone®, the proprietary name, whereas laurocapram is the INN. From a molecular viewpoint Azone® is a combination of a cyclic amide and a linear sulphoxide without the reactive sulphoxide group (Wiechers and De Zeeuw, 1990). Azone® is a clear, colourless liquid with a molecular weight of 281. It has a low acute toxicity and can be applied neat to human skin without any apparent irritation (Stoughton, 1982). Azone® is miscible with most organic solvents, including alcohols, ketones and hydrocarbons. It is, however, immiscible with water. Like oleic acid, it is thought to increase the permeability of the stratum corneum to penetrants via a fluidising effect on stratum corneum lipid bilayers (Ward and Tallon, 1988; Bouwstra *et al.*, 1989).

Azone® has been reported to enhance the percutaneous penetration of a wide range of compounds. Wiechers and de Zeeuw (1990) list over 40 compounds that show enhancement factors from single figures up to 3000. Generally, enhancement appears to be greater for compounds of higher polarity. Since the enhancer is insoluble in water, this presents some additional formulation problems. A suitable co-solvent system, or the formation of an o/w emulsion incorporating the enhancer in the internal phase, is required if the formulation is to be pharmaceutically elegant and stable. Interestingly, however, Stoughton and McClure (1983) report that a good enhancement effect can be observed when Azone® is employed only as a shaken emulsion with water. A possible inference from this is that the compound may actually penetrate the stratum corneum directly, thereby exerting its effect on the lipid bilayer structure, though there appears to be no definite information on this aspect of the use of Azone®.

5.6.2   Use of penetration enhancers with local anaesthetics

With most enhancers, a difficulty is caused by the time required for the enhancement effect to occur. For percutaneous local anaesthesia to gain widespread clinical acceptance an improvement in the speed of onset of the anaesthetic effect would be desirable. The fastest available route appears to be via iontophoretic delivery, but the drawback with this method is the very short duration of the anaesthetic effect. Presently, the fastest-acting percutaneous local anaesthetic preparation of those commercially available or under development appears to be the amethocaine phase-change system. This will produce effective local anaesthesia of the skin in most children within 30 minutes. Thus, any enhancement effect will have to be seen within this time period. This is clearly a difficult challenge. Azone®, the most effective percutaneous enhancer presently commercially available, is known to be relatively slow-acting. Further work in developing new, non-toxic chemical entities with percutaneous penetration enhancer properties will be aimed at producing a more rapid effect and still at least matching the enhancement capabilities of Azone®. Thus, for example, Wong *et al.* (1989) report the synthesis of a series of N,N-dialkyl-substituted amino acetates with a superior enhancement profile to Azone® with respect to indomethacin. These enhancers have a relatively rapid onset of action but are nevertheless still on a systemic transdermal drug delivery time scale which can extend to several days compared to the short delivery period required for the percutaneous delivery of a local anaesthetic.

An *in vivo* evaluation of Azone®, oleic acid and propylene glycol as potential penetration enhancers for the amethocaine phase-change system was undertaken by McCafferty and Woolfson (1991). The penetration enhancers were used at a concentration of 5% w/v, with the standard formulation, without any enhancer, acting as a control. A double-blind clinical trial was performed using a panel of 20 young, healthy volunteers (12 female) having an age range of 20 - 26 years. The four preparations (two per arm) were applied randomly to each volunteer on the ventral surface of the forearm at, or just below, the anticubital fossa. Each application (0.5 g) was covered with a film dressing and left in contact with the skin surface for 20 minutes. On removal of the preparation, onset of anaesthesia was determined at 5 minute intervals by pin-prick challenge. The results (Fig. 5.16) indicated that there was a slight increase in onset time when either Azone® (38.1 minutes) or propylene glycol (39.4 minutes) were used as penetration enhancers when compared to the control (37.2 minutes). In contrast, the formulation containing oleic acid caused some reduction in onset time (33.6 minutes). Overall, oleic acid enhanced the percutaneous absorption of amethocaine, but the effect was marginal and probably not sufficient to justify its inclusion in the formulation.

Sipos (1980) reported enhanced absorption of local anaesthetics through the stratum corneum when combined with a number of novel synthetic enhancers. The enhancers were classified structurally as (a) primary, secondary or tertiary straight- or branched-chain monohydric aliphatic alcohols (b) substituted cyclohexylalkanols and (c) substituted phenyl alkanols. Lignocaine, benzocaine and amethocaine were all considered to be suitable anaesthetic agents that could be combined with these enhancers. The local

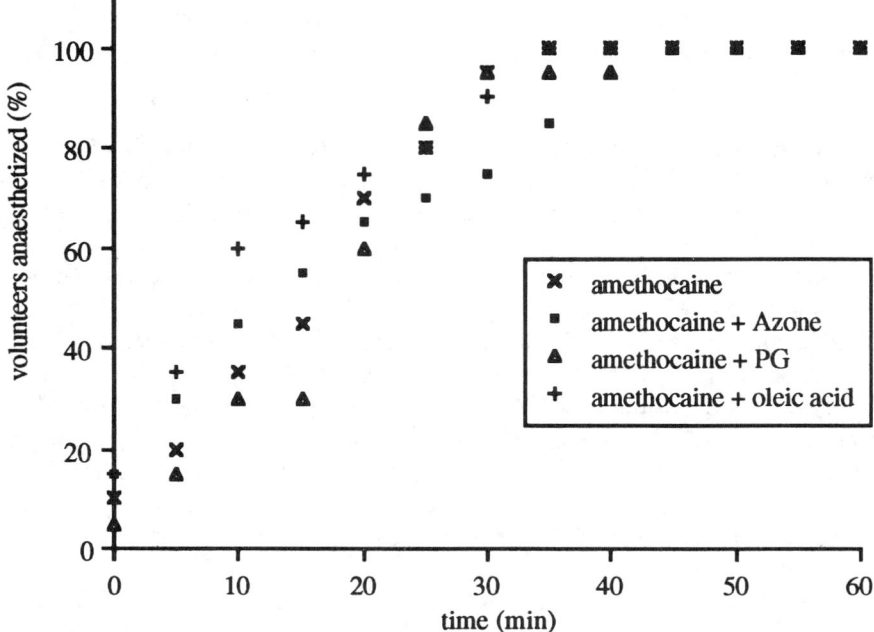

Fig. 5.16 — The effect of various penetration enhancers on the onset of local anaesthesia to pin-prick challenge following application of the amethocaine phase-change system: double-blind volunteer trial with a panel of 20 healthy volunteers (12 female) having an age range of 20-26 years

anaesthetic was formulated in the concentration range of 1 - 10% with the enhancer present at up to 15% by weight. The vehicle could be either excess enhancer or any conventional topical dosage form such as a semi-solid. A typical semi-solid formulation was (% w/w): ethanol 50, penetration enhancer 12, local anaesthetic 4, viscosity builder 3, water 31.

Formulations containing the various penetration enhancers were applied to intact human skin and were claimed to produce deep anaesthesia of the treated site within 15 - 60 minutes, such anaesthesia lasting for several hours. However, no further developments of this work have been reported. Significantly, no comments were made on possible adverse reactions to the formulations. Given the nature of the formulations, it is probable that they proved toxic to the skin, and could therefore not be developed further. This episode illustrates rather well the dilemma of the formulator in respect of producing what is really a prophylactic product for use on a healthy patient. An aggressive formulation will, in all likelihood, produce the desired rapid onset of deep cutaneous anaesthesia but, in so doing, will almost certainly damage healthy skin.

Aggressive formulations of lignocaine and its hydrochloride salt were also investigated as possible percutaneous local anaesthetics (Akerman *et al.*, 1979). Interestingly, despite the ease of assessment in humans of percutaneous anaesthetic preparations, an animal model (guinea pig) was used in this study. Pain was determined by the presence or absence of the twitching response to six pin-pricks of the skin.

Lignocaine hydrochloride was used as its aqueous solution. As would now be expected, it proved ineffective even in an animal model. The free base was formulated either in an aqueous alcoholic solvent mixture or in aqueous solutions of dipolar aprotic solvents. These included simple tertiary aliphatic amides, amides related to dimethylacetamide, some cyclic amides and a number of miscellaneous compounds. The free base was used throughout at a concentration of 20% and a one hour application period was used.

Assessment of the pain-blocking efficacy of the various formulations was made during a 25 minute period immediately following removal of the drug from the site, the results being expressed as a percentage anaesthetic score. The most effective formulations were solutions of lignocaine base in either aqueous dimethylformamide or aqueous dimethylacetamide. A poorer response was obtained with dimethylsulphoxide as the enhancer. Of other agents tested, lactam derivatives (substituted pyrrolidones and morpholones) appeared promising, with the best enhancer of this type being 2-pyrrolidone. With these compounds, increasing the size of the substituent at the nitrogen atom appeared to adversely affect their ability to enhance percutaneous penetration.

Radiolabelled (^{3}H) lignocaine base in isopropanol or dimethylacetamide aqueous solutions, or an aqueous solution of the salt, were applied to guinea pig skin. The local distribution of radioactivity in harvested skin samples was subsequently assessed (Fig.

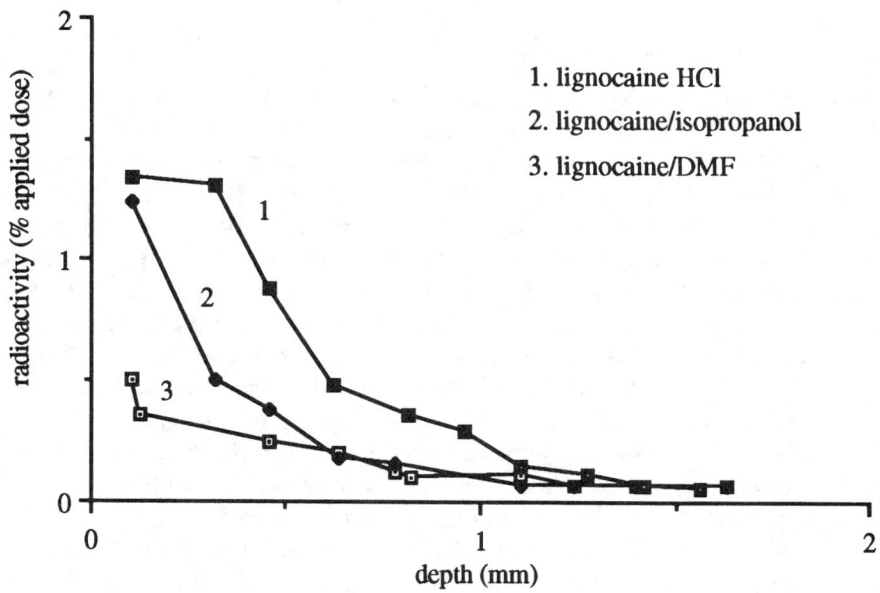

Fig. 5.17 — Distribution of tritiated lignocaine following epicutaneous application of three differing compositions of 20% ^{3}H-lignocaine to guinea pig skin. Each point represents the average activity as a percentage of the applied dose recovered in 0.16 mm sections. The solutions (0.4 ml) were applied for one hour under occlusion to groups of four animals. Reproduced from Akerman *et al.* (1979) with permission of the copyright owner, *Pharmacology and Toxicology*

5.17). In each case the highest activity was found in the superficial horizontal section consisting of the stratum corneum and viable epidermis. The activity decreased rapidly in the deeper sections. This is an ideal distribution profile for maximising the required local effect of the drug and minimising its possible systemic absorption.

The mechanism of action of lignocaine penetration enhancement by dimethylacetamide was considered in respect of the tendency of dipolar aprotic solvents to accept rather than donate protons. They can thus compete effectively for hydrogen donor molecules and may be capable of adversely affecting the stability of the stratum corneum, probably by displacing bound water from the tissue and substituting it with a looser structure offering an increased permeability to penetrants. The maintenance of a high electron density at the amide carbonyl appeared to be a structural requirement for efficient penetration enhancement, further supporting the proposed mechanism. Electron-withdrawing substituents decreased the electron density at the amide carbonyl, and such derivatives were less effective as penetration enhancers. Similar effects to those seen with lignocaine enhancement by dipolar aprotic solvents had also been previously reported by Brechner *et al.* (1967) for the enhancement of amethocaine percutaneous penetration by dimethylsulphoxide. However, the nature of the enhancing mechanism in both cases is probably also responsible for adverse topical reactions seen when such compounds are applied to intact healthy skin. For this reason, although studies of this type were valuable in their mechanistic approach to the problem, they have not yielded clinically safe preparations.

5.7   STABILITY CONSIDERATIONS

Common topical formulations of local anaesthetics invariably incorporate the drug as its water-soluble salt. In addition to simplifying the formulation this also largely eliminates any stability problems with the active component. Unfortunately, percutaneous local anaesthesia requires the use of a local anaesthetic in the lipophilic free base form. Stability problems resulting from this requirement would normally be controlled by formulating the free base in an ointment or other oily vehicle. However, a further requirement for clinical efficacy is the use of an aqueous vehicle in order not to retard drug penetration of the skin. Thus, the formulator is presented with the unenviable task of presenting, in a stable form, a topical local anaesthetic free base in an aqueous vehicle. In this context "stable" can be defined conventionally as the loss of no more than 10% of the active drug over a two year storage period at ambient temperature. Stability, of course, refers to the physical integrity of the preparation in addition to the chemical integrity of any active components. Dukes (1990) has reviewed general considerations for the stability testing of topical pharmaceutical formulations.

The chemical stability problems associated with local anaesthetic free bases are almost completely confined to consideration of the ester group of drugs. Amides such as lignocaine are reasonably stable chemically provided the storage temperature is below about 30°C. Published information on the stability of ester local anaesthetics in aqueous environments has been summarised by Connors *et al.* (1986) and refers mainly to benzocaine or procaine as model compounds in this class. Ester local anaesthetics degrade primarily by specific base catalysis resulting in hydrolysis of the ester group and formation of the corresponding acid and alcohol. For the esters, the acid hydrolysis product is either para-aminobenzoic acid or an analogue of this acid. Both the protonated and unprotonated species are subject to specific base catalysis, and specific acid catalysis also occurs. The exact degradation pathway is thus highly dependent on pH, and on the pK_a of the drug. However, at pH values high enough to precipitate the free base *in situ* , or for formulations prepared directly with the free base, the dominant degradation route is specific base catalysis.

A number of formulation options are available to increase the stability of aqueous local anaesthetic free base formulations. These methods of stabilisation, which all involve shielding the drug to some extent from water, either by physical or chemical means, include:

(i)   formulation of the drug as a topical suspension,

(ii)   complexation with caffeine (Higuchi and Lachman, 1955), β-cyclodextrin (Lach and Chin, 1964) or various other complexing agents (Lach and Pauli, 1959),

(iii) micellar solubilisation,

(iv)   stabilisation in liposomes,

(v)   adjustment of formulation pH to the optimum value for maximum stability compatible with the continuing clinical efficacy of the formulation,

(vi)   formulation as a reconstitutable (at the point of use) preparation, allowing the drug to be protected from an aqueous environment during storage.

Complexation does not sufficiently increase drug stability for it to be considered a worthwhile method in this case. In any case, further disadvantages associated with chemical complexation include the need to ensure that the complex is readily reversible at the site of action and the effect of the complexing agent on the inherent percutaneous penetration properties of the drug.

Benzocaine and procaine stability is enhanced in micellar systems using both ionic and non-ionic surfactants (Connors *et al.*, 1986). Again, the effect on percutaneous penetration properties is unpredictable. As with chemical complexation, the apparent solubility of the drug is also increased but the extent of stabilisation achieved is not particularly impressive.

Given that the efficacy of liposomal amethocaine preparations as percutaneous anaesthetics has already been established, the stabilisation of local anaesthetic free bases in liposomes seems a more promising route to follow. Similarly, the amethocaine phase-change system can be stabilised by a number of approaches, including presentation in a reconstitutable form or formulation as a topical suspension (McCafferty and Woolfson, 1988).

5.7.1   Stabilisation of local anaesthetics in liposomes

Stabilisation of hydrolytically susceptible drugs can be achieved by their incorporation into the phospholipid bilayers of liposomes. The stabilities of benzocaine and several other local anaesthetic drugs were measured both in liposomes and in aqueous buffer solutions by Habib and Rogers (1989). Stability was assessed by determining the first-order hydrolysis rate constants in both media, together with the fraction of drug associated with the lipid phase and the partition coefficient between aqueous and lipid phases. Several different phospholipid liposomal compositions, which differed in their gel-to-fluid phase transition temperatures, were investigated as potential stabilisation systems.

A number of factors could be identified as predisposing a local anaesthetic to enhanced stability in certain liposomal formulations. A prerequisite for stability enhancement appeared to be significant association of the drug with the lipid phase. This may lead to a reduction in the rate of drug hydrolysis due to a reduced reactivity in the lipid phase, possibly because much of the drug is partitioned deep in the lipid bilayers. Thus, those local anaesthetics which have a low rate constant and high association constant with respect to the lipid phase are most likely to show a significant improvement in drug stability when formulated in liposomal systems.

A further important parameter in determining the likelihood of drug stabilisation in liposomal formulations appears to be the partition coefficient between the lipid and aqueous buffered phases, with the greatest increases in stability achieved by those local anaesthetics with the greatest partition coefficients in favour of the lipid phase. Amethocaine, a very lipophilic agent, showed a 69% increase in drug stability in an L-α-dimyristoylphosphatidylcholine liposomal system compared to a 41% stability improvement achieved with the less lipophilic procaine. Overall, a correlation of predictive quality can be achieved by regression of the logarithm of the partition coefficient on the percentage increase in drug stability (Fig. 5.18).

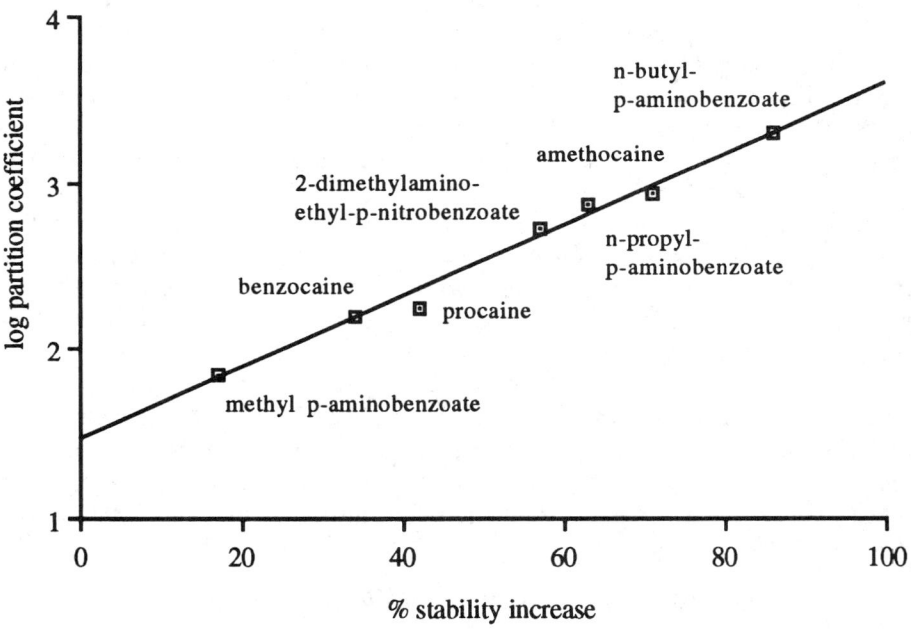

Fig. 5.18 — Correlation of the lipid-aqueous partition coefficient with the observed stability increase for ester local anaesthetics and related solutes in DMPC liposomes at pH 12.2 and 30°C. Reprinted from Habib and Rogers (1987) by courtesy of the copyright owner, Marcel Dekker Inc.

5.7.2   Stabilisation of the amethocaine phase-change system

The amethocaine phase-change system presents particular formulation problems in respect of hydrolytic stability since the formulation requires amethocaine free base to be in intimate contact with an aqueous vehicle. Stabilisation of the active drug can be achieved by formulating the preparation as a topical suspension in a vehicle of sufficient viscosity to hold the drug particles in an even distribution (McCafferty and Woolfson, 1988). The high viscosity, together with an appropriate buffering system, also retards the rate of drug dissolution and subsequent hydrolysis. However, the solid-liquid phase change that occurs above 30°C requires that the storage temperature for the preparation must remain below this point since the dissolution characteristics of the oil phase are substantially enhanced compared to the solid free base. In practice, this means that the preparation must be stored under cool conditions below 25°C.

Stability assessment of the amethocaine free base system presents some problems. Accelerated storage testing, in which the product is stressed at higher temperatures, is inappropriate due to the change in the physical nature of the system at elevated temperatures. This produces a substantially greater rate of hydrolysis and a very short predicted shelf life of only a few months (Fig 5.19). The unsuitability of the isothermal Arrhenius method for the system may readily be seen by comparing the data in Fig. 5.19 to the actual storage data under cool conditions given in Fig. 5.20.

The stability of the amethocaine phase-change system can most readily be enhanced by removal of water from the formulation. This necessitates its presentation in a reconstitutable form, and this can readily be achieved without affecting the clinical efficacy of the preparation (Woolfson and McCafferty, 1988).

5.8   PRESERVATION OF PERCUTANEOUS LOCAL ANAESTHETIC SYSTEMS

The ability of microorganisms to survive or multiply in many aqueous pharmaceutical preparations is well documented. Consequently, there is a general requirement to preserve such products against microbial challenge, both to protect the chemical and physical integrity of the product, and also, of course, to protect the patient from the risk of product-mediated infection. Percutaneous local anaesthetic systems, other than those that are formulated in the dry state for reconstitution, have a high water content. Their preservation against microbial attack must be considered as part of the overall formulation exercise.

Percutaneous local anaesthetic formulations are applied only to intact, healthy skin, unlike many conventional topical products, which are in contact with damaged or infected areas. Thus, the risk of microbial damage due to inadequate preservation is probably greater to the product than to the patient in these cases. This observation does not, of course, alleviate the need for adequate preservation of percutaneous local anaesthetic preparations. Adequate preservation may conveniently be defined in terms of the current recommendations of the British Pharmacopoeia, an amended version of the test for "Efficacy of Antimicrobial Preservatives in Pharmaceutical Products" first published in 1980. Interestingly, many pharmacopoeial preparations do not actually comply with the pharmacopoeial preservation test, yet they are known, on the basis of long experience, to be adequately preserved. Thus, the pharmacopoeial standard for preservation of aqueous pharmaceutical systems cannot be regarded as absolute.

For local anaesthetic preparations, the need for adequate preservation does not necessarily imply the need for a specific preservative agent to be included in the

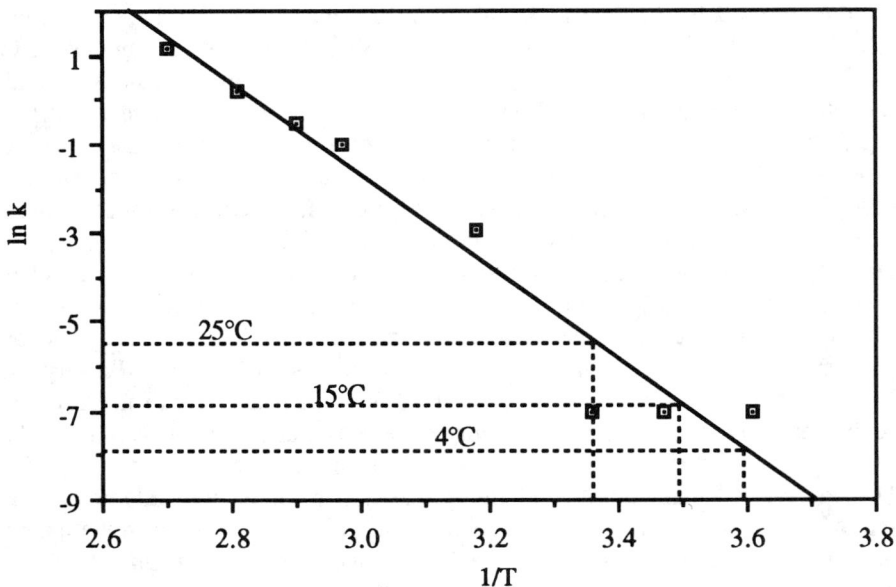

Fig. 5.19 — Arrhenius plot for the amethocaine phase-change system

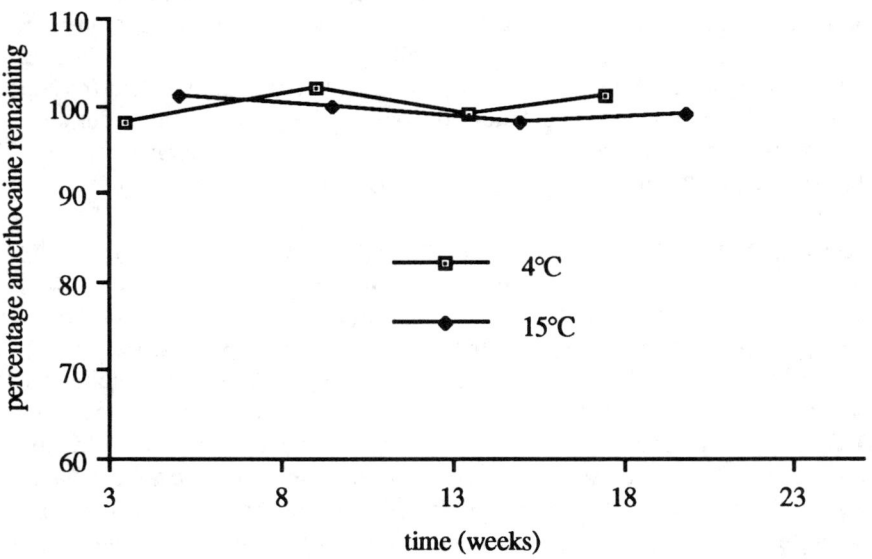

Fig. 5.20 — Storage data at 4°C and 15°C for the amethocaine phase-change
system

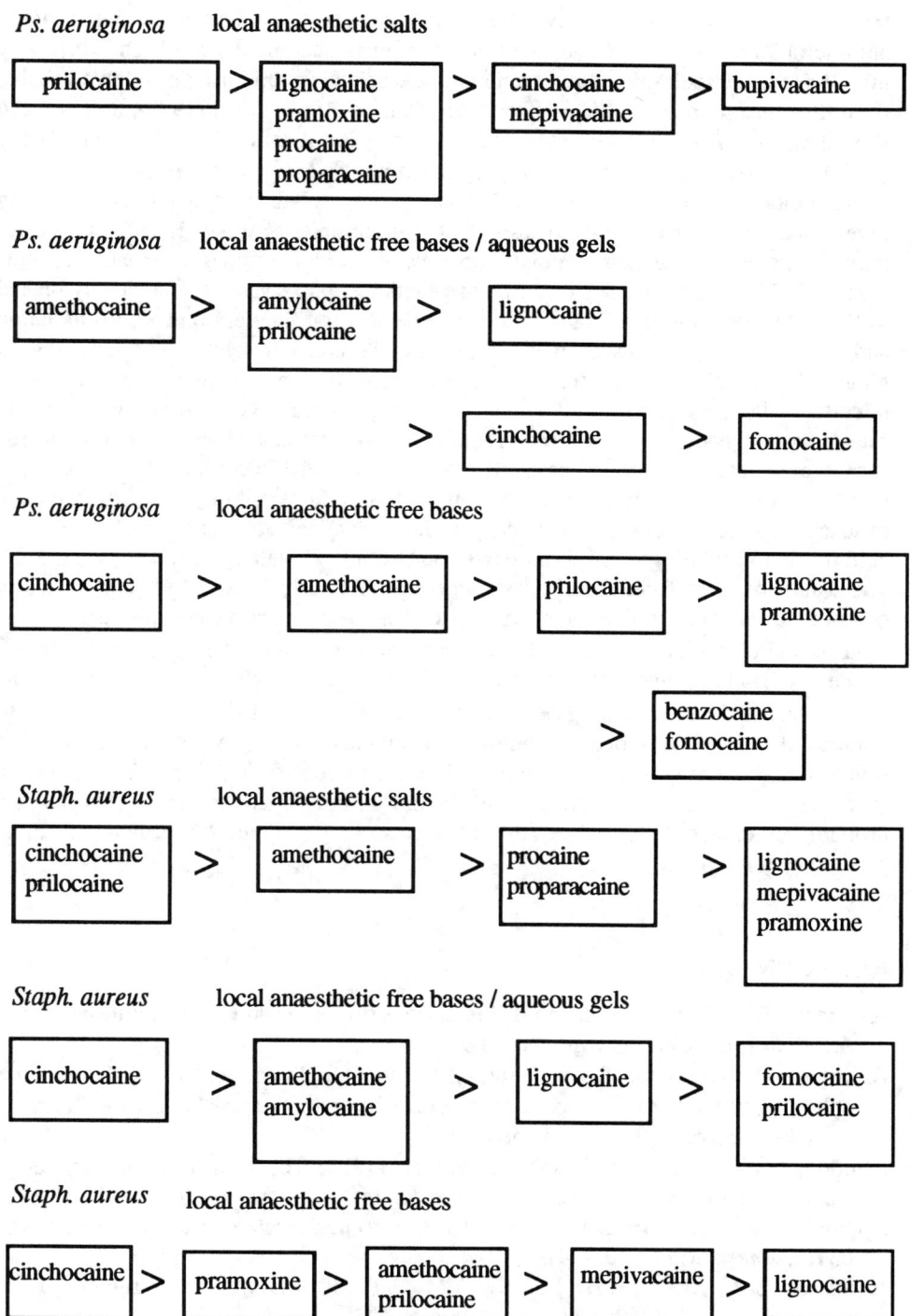

Fig. 5.21 — Order of antimicrobial inhibitory activities of local anaesthetic salts, free bases and free base aqueous gel formulations

formulation. This is because local anaesthetic agents themselves possess substantial antimicrobial properties. The mode of action of local anaesthetics has been extensively investigated, and their minimum inhibitory and cidal concentrations are widely available from literature sources, including Kleinfeld and Ellis (1967), Ohki (1970), Schmidt and Rosenkranz (1970), Weinstein *et al.* (1975), Leung and Rawal (1977), Zaidi and Healy (1977), Salt and Traynor (1979), and Fazly Bazaz and Salt (1983a and 1983b).

Amethocaine and its hydrochloride salt have probably been the most widely investigated local anaesthetics in respect of antimicrobial activity. Local anaesthetics may also potentiate the antimicrobial properties of antibiotics and other chemical agents (Labedan, 1988). The efficacy of local anaesthetics as preservatives is obviously related to their concentration in solution. This is dependent on the nature of the formulation and its pH. Clearly, local anaesthetic free bases will have low solution concentrations at higher pH values and less preservative activity. The drug may be present in emulsified, micellar or liposomal forms and in such cases its preservative efficacy may be limited. Therefore, it is necessary to test each formulation for compliance with current standards for the preservation of topical products, and on this basis to decide whether additional preservatives should be included in the formulation. The variability in the preservative efficacy of local anaesthetics in respect of their chemical state, and the effect on this activity of formulating the free bases as semi-solids, is well illustrated by Fig. 5.21. The data shown are from the authors' laboratory and ranks local anaesthetic agents in order of antimicrobial inhibitory efficacy in response to a standard challenge test.

The antimicrobial activity of the lidocaine-prilocaine eutectic system as EMLA® cream has also been investigated (Powell *et al.*, 1991). After exposure of *Staphylococcus aureus* suspensions containing between 10^2 and 10^5 cfu/ml to EMLA® cream for 30 minutes, there were significant decreases in the number of viable bacteria compared to saline controls. Growth inhibitory effects detected by zone of inhibition experiments on inoculated agar plates also showed substantial antimicrobial activity. This activity probably precludes the need for additional preservation of the lignocaine-prilocaine eutectic system.

REFERENCES

Akerman, B. (1978) Percutaneous local anaesthesia: problems - solutions. *Acta Anaesthesiol. Scand.* **Suppl. 70** 90-91.

Akerman, B., Haegerstam, G., Pring, B.G. and Sandberg, R. (1979) Penetration enhancers and other factors governing percutaneous local anaesthesia with lidocaine. *Acta Pharmacol. et Toxicol.* **45** 58-65.

Amidon, G.E., Higuchi, W.I. and Ho, N.F.H. (1982) Theoretical and experimental studies of transport of micelle-solubilised solutes. *J. Pharm. Sci.* **71** 77-84.

Appiani, L. and Laveneziana, D. (1966) Il blocko peridurale con chetocaina (rec. 7-0518). *Anest. Rianim.* **3** 441.

Arvidsson, S.B., Ekroth, R.H., Hansby, A.M.C., Lindholm, A.H. and William-Olsson, G. (1984) *Acta Anaesthesiol. Scand.* **28** 209-210.

Aungst, B.J., Rogers, N.J. and Shefter, E. (1986) Enhancement of naloxolone penetration through human skin *in vitro* using fatty acids, fatty alcohols, surfactants, sulfoxides and amides. *Int. J. Pharm.* **33** 225-234.

Banga, A.K. and Chien, Y.W. (1988) Iontophoretic delivery of drugs: fundamentals, developments and biomedical applications. *J. Contr. Rel.* **7** 1-24.

Barry B.W. (1983) *Dermatological Formulations.* Marcel Dekker, New York, pp. 160-161.

Bellantone, N.H., Rim, S., Francoeur, M.L. and Rasadi, B. (1986) Enhanced percutaneous absorption via iontophoresis. I. Evaluation of an *in vitro* system and transport of model compounds. *Int. J. Pharm.* **30** 63-72.

Brechner, V.L., Cohen, D.D. and Pretsky, I. (1967) Dermal anaesthesia by the topical application of tetracaine base dissolved in dimethylsulphoxide. *Ann. New York Acad. Sci.* **141** 524-531.

Bouwstra, J.A., Peschier, L.J.C., Brussee, J. and Bodde, H.E. (1989) Effect of N-alkyl-azocycloheptan-2-ones including Azone® on the thermal behaviour of human stratum corneum. *Int. J. Pharm.* **52** 47-54.

Broberg, B.F.J. and Evers, H.C.A. (1981) European patent 0 002 425.

Brodin, A., Nyqvist-Mayer, A., Wadsten, T., Forslund, B. and Broberg, F. (1984) Phase diagram and aqueous solubility of the lidocaine-prilocaine binary system. *J. Pharm. Sci.* **73** 481-484.

Bucks, D.A.W., Maibach, H.I. and Guy, R.H. (1989) Occlusion does not uniformly enhance penetration *in vivo*. In: Bronaugh, R.L. and Maibach, H.I. (eds). *Percutaneous Absorption, 2nd. edn.* Marcel Dekker, New York, pp. 77-94.

Burnette, R.R. and Marrero, D. (1986) Comparison between the iontophoretic and passive transport of thyrotropin releasing hormone across nude mouse skin. *J. Pharm. Sci.* **75** 738-743.

Burnette, R.R. and Ongpipattanakul, B. (1988) Characterisation of the pore transport properties and tissue alteration of excised human skin during iontophoresis. *J. Pharm. Sci.* **77** 132-137.

Cameroy, B.M. (1966) Ultrasound enhanced local anaesthesia. *Am. J. Ortho.* **8** 47.

Chien, Y.W., Siddiqui, O., Sun, Y., Shi, W.M. and Liu, J.C. (1988) Transdermal iontophoretic delivery of therapeutic peptides and proteins: I. Insulin. *Ann. N. Y. Acad. Sci.* **507** 32-51.

Comeau, M., Brummett, R. and Vernon, J. (1973) Local anaesthesia of the ear by iontophoresis. *Arch. Otolaryngol.* **98** 114-120.

Connors, K.A., Amidon, G.L. and Stella, V.J. (1986) *Chemical Stability of Pharmaceuticals.* Wiley-Interscience, New York, pp. 264-273 and 693-703.

Dohner, J.W. (1987) Development of process and equipment for rate-controlled transdermal therapeutic systems. In: Chien, Y.W. (ed.). *Transdermal Controlled Systemic Medications.* Marcel Dekker, New York, pp. 349-364.

Dukes, G.R. (1990) General considerations for stability testing of topical pharmaceutical formulations. In: *Topical Drug Delivery Formulations.* Marcel Dekker, New York, pp. 197-211.

Egbaria, K. and Weiner, N. (1990) Topical drug delivery systems using liposomes. *Pharm. Res.* **7** Suppl. 7254.

Ehrenstrom-Reiz, G.M.E. and Reiz, S.L.A. (1982) EMLA - a eutectic mixture of local anaesthetics for topical anaesthesia. *Acta Anaesthesiol. Scand.* **26** 596-598.

El Banna, H.M., Khalil, S.A. and Gouda, M.W. (1978) Solid dispersion of pharmaceutical ternary systems. II: Dispersion studies on aspirin-acetaminophen-urea systems. *J. Pharm. Sci.* **67** 1112-1117.

Fazly Bazaz, B.S. and Salt, W.G. (1983a) Local anaesthetics as antimicrobial agents: structure-action considerations. *Microbios* **37** 45-64.

Fazly Bazaz, B.S. and Salt, W.G. (1983b) Local anaesthetic induced turbidity increases: implications of interactions with intact bacterial cells with subcellular fractions. *Microbios* **37** 135-147.

Fellinger, K. and Schmid, J. (1954) *Klinik und Therapie des chronischen, Gelenkreumatismus.* Maudrich, Vienna, pp. 549-552.

Flynn, G.L. (1979) Topical drug absorption and topical pharmaceutical systems. In: Banker, G.S. and Rhodes, C.T. (eds). *Modern Pharmaceutics.* Marcel Dekker, New York, pp. 227-262.

Foldvari, M., Gesztes, A. and Mezei, M. (1990) Formulation and evaluation of topical liposomal drug delivery systems containing local anaesthetic agents. *Pharm. Res.* **7** Suppl. 7255.

Francoeur, M.L., Golden, G.M. and Potts, R.O. (1990) Oleic acid: Its effect on stratum corneum in relation to (trans)dermal drug delivery. *Pharm. Res.* **7** 621-627.

Fuhrer, C. (1982) The classification of agents used in dermatology. In: Brandau, R. and Lippold, B.H. (eds). *Dermal and Transdermal Absorption.* Wissenschaftliche Verlagsgesellschaft GmbH, Stuttgart, pp. 14-26.

Ganesan, M.G., Weiner, N.D., Flynn, G.L. and Ho, N.F.H. (1984) Influence of liposomal drug entrapment on percutaneous absorption. *Int. J. Pharm.* **20** 139-154.

Gangarosa, L.P., Park, N.H., Fong, B.C., Scott, D.F. and Hill, J. (1978) Conductivity of drugs used for iontophoresis. *J. Pharm. Sci.* **67** 1439-1443.

Gangarosa, L.P. (1981) Defining a practical solution for iontophoretic local anesthesia of the skin. *Meth. and Find. Exptl. Clin. Pharmacol.* **3** 83-94.

Gesztes, A. and Mezei, M. (1988) Topical anesthesia of the skin by liposome-encapsulated tetracaine. *Anesth. Analg.* **67** 1079-1081.

Green, P.G., Guy, R.H. and Hadgraft, J. (1988) *In vitro* and *in vivo* enhancement of skin penetration with oleic and lauric acids. *Int. J. Pharm.* **48** 103-111.

Groning, R. (1987) Electrophoretically controlled dermal or transdermal application systems with electronic indicators. *Int. J. Pharm.* **36** 37-40.

Habib, M.J. and Rogers, J.A. (1987) Stabilisation of local anaesthetics in liposomes. *Drug. Dev. Ind. Pharm.* **13** 1947-1971.

Habib, M.J. and Rogers, J.A. (1989) Stabilisation of local anaesthetics in liposomes. In: Rubinstein, M.H. (ed.) *Pharmaceutical technology: Drug Stability.* Ellis Horwood, Chichester, pp. 24-39.

Higuchi. T. and Lachman, L. (1955) *J. Am. Pharm. Assoc., Sci. Ed.* **44** 521.

Hori, M., Satoh, S. and Maibach, H.I. (1989) Classification of percutaneous penetration enhancers: A conceptual diagram. In: Bronaugh, R.L. and Maibach, H.I. (eds). *Percutaneous Absorption: Mechanisms, Methodology and Drug Delivery.* Marcel Dekker, New York, pp. 197-209.

Jain, M.K. and Wu, N.M. (1977) Effect of small molecules on the dipalmitoyl lecithin lipid bilayer III. Phase transitions in lipid bilayer. *J. Memb. Biol.* **34** 157-201.

Kleinfeld, J. and Ellis, P.P. (1967) Inhibition of microorganisms by topical anaesthetics. *Appl. Microbiol.* **15** 1296-1298.

Kligman, A.M. (1965) Topical pharmacology and toxicology of dimethylsulphoxide. *J. Amer. Med. Ass.* **193** 140-148.

Kligman, A.M. and Papa, C.M. (1966) *J. Invest. Dermatol.* **47** 1-9.

Labedan, B. (1988) Increase in the permeability of *E. coli* outer membrane by local anesthetics and penetration of antibiotics. *Antimicrob. Agents. Chemother.* **32** 153-155.

Lach, J.L. and Pauli, W.A. (1959) *Drug. Std.* **27** 104.

Lach, J.L. and Chin, T.F. (1964) Schardinger dextrin interaction. IV. Inhibition of hydrolysis by means of molecular complex formation. *J. Pharm. Sci.* **53** 924-931.

Lee, J.A. and Nobles, W.L. (1959) Pharmaceutical applications of the sodium salt of Carbopol 934. *J. Am. Pharm. Ass. Sci. Ed.* **48** 92-94.

Leung, Y-W. and Rawal, B. (1977) Mechanism of action of tetracaine hydrochloride against *Pseudomonas aeruginosa. J. Infect. Dis.* **136** 679-683.

McCafferty, D.F. and Woolfson, A.D. (1988) Percutaneous local anaesthetic composition for topical application and associated method. U. K. Patent 2163956.

McCafferty, D.F. and Woolfson, A.D. (1991) Effect of penetration enhancers on the onset time of percutaneous local anaesthesia. *Int. Pharm. J.* **Suppl. 151** 2.

McCafferty, D.F., Woolfson, A.D., McClelland, K.H. and Boston, V. (1988) Comparative *in vivo* and *in vitro* assessment of the percutaneous absorption of local anaesthetics. *Br. J. Anaesth.* **60** 64-69.

McClelland, K.H. (1986) *Studies on percutaneous local anaesthesia.* Ph.D. thesis. The Queen's University of Belfast.

McElnay, J.C., Mathews, M.P., Harland, R. and McCafferty, D.F. (1985) The effect of ultrasound on the percutaneous absorption of lignocaine. *Br. J. Clin. Pharmacol.* **20** 421-424.

McGowan, K.E. (1990) *Percutaneous local anaesthesia with amethocaine.* Ph.D. thesis. The Queen's University of Belfast.

Mezei, M. and Gulasekharam, V. (1980) Liposomes - a selective drug delivery system for the topical route of administration. I. Lotion dosage form. *Life Sci.* **26** 1473-1477.

Mezei, M. and Gulasekharam, V. (1982) Liposomes - a selective drug delivery system for the topical route of administration: gel dosage form. *J. Pharm. Pharmacol.* **34** 473-474.

Mezei, M. and Nugent, F.J. (1984) Method of encapsulating biologically active materials in multilamellar lipid vesicles. U.S. Patent 4,485,054.

Miller, K.J. Jnr., Rao, Y.K., Shah, D.O. and Goodwin, S.R. (1991a) *In vitro* transdermal diffusional properties of tetracaine from a topical formulation. In: Scott, R.C., Guy, R.H., Hadgraft, J. and Bodde, H.E. (eds) *Prediction of Percutaneous Penetration, Vol. 2.* IBC, London, pp.105-112.

Miller, K.J. Jnr., Westermann-Clark, G.B. and Shah, D.O. (1991b) Quasi-steady-state model for percutaneous absorption of local anaesthetics. In: Scott, R.C., Guy, R.H., Hadgraft, J. and Bodde, H.E. (eds) *Prediction of Percutaneous Penetration, Vol. 2.* IBC, London, pp. 336-349.

Moll, M. (1979) A new approach to pain: Lidocaine and decadron with ultrasound. *U.S.A.F. Med. Serv. Dig.* **30** 8-11.

Novak, E.J. (1964) Experimental transmission of lidocaine through intact skin by ultrasound. *Arch. Phys. Med. Rehab.* **64** 331-332.

Nyqvist-Mayer, A., Brodin, A.F. and Frank, S.G. (1985) Phase distribution studies on an oil-water emulsion based on a eutectic mixture of lidocaine and prilocaine as the dispersed phase. *J. Pharm. Sci.* **74** 1192-1195.

Nyqvist-Mayer, A., Brodin, A.F. and Frank, S.G. (1986) Drug release studies on an oil-water emulsion based on a eutectic mixture of lidocaine and prilocaine as the dispersed phase. *J. Pharm. Sci.* **75** 365-373.

Ohki, S. (1970) Effects of local anesthetics on phospholipid bilayers. *Biochim. Biophys. Acta.* **219** 1827.

Ohlsen, L. and Englesson, S. (1980) New anaesthetic formulation for epicutaneous application tested for cutting split skin grafts. *Br. J. Anaesth.* **52** 413-417.

Okabe, K., Yamaguchi, H. and Kawai, Y. (1986) New iontophoretic transdermal administration of the beta blocker metoprolol. *J. Cont. Rel.* **4** 79-85.

Pena, L.E. (1990) Gel dosage forms: Theory, formulation and processing. In: Osborne, D.W and Amann, A.H. (eds). *Topical drug delivery formulations.* Marcel Dekker, New York, pp. 381-388.

Petelenz, T., Axenti, I., Petelenz, T.J., Iwinski, J. and Dubel, S. (1984) Mini set for iontophoresis for topical analgesia before injection. *Int. J. Clin. Pharmacol. Ther. Toxicol.* **22** 152-155.

Pettersson, L.O. (1978) Percutaneous anaesthesia for some minor surgical procedures. *Scand. J. Plastic Reconstruct. Surg.* **12** 283-286.

Pettersson, L. and Strombeck, J.O. (1978) Percutaneous anaesthesia for dermabrasion. *Scand. J. Plast. Reconstr. Surg.* **12** 287-290.

Ponten, B. and Ohlsen, L. (1977) Skin surface application of ketocaine to provide local anaesthesia for cutting split skin grafts. *Brit. J. Plastic Surgery* **30** 251-254.

Powell, D.M., Rodeheaver, G.T., Foresman, P.A., Hankins, C.L., Bellian, K.T., Zimmer, C.A., Becker, D.G. and Edlich, R.F. (1991) Damage to tissue defenses by EMLA cream. *J. Emerg. Med.* **9** 205-209.

Rapperport, A.S., Larson, D.L., Hengel, D.F., Lynch, J.B., Blocker, T.G. and Lewis, R.S. (1965) Iontophoresis: A method of antibiotic administration in the burn patient. *Plastic Reconstruct. Surg.* **36** 547-552.

Rosendal, T. (1942) Studies on the conducting properties of the human skin to direct current. *Acta Physiol. Scand.* **5** 130.

Russo, J., Lipmann, A.G., Comstock, T.J., Page, B.C. and Stephen, R.L. (1980) Lignocaine anaesthesia: Comparison of iontophoresis, injection and swabbing. *Dermatol. Scand.* **60** 544-546.

Salt, W.G. and Traynor, J.R. (1979) Interactions between amethocaine and non-growing cultures of *Escherichia coli*. *J. Pharm. Pharmacol.* **31** 41-42.

Sasaki, H., Kojima, M., Yoshiyuki, M., Nakamura, J. and Shibaski, J. (1988) Enhancing effect of pyrrolidone derivatives on transdermal drug delivery. *Int. J. Pharm.* **44** 15-24.

Schaeffer, H.E. and Krohn, D.L. (1982) Liposomes in topical drug delivery. *Invest. Opthalmol. Vis. Sci.* **22** 220-227.

Schmidt, R.M. and Rosenkranz, H.S. (1970) Antimicrobial activity of local anaesthetics: lidocaine and prilocaine. *J. Infect. Dis.* **121** 597-607.

Siddiqui, O., Roberts, M.S. and Polack, A.E. (1985) The effect of iontophoresis and vehicle pH on the *in vitro* permeation of lignocaine through human stratum corneum. *J. Pharm. Pharmacol.* **37** 732-735.

Silva, M.T., Sousa, J.C.F., Polonia, J.J. and Macedo, P.M. (1979) Effects of local anesthetics on bacterial cells. *J. Bacteriol.* **137** 461-468.

Sipos, T. (1980) Topical medicaments. U.K. patent 1, 569, 424.

Sisler, H.A. (1978) Iontophoretic local anesthesia for conjunctival surgery. *Ann. Ophthalmol.* **10** 597-598.

Southwell, D. and Barry, B.W. (1983) Penetration enhancers for human skin: Mode of action of 2-pyrrolidone and dimethylformamide on partition and diffusion of model compounds, water, n-alcohols and caffeine. *J. Invest. Dermatol.* **80** 507-514.

Stoughton, R.B. (1982) Enhanced percutaneous penetration with 1-dodecylazacycloheptan-2-one. *Arch. Dermatol.* **118** 474-477.

Stoughton, R.B. and McClure, W.O. (1983) Azone®: A new non-toxic enhancer of cutaneous penetration. *Drug. Dev. Ind. Pharm.* **9** 725-744.

Uster, P.S. (1990) Liposome-based vehicles for topical delivery. In: Osborne, D.W. and Amann, A.H. (eds). *Topical Drug Delivery Formulations.* Marcel Dekker, New York, pp. 327-348.

Walters, K.A. (1989) Penetration enhancers and their use in transdermal therapeutic systems. In: Hadgraft, J. and Guy, R.H. (eds). *Transdermal Drug Delivery.* Marcel Dekker, New York, pp. 197-246.

Ward, A.I.J. and Tallon, R. (1988) Penetration enhancer incorporation in bilayers. *Drug. Dev. Ind. Pharm.* **14** 1155-1166.

Weinstein, M.P., Maderazo, E., Tilton, R., Maggini, G. and Quintiliani, R. (1975) Further observations on the antimicrobial effects of local anaesthetic agents. *Curr. Ther. Res.* **17** 369-374.

Wiechers, J.W. and De Zeeuw, R.A. (1990) Transdermal drug delivery: Efficacy and potential applications of the penetration enhancer Azone®. *Drug. Des. Del.* **6** 87-100.

Wong, O., Huntington, J., Nishihata, T. and Rytting, J.H. (1989) New alkyl N,N-dialkyl-substituted amino acetates as transdermal penetration enhancers. *Pharm. Res.* **6** 286-295.

Woodford, R. and Barry, B.W. (1986) Percutaneous enhancers and percutaneous absorption of drugs: An update. *J. Toxicol.- Cut. Ocul. Toxicol.* **5** 165-175.

Woolfson, A.D. and McCafferty, D.F. (1988) Preparation of amethocaine-containing unit-dose film compositions for percutaneous local anaesthesia, and process for their application. PCT Int. Appl. WO 8809169.

Woolfson, A.D., McCafferty, D.F., McClelland, K.H. and Boston, V. (1988) Concentration-response analysis of percutaneous local anaesthetic formulations. *Brit. J. Anaesth.* **61** 589-592.

Woolfson, A.D., McCafferty, D.F. and McGowan, K.E. (1991) Differential scanning calorimetry of a novel amethocaine preparation and its effect on human stratum corneum. *Proc. 10th. Pharm. Tech. Conf.*, Bologna, Italy, pp. 405-423.

Wurster, D.E. and Kramer, S.F. (1961) Investigation of some factors influencing percutaneous absorption. *J. Pharm. Sci.* **50** 288-293.

Zaidi, S. and Healy, T.E.J. (1977) A comparison of the antibacterial properties of six local anaesthetic agents. *Anaesthesia* **32** 69-70.

6

Clinical applications of percutaneous local anaesthesia

Many people, especially children, have a horror of needles. This combination of fear and pain can make the insertion of intravenous needles and cannulae a traumatic experience. Some children may have to be restrained, a distressing experience for parents, nurses, doctors and the child. In one study hospitalised children, aged 4 - 10 years, were asked what, of all the things that had ever happened to them, had hurt the most. Of those responding to this enquiry 55% (65 of 119) perceived an injection to be more painful than even the events leading up to their admission (Elland and Anderson, 1977).

The insertion of a needle can take many forms such as venepuncture, lumbar puncture, arterial cannulation, haemodialysis cannulation and i.v. catheterisation. Percutaneous local anaesthesia offers a means of eliminating or substantially reducing the pain associated with these procedures. Of course, there are many cases where adults can also benefit from this type of pain relief. The clinical applications of percutaneous local anaesthesia are therefore not restricted solely to children, nor are they applicable simply to those procedures involving some form of needle insertion. Indeed, an increasing variety of clinical uses for percutaneous local anaesthesia has now been reported, extending the value of the method to many minor surgical procedures.

6.1   VENEPUNCTURE IN CHILDREN

Fear and pain can make the insertion of intravenous needles in children a traumatic experience. The insertion technique itself is described in detail by Spitz and Thomas (1992). Intravenous induction of general anaesthesia in paediatric practice, even by experienced paediatric anaesthetists, may produce severe distress and lead to the development of "needle-phobia". This is particularly so where the child requires subsequent repeat surgery. The problem is not completely solved by the use of a fine needle or by the administration of opiate premedication.

Reducing the pain of venepuncture in children at induction of anaesthesia has been investigated by Cooper *et al.* (1987). In a double-blind, randomised trial, 40 children, aged from three to thirteen years, were assessed for the reduction of pain and the technical difficulty of venepuncture. All were to undergo day case surgery under general anaesthesia. A percutaneous local anaesthetic cream (EMLA®) and a placebo preparation were applied for at least one hour over an area of 2 cm². About 2 g of cream were applied to the dorsum of one hand and covered with an adhesive plastic dressing. A fine 25-gauge butterfly needle was used for venepuncture.

Pain assessment in the study was by four methods. The patient used a verbal rating scale and a visual analogue scale, and the anaesthetist employed a four-category observation scale and a visual analogue scale (Table 6.1). A subjective assessment was made by the anaesthetist of the actual technical difficulty of venepuncture compared with that which would be expected in a particular patient. This was graded as easier, the same or harder than expected. Account was taken of subjective factors such as ease of location of the vein, reflex movements and general behavioural status of the patient.

Table 6.1 — Patient and observer assessment scales for pain due to venepuncture

Patient assessment scales		Observer assessment scales	
Verbal Rating	Linear Analogue	Observer Rating	Linear Analogue
1 Did not hurt	10 cm horizontal	1 No reaction	10 cm horizontal
2 Hurt a little	line labelled at one	2 Slight reaction	line labelled at one
3 Hurt quite a lot	end "no pain" and	and minor	end "no reaction"
4 Hurt very much	at the other "very	movement	and at the other
	bad pain"	3 Moderate	"marked distress"
		reaction	
		and verbal protest	
		4 Marked distress	

Reproduced from Cooper *et al.* (1987) with permission of the copyright holder, Blackwell Scientific Publications Ltd

Two groups, each of twenty children, were used in the study with one group receiving percutaneous local anaesthesia and the other placebo. The percutaneous anaesthesia group experienced significantly less pain than the placebo group using all four methods of pain assessments. When assessed by patient verbal rating and observer rating scales the effect of age on pain scores approached significance. Generally, older children recorded lower pain scores, although this was not the case when visual analogue scales were used.

Significantly more venepunctures were recorded as easier than expected in the percutaneous anaesthesia group, though this finding may have been influenced by the

Table 6.2 — Assessment of the technical difficulty of venepuncture with, and without, percutaneous local anaesthesia

treatment	easier than expected	the same as expected	more difficult than expected
percutaneous local anaesthesia (n = 20)	17	3	0
Placebo (n = 20)	9	11	0

The figures are the number of replies in each category.

Reproduced from Cooper *et al.* (1987) with permission of the copyright holder, Blackwell Scientific Publications Ltd

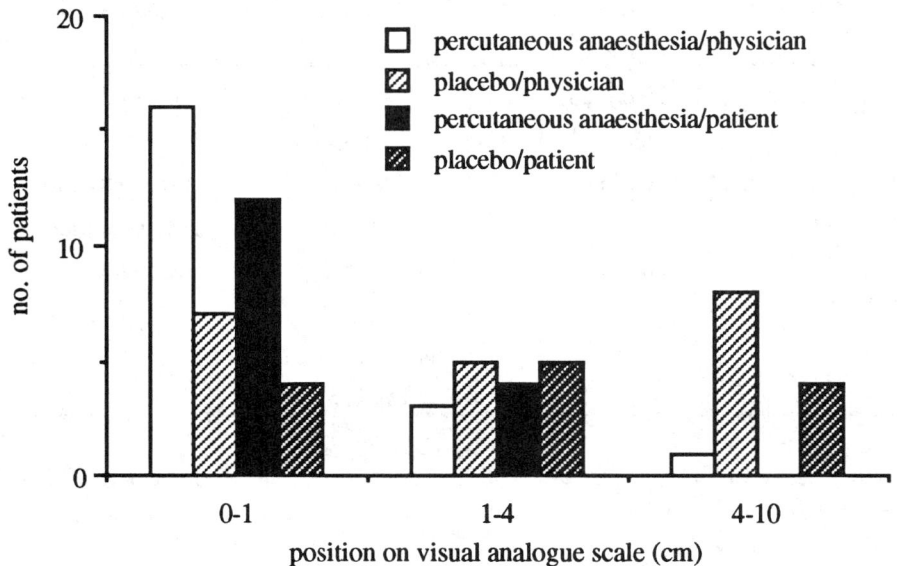

Fig. 6.1 — Number of patients recorded in each section of the physician's or patient's visual analogue scale (VAS) following venepuncture with percutaneous local anaesthesia or placebo pretreatment. Data from Cooper *et al.* (1987)

fine gauge of the needle used in the study (Table 6.2). The percutaneous anaesthetic group felt significantly less pain from the procedure than the placebo group (Fig. 6.1). This was true for all four pain assessment scales. The only local reaction noted was pallor, which was recorded by some patients in both groups with no statistically significant difference between them.

The study by Cooper *et al.* (1987) considered children over three years old. Hopkins *et al.* (1988) considered 120 children, in the age group from one to five years, in an otherwise similar study using percutaneous local anaesthesia prior to intravenous induction of general anaesthesia. The study was a randomised, double-blind comparison of percutaneous local anaesthesia with EMLA® cream, applied to 80 children, versus placebo, which was received by the remaining 40 participants. Some children received premedication administered one hour pre-operatively and consisting of a mixture of mefenamic acid 8.3 mg ml^{-1}, trimeprazine 1.0 mg ml^{-1} and atropine 30 µg ml^{-1} in a dose of 1.0 ml kg^{-1}. The cream was applied to the dorsum of the hand and covered with an occlusive dressing for at least 30 minutes prior to each operation. The emotional state of the child was assessed on a visual analogue scale (VAS) from asleep (0) to agitated (100). Venepuncture was performed using a fine 27-gauge needle. The operating department assistant assessed the child's reaction at the moment of venepuncture using a visual rating system (VRS) which had four points ranging from no pain to severe pain. The VAS was statistically analysed using the Wilcoxon rank sum test and the VRS with a chi-square test.

Of the percutaneous local anaesthetic group, 32% had been premedicated, as had 39% of the placebo group. There was no statistical difference between those patients who received either premedication or no premedication, with reference to condition on arrival in theatre between the active and placebo groups as determined by VAS comparison. There was a statistically significant difference within each group between those patients who had been premedicated and those who had not, as might be expected. The premedicated group also had lower pain scores with both VAS and VRS assessments.

Pretreatment with the percutaneous local anaesthetic was found to result in significantly less subjectively assessed pain on venepuncture (Fig. 6.2). Separate analysis of premedicated and unpremedicated subgroups also revealed a similar reduction in assessed pain (Fig. 6.3). In common with Cooper *et al.* (1987) pretreatment with a percutaneous local anaesthetic was found to significantly reduce noxious stimulation due to venepuncture. This was beneficial to children from one year upwards, and, consequently, also to the anaesthetist. Hopkins *et al.* (1988) recommended an application time of at least 30 minutes for children under four years, 60 minutes application for children from four to seventeen years and 45 minutes for adults. This differs from most other studies using EMLA® and may have been a consequence of relying on observer rather than patient assessment of pain. The authors concluded that percutaneous local anaesthesia should form part of the pre-operative preparation of every child who is to undergo intravenous induction of general anaesthesia, as well as other procedures such as the insertion of intravenous cannulae or venous blood sampling.

Ehrenstrom-Reiz and Reiz (1982) investigated percutaneous local anaesthesia with EMLA® and a placebo preparation using a group of 60 children with an age range of 6-15 years. The site was again the dorsum of the hand with an application time of approximately one hour under occlusion. The scheduled treatment was either intravenous general anaesthesia or intravenous cannulation for fluid or drug therapy. Pain was

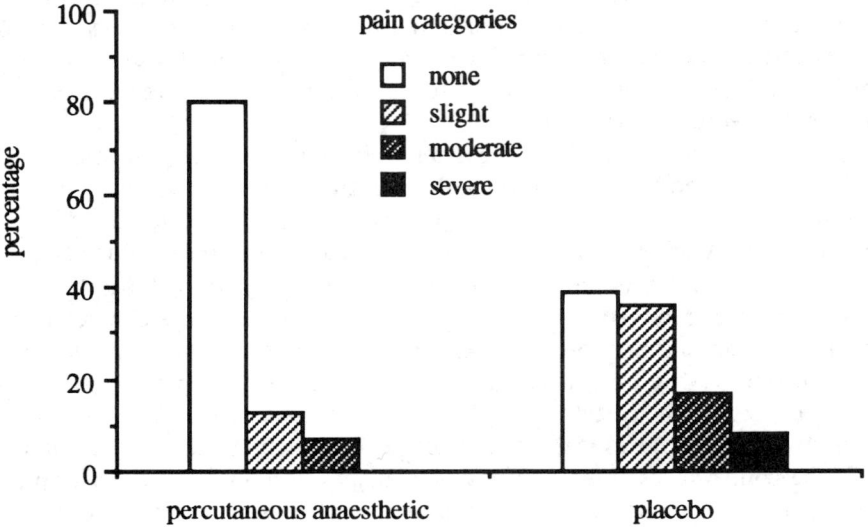

Fig. 6.2 — Comparison of verbal rating pain scale (VRS) scores for all patients, percutaneous local anaesthetic treated versus placebo treated. Reproduced from Hopkins *et al.* (1988) with permission of the copyright holder, Academic Press Inc. (London) Ltd

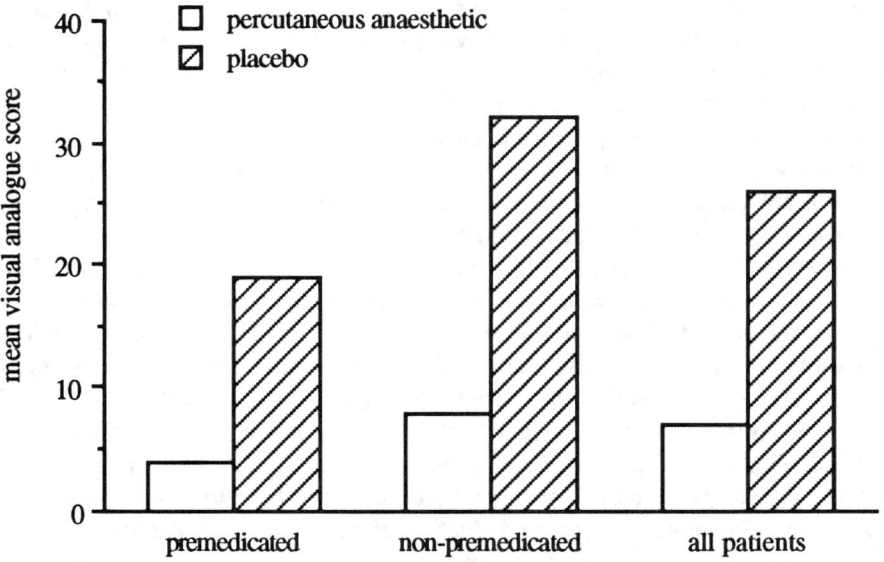

Fig. 6.3 — Mean visual analogue scale (VAS) scores for percutaneous anaesthetic and placebo groups subdivided into premedicated and medicated groups. Reproduced from Hopkins *et al.* (1988) with permission of the copyright holder, Academic Press Inc. (London) Ltd

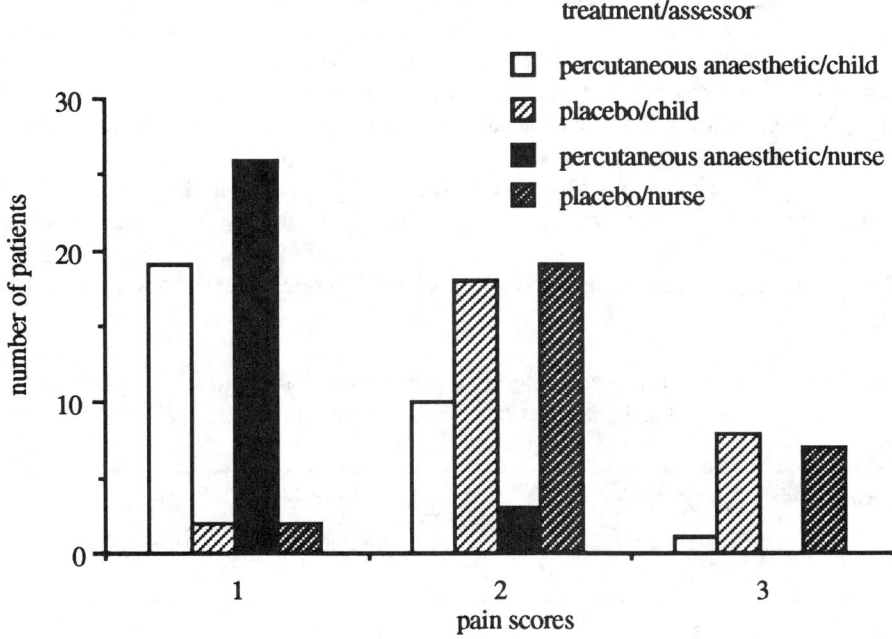

Fig. 6.4 — Pain scores judged by (i) children treated with a percutaneous local anaesthetic or placebo prior to venous cannulation and (ii) by the nurse inserting the catheter. Data from Ehrenstrom-Reiz and Reiz (1982)

evaluated by the child on a scale of 1 (no pain), 2 (slight to moderate pain) or 3 (painful to very painful). The nurse anaesthetist evaluated the child's reaction to cannulation according to the same scale and all results (Fig. 6.4) were evaluated statistically by a non-parametric hypothesis test.

The difference in recorded pain scores between the treated and untreated groups was statistically significant. The judgement of the nurse was slightly more favourable than that of the children with the active treatment, whereas both judgements were in agreement when the placebo was used. No pain was experienced by 63% of children on venous cannulation with percutaneous anaesthetic pretreatment. In the placebo group the corresponding figure was 10%. Numerically, this comprised only 3 children, one of whom was heavily premedicated. Slight pain was felt in 33% of the percutaneous anaesthetic group. This was described as a dull discomfort or pain due to penetration of the subcutaneous tissue or venous wall rather than to the penetration of the skin. The study concluded that the side effects of EMLA® were few and that pretreatment with this percutaneous local anaesthetic preparation can effectively reduce the pain associated with venous cannulation in children.

Wahlstedt *et al.* (1984) investigated the use of percutaneous anaesthesia for venepuncture at the cubital fossa rather than the dorsum of the hand. The number of children considered was 60, aged from five to fifteen years. An active preparation (EMLA®) and a placebo were used in this double-blind study. Pain was assessed by staff, for ease of venepuncture, and patients, for evaluation of severity. Differences were tested by a non-parametric hypothesis test, with the results shown in Table 6.3. Although a different treatment site was used in this study, staff again judged venepuncture to be easier when the child had been pretreated with the percutaneous anaesthetic preparation. The size of needle used in the procedure, an important factor in the severity of pain experienced, was not stated.

Most studies designed to evaluate the efficacy of percutaneous local anaesthesia at preventing or reducing pain due to venepuncture are of double-blind design using a placebo preparation. Although this is sound clinical experimental practice, percutaneous local anaesthesia is often used in place of intradermal lignocaine infiltration. Soliman *et*

Table 6.3 — Assessment of venepuncture at the cubital fossa with either percutaneous local anaesthetic or placebo pretreatment

descriptor	percutaneous anaesthetic (n = 25)	placebo (n = 26)
male/female	9/16	12/14
median age (and range) (yr)	13 (9-17)	13 (8-17)
median application time (and range) (min)	75 (55-135)	75 (60-130)
Child's rating of pain		
none	16	2
slight	9	23 (P < 0.001)
severe	0	1
Staff rating of ease of procedure		
easier	13	5
as usual	12	19 (P< 0.01)
more difficult	0	2
Adverse effects		
oedema	0	0
redness	8	1 (P < 0.01)
paleness	3	1

Reproduced from Wahlstedt *et al.* (1984) with permission of the copyright holder, The Lancet Ltd

al. (1988) considered whether EMLA® was more effective than lignocaine infiltration prior to venous cannulation in awake, unpremedicated children. The test site was the dorsum of the non-dominant hand in children aged from seven to twelve years. The topical treatment was applied under occlusion for 60 minutes. The alternative pretreatment was infiltration with 0.2 ml of 1% lignocaine (skin weal) using a 30 gauge needle. All venepunctures were performed by the same investigator. The patient's response was assessed first during the performance of a skin "nick" using the bevel of a 19-gauge needle and again during i.v. cannulation using a 20 gauge catheter in all cases. An anaesthetist and an independent observer assessed the child using a VAS (0-10). The cooperation of the child was noted on a 5 point scale from 1 (restraint) to 5 (crying) and the resultant data were analysed by Spearman's rank correlation test The results of this study (Table 6.4) showed that children in both groups rated their pain and discomfort significantly higher than the anaesthetist or the observer.

Table 6.4 — Comparison of percutaneous local anaesthesia and intradermal lignocaine infiltration for pain relief during i.v. cannulation

assessment	pain score percutaneous anaesthetic (n = 20)	pain score intradermal infiltration (n = 20)
Child		
median	3.0	3.5
range	(0-10)	(0-10)
Anaesthetist		
median	0.5	1.0
range	(0-8)	(0-8)
Observer		
median	0.5	0.5
range	(0-8)	(0-8)

Reproduced from Soliman *et al.* (1988) with permission of the copyright holder, J. P. Lippincott Co.

Interestingly, in this particular study the degree of cooperation of the child with the procedure, as determined by the observer, showed a poor correlation (r = 0.43) with the degree of pain perceived by the child. Cooperation did not improve with lower pain scores. Itching and transient blanching were observed in 7 patients, though both problems resolved spontaneously. A further practical observation concerned the greasy quality retained by the skin after removal of EMLA®. This made it slightly difficult to apply adhesive tape to the skin and required special care in securing the i.v. catheter. Percutaneous anaesthesia was found to be equally effective with traditional skin weal infiltration. However, in unpremedicated children, cooperation did not improve with the attainment of a pain-free state. This adds further emphasis to the significance of the emotional component of pain anticipation which children associate with needles and venepuncture.

Intravenous induction of anaesthesia is often chosen by older children and teenagers who prefer onset of sleep to the slower induction provided by inhaled anaesthetics. Intravenous induction is also preferred in children who need emergency surgery and are thought to have a full stomach. EMLA® was effective if occluded for 1 hour, but the prolonged application period probably makes the use of this particular product unsuitable in an emergency situation. Soliman *et al.* (1988) did conclude that percutaneous local anaesthesia was appropriate for ensuring pain-free i.v. cannulation in children who are scheduled for elective surgery. The prolonged application period required with EMLA® can, however, present a problem, even in an elective situation, in the event of an unsuccessful i.v. cannulation at a prepared site. Since waiting for a further hour to prepare a second site is not practical, the initial pretreatment of two possible cannulation sites would therefore seem advisable.

Most clinical studies on percutaneous local anaesthesia have tended to involve relatively small numbers of patients. However, a much larger open study on the use of this technique for the prevention of venepuncture pain in children has been reported by Woolfson *et al.* (1990). A total of 1241 children up to the age of sixteen were involved in this trial. The percutaneous anaesthetic preparation was derived from the amethocaine phase-change system. Each patient received 500 mg of this percutaneous anaesthetic with an application period of 30 minutes. The presence of anaesthesia was confirmed in some cases by pin-prick prior to performing the venepuncture.

Given the open nature of the study and large-scale routine clinical use of the percutaneous anaesthetic preparation, pain classification was necessarily based on a simple system of no pain (a score of 1), minimal sensation (2), moderate pain (3) and severe pain corresponding to no anaesthesia (4). Scores of 1 and 2 were taken to represent successful anaesthesia and scores of 3 and 4 were classified as failure of the technique. The detailed statistical analysis of the data was by the chi-square test and the effect of a number of variables on the efficacy of the procedure was investigated. These were patient sex and age, application time, and hospital unit. The latter variable was included since initial evidence suggested that training and experience of clinical staff in the procedure was of some significance to its successful outcome. Some patients received more than one application of the percutaneous anaesthetic. Consequently, statistical analysis of the data, summarised in Table 6.5, was performed with both the inclusion and exclusion of repeat data.

On analysis of the data, 879 cases (70.8%) reported no pain on or following venepuncture and 222 cases recorded a minimal sensation (17.9%), this latter being almost certainly due to the actual pressure on the skin exerted by the needle. Thus, 88.7% of all cases recorded satisfactory anaesthesia to the procedure. Of the remainder 86 cases (6.9%) experienced moderate pain and 54 (4.4%) had no apparent pain relief.

There were rather more males in the study than females, but there was no significant difference between the sexes with respect to anaesthetic efficacy. However, the age of the child did prove to be statistically significant when this factor was tested against efficacy. Subsequent investigation of the data demonstrated that this was due entirely to the inclusion of results from the 0-2 age group, some 68 cases. There was no significant difference in data from any of the older age groups. It is, perhaps, not surprising that very young children appear to benefit less from percutaneous local anaesthesia, given the trauma of hospitalisation and the inherent difficulties of pain assessment. A child of this age may well show distress counting as failure of the technique, but such distress may be present in any case, even in the absence of venepuncture or other painful procedures. Nevertheless, even in this very young age group, 82% of cases were judged to have satisfactory anaesthesia to venepuncture.

Table 6.5 — Effect of variables on the efficacy of percutaneous local anaesthesia with the amethocaine phase-change system to venepuncture challenge in children

| | significance (chi-square) | |
| | inclusion of repeat | exclusion of repeat |
test	applications	applications
efficacy vs. sex	$0.5 < P \leq 0.7$	$0.7 < P \leq 0.8$
efficacy vs. age	$0.02 < P \leq 0.05$	$0.05 < P \leq 0.1$
efficacy vs. application time	$P \leq 0.001$	$0.001 < P \leq 0.01$
efficacy vs. hospital unit	$P \leq 0.001$	$P \leq 0.001$

Modified from Woolfson *et al.* (1990)

Application time is of prime importance with percutaneous local anaesthetic preparations. Clinical convenience dictates as short a time as possible but efficacy requires a minimum period to be established. In the case of the amethocaine phase-change system, a 30 minute regimen in children was recommended. In clinical practice, this was frequently not adhered to, a real and important difference from results obtained with carefully controlled clinical trials. Application periods varying from less than 20 minutes to greater than 120 minutes were recorded, a practical test of the ruggedness of the procedure. Application period had a significant effect on anaesthetic efficacy but this was due entirely to inclusion of data from application periods less than 20 minutes. Although a 20 minute application time is less than that recommended for the amethocaine phase-change system, almost 70% of applications produced successful anaesthesia even within this short time. This observation, compared to those from adult volunteer trials on the same preparation (McCafferty *et al.*, 1989), suggested that this preparation acts more rapidly in children than in adults, where the mean onset time for anaesthesia was about 40 minutes. The main effect of increasing the application period is to increase the duration of anaesthesia (McCafferty *et al.*, 1989).

The analysis of the anaesthetic efficacy reported by different hospital units using the procedure was designed to allow for the different number of applications made by each unit and therefore the differences in experience gained by the relevant nursing staff. There was a trend towards an increased reported anaesthetic efficacy in those units which made the greatest use of the procedure, reflecting an increased experience both in using the preparation and gauging the reaction of the child to venepuncture challenge. Interestingly, trials on adult volunteers with the amethocaine phase-change system confirm a 100% anaesthetic efficacy with this preparation compared with an overall efficacy of 90% obtained with children in a real clinical situation. It seems likely, given the trauma and anxiety associated with hospital, together with previous painful experiences and the use of perceived threatening equipment such as needles, that there will always be a small but finite percentage failure with percutaneous local anaesthetic preparations in children. This failure will be psychological rather than physical in origin, but its extent can be substantially reduced by staff taking time to reassure both child and parents. In one paediatric outpatient department the procedure is described to the child in terms of the application of a "magic" cream which will make the procedure less painful. Arguably, the child should not be told that the procedure will be totally painless since, in the event of failure due, for example, to an insufficient application period, the child may feel betrayed and may harbour a continuing mistrust of medical and nursing staff. (Spitz and Thomas, 1992).

6.2   VENEPUNCTURE IN ADULTS

Although the initial interest in the clinical applications of percutaneous local anaesthesia was largely confined to children, it was soon realised that many adults also have a pronounced fear of procedures involving the use of needles. Hallen *et al.* (1985) investigated the efficiency of percutaneous local anaesthesia in preventing the pain of venepuncture in adults. The study was double-blind, randomised and of crossover design with a placebo preparation and EMLA®. Each volunteer received five applications of the active formulation and three of the placebo, under occlusion, at the cubital fossa or, as a second choice, the dorsum of the hand, prior to venous blood sampling. The application time was one hour and the clinical procedure was i.v. cannulation. Pain was assessed using a VAS (0-100 mm). Local reactions were noted on a four point scale as none, slight, moderate, or severe and the results were analysed by the Wilcoxon signed rank test.

The median age of volunteers in this study was thirty-one years and the range, eighteen to forty-eight years. Of 220 applications, 81% were in the cubital fossa, 15% on the dorsum of the hand and 4% on the lower arm. The number of volunteers who received the active treatment was 140 with 80 patients receiving the placebo. The percutaneous local anaesthetic was superior to placebo in all but 3 volunteers in whom both preparations produced similar effects. The pain scores were scattered (Fig. 6.5) but the majority of those treated with the percutaneous anaesthetic were near the "no pain" end of the scale. This treatment resulted in significantly lower mean pain scores compared to placebo.

Transient local skin reactions for both percutaneous local anaesthetic and placebo preparations consisted of skin blanching, erythema and oedema in a few patients. The reactions were almost equally distributed between the two treatment groups and did not increase in severity with repeated application. The study concluded that percutaneous

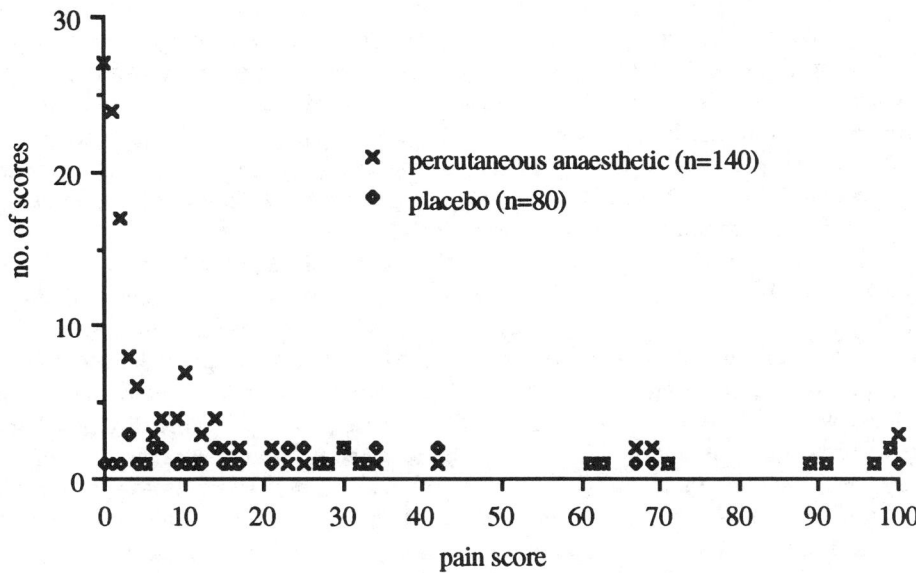

Fig. 6.5 — Scattergram of pain scores recorded by adult volunteers using a visual
analogue scale (VAS). The procedure used was i.v. cannulation following
pretreatment with a percutaneous local anaesthetic preparation or a placebo. Data
from Hallen *et al.* (1985)

local anaesthetic pretreatment of the site substantially decreased the pain produced by
routine venous cannulation in adults. As a consequence, the first experience of an
anxious patient in the operating room need no longer be that of a painful venepuncture.

The time delay between initial application and onset of skin anaesthesia following
the application of a percutaneous local anaesthetic preparation is obviously a major
drawback with this method of pain relief, particularly when the procedure has not been
anticipated. In the case of EMLA® this time delay is generally one hour. Nott and
Peacock (1990), in an attempt to dramatically shorten this period, used inunction
(rubbing in) with EMLA® cream, which was applied only 5 minutes before
venepuncture. The study consisted of 120 patients due for morning blood tests. There
were four treatment groups. In one group the percutaneous anaesthetic was applied
conventionally to either convenient anticubital fossa under an occlusive dressing for 60
minutes. Another group received the percutaneous anaesthetic at the same site.
However, in this case the preparation was rubbed into the skin and the elbow flexed for
five minutes. A third group received a placebo preparation in an otherwise identical
treatment and the final group had no treatment prior to venepuncture. Patients were
asked to assess needle puncture pain on a 10 cm line marked "no pain" (0) and "severe
pain" (10). They were also asked to assess any pain as "none", "slight", "moderate" or
"severe". The results (Table 6.6) were examined by analysis of variance of the
transformed linear scores (logarithm of [score + 1]), and by a less detailed examination of
the verbal ratings.

Pain was found to decrease from no previous treatment, recording the highest pain score, through placebo to treatment with the active preparation which was applied for both 5 minutes and, finally, for 60 minutes. Needle puncture following the 5 minute application was significantly less painful than either the placebo or no treatment. The apparent response to placebo only was not significantly different from no treatment. The active preparation was effective whether the needles used for venepuncture were large or small. Not surprisingly, patients who had the largest needles (18 gauge) reported the most pain while those who were subjected to the smallest needle size (22 gauge) reported the least pain, the difference being statistically significant.

Age also affected pain perception in this study. Male patients were aged from eighteen to eighty-six years (mean sixty-six years) and females from nineteen to ninety-four years (mean sixty-four years). The youngest and oldest patients reported the most pain, while those in between reported the least. This effect was significant and was not due to a biased needle allocation. Also, male patients reported less pain than female patients with median pain scores of 0.9 and 1.3 respectively. This difference was significant ($P = 0.02$). Of the male patients, 52% stated that they felt no pain, compared with 40% of female patients. Left-handed patients reported less pain than those who were right-handed and less pain was reported by 57 patients in whom the non-dominant side was used compared with 63 patients in whom venepuncture was carried out on the dominant side. However, these results, although interesting, were not clinically significant. The study concluded that EMLA® cream was effective when applied 5 minutes prior to venepuncture. It is likely that a combination of inunction and vigorous movement at the site promoted some degree of percutaneous absorption of the local anaesthetics compared to the normal passive application. In general, however, a 60 minutes application time still produced superior results and is probably required to ensure reliable and effective pain relief.

One of the more unusual combinations prior to venepuncture is local application of a percutaneous anaesthetic (EMLA®) and glyceryl trinitrate (GTN) as a 2% ointment,

Table 6.6 — Median combined pain scores on a linear scale from adult patients receiving a percutaneous anaesthetic (EMLA®) for 5 or 60 minutes, placebo (5 minutes) or nil treatment. The procedure in all cases was venepuncture

treatment	needle size 22 g	needle size 20 g	needle size 18 g	all
PA 60	0.3	0.2	1.2	0.4
PA 5	0.4	0.5	1.1	1.0
placebo 5	0.8	1.4	2.3	1.9
nil	1.6	1.2	2.8	2.3
all	0.5	0.9	1.9	

Key: PA 60 - percutaneous anaesthetic preparation for 60 minutes
          PA 5 - percutaneous anaesthetic preparation for 5 minutes

Reproduced from Nott *et al.* (1990) with permission of the copyright holder, Academic Press Inc. (London) Ltd

reported by Gunawardene *et al.* (1990). GTN causes local vasodilation which is thought to facilitate venepuncture. Adult patients (a total of 100 with an age range of twenty-seven to sixty-eight years) who were to undergo day care surgical procedures, were entered into a double-blind and randomised study. No patient was premedicated and each patient was randomly allocated to one of four groups receiving the percutaneous anaesthetic/GTN combination, a placebo, a percutaneous anaesthetic only or GTN ointment only. The percutaneous anaesthetic was conventionally applied in all cases for one hour before a 23-gauge butterfly needle was inserted prior to induction of anaesthesia. A tourniquet was applied above the wrist. The patient evaluated pain using a verbal rating scale of 1 to 10. The anaesthetist evaluated the venepuncture subjectively as very easy, usual, difficult or very difficult. Data was analysed by the Kruskal-Wallis test for non-parametric data.

Results from this study demonstrated highly significant differences between the groups with respect to both pain scores and ease of venepuncture. Further, an analysis of the pain scores demonstrated that the differences between EMLA® alone and EMLA®/GTN were not statistically significant from each other. However, the data from these two groups were statistically different from the placebo and GTN-only groups. Ease of venepuncture data revealed no significant difference between the EMLA®/GTN group and GTN alone.

Vasoconstriction of the skin has been suggested as the cause of pallor after EMLA® applications, but only 2 out of 25 patients in the EMLA®/GTN group showed pallor in this study. The blanching, it was suggested, could be caused by moisture under the occlusive dressing. Also, anxiety and cold weather (the study was performed in the winter) could contribute to the pallor. Patients who received GTN/EMLA® or GTN ointment had warm hands with prominent veins. Lower pain scores and easier venepuncture were achieved with EMLA®/GTN when this treatment was applied to the dorsum of the hand. The technique may have some value in patients where there is a likelihood of particular difficulty in performing a venepuncture.

6.3 PERCUTANEOUS LOCAL ANAESTHESIA WITH PREMEDICATION

Given the psychological aspects to venepuncture pain, particularly in very young children, there is some merit in considering the use of a premedication sedative in combination with a percutaneous local anaesthetic. Page and Morgan-Hughes (1990) considered whether triclofos sodium (70 mg/kg), in combination with percutaneous local anaesthesia and a reassuring parental presence, altered the frequency of calm behaviour in young children before induction anaesthesia. Although trimeprazine is generally favoured in the UK for premedication, it is documented as increasing the frequency of crying and struggling at induction. Benzodiazepines are widely used for sedation preoperatively in children but the authors found that triclofos produced more satisfactory behaviour at induction than either diazepam or flunitrazepam.

Children aged from one to five years were recruited into this study. They were scheduled for general, genito-urinary, plastic, orthopaedic, ophthalmic or dental surgery under general anaesthesia as day cases or in-patients. Premedication was allocated randomly and consisted of either atropine or triclofos (100 mg) with atropine. Both solutions were similar in taste and appearance and each was administered orally 90 minutes before the operation. A percutaneous anaesthetic (EMLA®) was applied to the dorsum of the hand.

The child's demeanour on arrival in the anaesthetic room was variously described as sleepy, cheerful, serious, apprehensive, tearful or noisy. The responses to intravenous induction were described as no response, winced, whimpered, cried or violent. Inhalation induction was described as smooth, minor objection or needed restrained. Behavioural results were analysed by a chi-square test, with both premedication and recovery times analysed by an unpaired t-test. The triclofos group contained 128 children and the placebo group had 135 children. The only significant difference occurred in respect of the frequency of unsatisfactory demeanour in the triclofos group, which was half that in the placebo group. More children were sleepy in the triclofos group, but this did not appear to influence the anaesthetist's choice of method of induction since equal numbers of intravenous inductions were performed in each group. The frequency of unsatisfactory response to induction was lower in the triclofos group both for intravenous and inhalation induction (Table 6.7).

Table 6.7 — Number of patients responding satisfactorily to intravenous induction following treatment with a percutaneous anaesthetic with or without premedication - comparison with inhalation induction

response	triclofos premedication	placebo
intravenous induction		
satisfactory		
no response	59	53
winced	14	10
unsatisfactory		
whimpered	11	15
cried	13	15
violent	2	3
inhalation induction		
satisfactory		
smooth	20	19
minor objection	4	5
unsatisfactory		
needed restraint	5	15

Data from Page and Morgan-Hughes (1990)

In the triclofos group 70% of children had both a satisfactory demeanour on arrival in the anaesthetic room and a satisfactory response to induction. This is significantly higher than the 54% frequency of overall satisfactory behaviour in the placebo group. Both groups of children spent equal time in the recovery ward. Perhaps the significance of this study is that, although a percutaneous anaesthetic satisfactorily relieves pain preoperatively with respect to venepuncture, it does not necessarily modify the behaviour of the child. Premedication may, therefore, also be required.

Venous cannulation can also be painful for children. Manner *et al.* (1987) studied 74 children, aged between four and ten years, in a double-blind, randomised trial involving percutaneous local anaesthesia with EMLA®. The study also attempted to use hormonal responses in the quantitative assessment in children of anxiety related to venous cannulation. In one such open study 5 children were treated with EMLA® and 5 had no treatment. The venous plasma catecholamine and arginine vasopressin (AVP) levels were compared. Lignocaine levels were also measured. Lignocaine samples were also taken from another group of 6 patients using different sampling sites, the dorsum of the hand, anticubital fossa and the contralateral extremity. The main bulk of the study, however, was the comparison between percutaneous local anaesthetic and placebo, 20 patients being given the active preparation and 20 a placebo. The control group consisted of 18 children who received no local treatment.

All patients in this study were premedicated with oral flunitrazepam about 90 minutes prior to venous cannulation. In addition, children scheduled for otolaryngology operations received glycopyrrolate orally. The anaesthetist assessed the patient's anxiety on a four point scale as calm, somewhat frightened, frightened or extremely frightened. After removal of the topical preparation, the skin was disinfected and an intravenous cannula (18 or 20 g) was inserted. The child was asked to assess this pain on a four point scale as none, slight, moderate or severe. Pain intensity was assessed on a VAS of 10 cm length. In the open study blood samples were drawn at 0, 2, 4, 10 and 20 minutes for catecholamine detection. For AVP determinations sampling was made at 0, 5, 10 and 20 minutes.

The range of EMLA® application times used in the study was 65-280 minutes with the median being 98.5 minutes. In the placebo group the range was 65-280 minutes with the median being 94.5 minutes. Most children were calm or just slightly frightened and there was no statistical difference between the two groups. No significant changes in venous plasma catecholamines were observed in either treated or untreated children. It was expected that there would be an increase in these concentrations. The suggested reasons for this lack of change were that the stress-induced alterations in catecholamine concentrations are less pronounced in peripheral venous blood compared with central venous or arterial sampling sites due to catecholamine uptake in peripheral tissues and, in addition, effective premedication may have blunted the catecholamine responses. All children in the active group expressed no or only slight pain at cannula insertion. In both the placebo cream and control groups half of the children reported moderate or severe pain. This study reinforced the efficacy of percutaneous local anaesthesia for pain relief in such minor procedures as catheterisation. Unfortunately, the attempt to determine anxiety by measuring hormonal levels was inconclusive, once again leaving pain assessment as a matter of experienced clinical judgement and interpretation.

A similar study was carried out by Wig and Johl (1990) to investigate the efficiency of EMLA® with premedication. In this case the premedication was morphine sulphate. The number of children considered was 75 between the ages of 18 months and ten years. The premedication was administered 90 minutes prior to surgery. Two groups were set up in this study. Group A (the placebo group) consisted of 25 children, 12 aged between 18 months and three years, and 13 aged between three and ten years. Group B, which received a percutaneous local anaesthetic treatment, consisted of fifty children, half of whom were aged between 18 months and three years and the other half between three and ten years. The study was double-blind and randomised. The patient's level of anxiety was assessed in the operating room as calm, somewhat frightened, frightened and extremely frightened. Pain was graded in 3 levels. Grade I represented no pain, no grimacing or whimpering and no reflex movement. Grade II was slight pain, slight grimacing and minor reflex movement. Finally, grade III was classified as severe pain, loud cry and intense reflex movement. The anxiety and pain scores were analysed statistically.

When considering anxiety scoring, no significant difference was observed between the groups (Table 6.8). In the group of children who received the active percutaneous anaesthetic 84% experienced no pain (grade I) and the remaining 16% had grade II - III pain. With the children who received the placebo 72% experienced grade III pain while only 10% experienced no pain. The difference between the two groups was highly significant. Pallor was observed in both groups but in this respect there was no significant difference between the active and placebo treatments.

In contrast to most previous investigations, the study by Wig and Johl (1990) concluded that premedication, when combined with percutaneous local anaesthesia, did

Table 6.8 — Anxiety scores prior to venous cannulation and grading of pain at cannulation in children treated with a percutaneous local anaesthetic or placebo

	placebo (n = 25)	percutaneous anaesthetic (n = 50)
anxiety scores		
calm	7	13
somewhat frightened	8	15
frightened	4	12
extremely frightened	6	10
grading of pain		
grade I	4	42
grade II	3	4
grade III	18	4

Reproduced from Wig and Johl (1990) with permission of the copyright owner, Indian Journal of Physiology and Pharmacology

not result in a lessening of anxiety compared with the use of a percutaneous anaesthetic alone. Patients were found to be evenly distributed in both active and placebo groups with respect to the degree of calmness before venous cannulation. The choice of premedication agent is clearly important and may not have been optimised in this particular study.

6.4   PAIN RELIEF DURING ARTERIAL CANNULATION

Although much work has been done in establishing the efficacy of percutaneous local anaesthesia for pain relief in venepuncture and related applications, comparatively little attention has been paid to the problems of pain associated with arterial cannulation. Indeed, only two studies have been published on this topic and, in one of these, Nilsson *et al.* (1990) considered the length of time that a percutaneous anaesthetic (EMLA®) had to be applied to the skin in order to achieve a satisfactory analgesic effect in arterial cannulation.

Cannulation of the radial artery is a frequently performed procedure in clinical medicine. It is used for repeated blood analysis and direct arterial pressure monitoring. Apart from relieving pain in the normal patient, pain relief is also specifically indicated for this purpose in patients with cerebral aneurysms and raised intracranial pressure. This pain relief is normally achieved using infiltration of a small volume of local anaesthetics. As the pain associated with arterial puncture and venepuncture is known to be different, the application time of the percutaneous anaesthetic preparation may well differ from the established norm.

A total of 90 patients were recruited into a double-blind and placebo-controlled study. All patients were scheduled for surgery where arterial cannulation for direct arterial pressure monitoring was indicated. The active or placebo preparations were applied on the radial artery at the wrist to 60 patients. All patients were premedicated with an opiate. An arterial cannula with an outer diameter of 1 mm was then inserted. Patient pain was assessed using a VAS. The pain reaction was graded on a verbal scale by the nurse as either no pain, slight, moderate or severe pain.

There was no statistically significant difference between the percutaneous anaesthetic and the placebo in VAS or observer scores for a 60 minute application period. The study was therefore extended to a 90 minutes application time. The mean values were analysed by Student's t-test for unpaired data and the observer scores, which were comparisons of proportions, by the Ansari-Bradley test.

When the application time exceeded 90 minutes, there was no statistical difference in the pain experienced as measured on a VAS but there was a statistically significant difference in the distribution of observer pain scores, with lower values being recorded in the percutaneous anaesthetic group (Fig. 6.6). The actual application time in the 90 minutes group averaged just over 120 minutes. The effect of EMLA® is probably at its maximum after this application time. The study concluded that neither 60 nor 120 minutes application of the percutaneous anaesthetic significantly reduced the subjective pain experienced, using a VAS scale, in arterial cannulation. However, observer scores of pain indicated a beneficial effect of percutaneous anaesthesia. With an application time for EMLA® exceeding 90 minutes, 85% of patients scored no pain. This figure fell to 37% when the application time was reduced to 60 minutes.

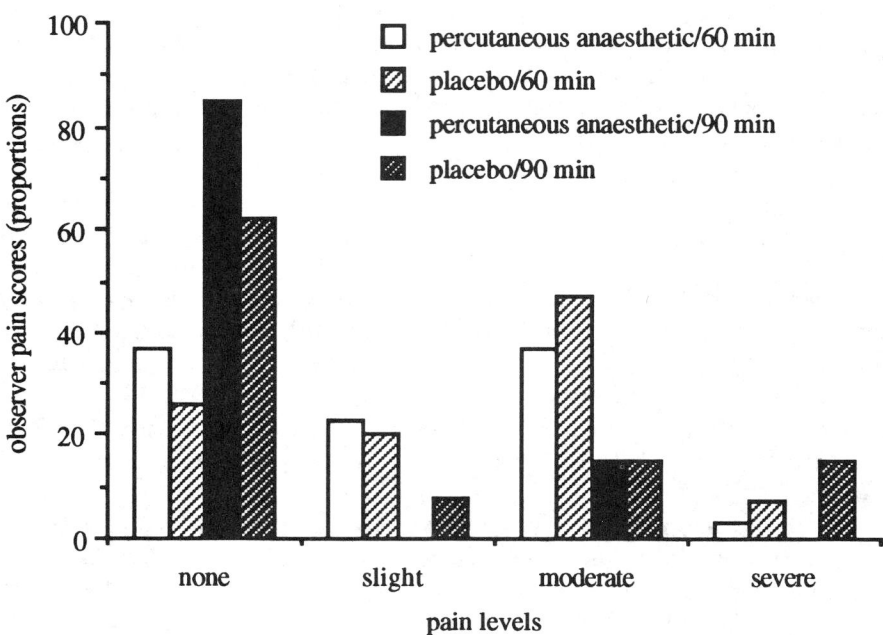

Fig. 6.6 — Observer pain ratings (proportions) after the application of percutaneous local anaesthetic and placebo preparations for 60 and 90 minutes respectively. Data from Nilsson *et al.* (1990)

The pain in arterial cannulation is normally relieved with lignocaine infiltration. Smith *et al.* (1990) compared the effectiveness of lignocaine infiltration to that of percutaneous anaesthesia with EMLA®. Infiltration may be painful and may not provide adequate analgesia. Premedicated patients may be able to tolerate arterial cannulation but in unpremedicated patients the experience may be unpleasant. The study was undertaken in 40 adults who were not premedicated. Neurosurgical patients who would not normally receive premedication were included. The patients were divided into four groups. These received the percutaneous anaesthetic alone or in combination with either lignocaine or saline infiltration, with the final group receiving placebo cream combined with lignocaine infiltration. The application time was 60 minutes with the sites of both radial arteries being treated. In those patients who were to receive infiltration the two agents used were either 0.9% saline or 1% lignocaine in a 0.2 - 0.3 ml volume, injected intradermally using a 35-gauge needle. Arterial cannulation was performed, using a 20-gauge cannula, 2 minutes after infiltration or immediately on removal of the cream in those who received percutaneous anaesthetic only.

Patients assessed pain on a VAS scale. An independent observer rated pain in four categories on a verbal rating scale (VRS) of 1 = no response, 2 = mild facial grimace, 3 = verbal response and 4 = withdrawal of the hand. VAS and VRS data were analysed using the Kruskal-Wallis one-way analysis of variance by ranks and the Mann-Whitney U test. The mean age of patients was forty-eight years, with a range of twenty-two to sixty-nine years.

VAS scores were significantly lower in the groups receiving a percutaneous anaesthetic than the placebo cream-lignocaine infiltration group. There was no significant difference between the percutaneous anaesthetic groups. The VRS scores in these groups were similar and significantly lower than those in the placebo cream/infiltration group. In contrast to the study by Nilsson *et al.* (1990), the percutaneous anaesthetic applied for 60 minutes was found to be useful in alleviating pain during arterial cannulation in unpremedicated adults. Smith *et al.* (1990) also concluded that EMLA® was more effective than lignocaine infiltration in arterial cannulation. However, both published studies on arterial cannulation are somewhat contradictory. This emphasises the need for further work in additional centres in order to fully establish the efficacy of percutaneous local anaesthesia in this particular application.

6.5   PAIN RELIEF DURING LUMBAR PUNCTURE

Lumbar punctures can cause intense anxiety, particularly in paediatric patients and, indeed, in their parents. This, in turn, places stress on the paediatrician performing the procedure. In leukaemia patients lumbar punctures unfortunately have to be repeated periodically in order to rule out CNS involvement and to administer chemotherapy.

One study which considered the efficacy of percutaneous local anaesthesia in lumbar puncture was undertaken by Kapelushnik *et al.* (1990). Both a double-blind, placebo-controlled study and an open, crossover, randomised study were carried out. This latter study, which consisted of 18 children with an age range from five to fifteen years, compared EMLA® with a no-treatment regimen. The percutaneous anaesthetic was applied to the puncture site between 45 minutes and 60 minutes prior to lumbar puncture. After this period the skin was disinfected. Pain was measured using a 100 mm VAS ranging from 0 (no pain) to 5 (the most intense pain imaginable). In the double-blind, placebo-controlled study the children were between four and eleven years of age. In addition to the VAS, the children graded their pain using a visual analogue scale showing facial expressions ranging from smiling (no pain) to crying (maximal pain). Nurses also used the same scoring system.

With the open crossover study, percutaneous anaesthetic treatment was superior in every case compared to no treatment. The pain scores were 2.55 ± 0.6 with no treatment and 1.66 ± 0.83 with the percutaneous anaesthetic. Nurse and parental assessments were identical and the differences between treatments were statistically significant. In the double-blind study using a 100 mm VAS the mean scores were 3.1 ± 1 with the placebo and 2.0 ± 1.4 with the percutaneous anaesthetic. The facial expression scores were 3.8 ± 1.2 with placebo and 2.9 ± 1.7 with EMLA®. This was similar to results recorded by nursing staff.

The double-blind trial revealed a significant correlation between the numerical and pictorial visual analogue scales used by the children. However, there was no correlation between the child's and the nurse/observer's scoring. This may mean that estimating pain in non-verbalising children can result in an inaccurate report. Although in the open study percutaneous anaesthesia was reported to be invariably effective, in the blinded study it was inferior to the placebo in two cases. If there had been a third such case, the effect of the percutaneous anaesthetic in lowering pain scores would not have reached statistical significance. These two cases of apparent failure in children were at the youngest age range and it was not established if they could actually report pain as a continuous variable. This observation is supported by the open venepuncture study reported by Woolfson *et al.* (1990).

Another investigation involving lumbar puncture was carried out by Halperin *et al.* (1989) and consisted of 14 children aged from five to fifteen years. The children were scheduled for intrathecal chemotherapy. Each patient had two lumbar punctures carried out 60 minutes after application of a placebo preparation or percutaneous local anaesthetic (EMLA®) using size-appropriate needles with a trocar. The study was a double-blind crossover design. Pain was scored by the patients using a 10 cm VAS from 0 (no pain) to 10 (maximal pain).

Percutaneous anaesthesia was preferred by 12 out of 14 children, with the mean pain score being 1.9 ± 1.9 compared to 5.6 ± 3.0 with the placebo, a statistically significant difference. However, there was no statistically significant difference in the pain scores of children who had received a previous lumbar puncture compared with those who had no previous experience of the procedure. The study concluded that EMLA® was effective at reducing pain in children at lumbar puncture.

Two further studies support the results obtained by Halperin *et al.* (1989). Young *et al.* (1987) say that the infiltration of local anaesthetic is painful, increases lumbar muscle tension and triggers flexar spasms in patients with lower limb spasticity. Thus, the patient may move from the correct position for the procedure. Infiltration of local anaesthetics may obliterate anatomical landmarks. Percutaneous local anaesthesia overcomes these problems but must be applied, in the case of EMLA®, at least 60 minutes prior to lumbar puncture. Young *et al.* (1987) concluded that, despite the additional cost involved in using a percutaneous anaesthetic, it was nevertheless worthwhile, even in adults, as the patient was more comfortable before the needle puncture. Price (1988) confirmed that percutaneous anaesthesia is effective for lumbar puncture in children and he suggested that it be widely available in the paediatric wards of developed countries.

6.6 PAIN RELIEF FOR THE INSERTION OF HAEMODIALYSIS CANNULAE AND PUNCTURES THROUGH SUBCUTANEOUS DRUG RESERVOIRS

Pain inflicted by the insertion of large cannulae into arteriovenous fistulas is a significant cause of concern for both children and adults on regular haemodialysis. At the University Children's Hospital in Berne, Switzerland, the procedure was always preceded by a subcutaneous injection of lignocaine. To avoid the pain produced by subcutaneous injection, Bianchetti *et al.* (1990) decided that patients should apply a percutaneous local anaesthetic cream (EMLA®) at home immediately before coming to the dialysis unit. The number of patients using this method on a regular basis were 5 aged between nine and seventeen years. This method has now completely replaced subcutaneous anaesthesia.

Another study performed by Wehle *et al.* (1989) considered repeated applications of EMLA® for the alleviation of cannulation pain in haemodialysis. The percutaneous anaesthetic was used prior to each haemodialysis, a total of two or three times weekly per patient. The study was a double-blind, crossover and placebo-controlled design. It consisted of 312 patients between the ages of forty-eight and seventy-five years. For blood access, arteriovenous fistulas were used, of which twelve were grafts. The fistulas/grafts were situated in the forearm (n = 28), the upper arm (n = 2) or the antecubital fossa (n = 1). The median amount of time on haemodialysis for patients entering into this trial was 9 months with a range of 0 to 12.5 years Patients applied the percutaneous anaesthetic to each cannulation site at home and the efficacy of pain relief was clinically assessed at every thirteenth application versus a placebo. The median application time was 95 ± 26.5 minutes. Immediately prior to haemodialysis two fistula-needles were inserted. EMLA® was applied to one site and a placebo cream to the other. Using a VAS of 100 mm, the patient was asked to rate the pain from a cannulation made without a percutaneous anaesthetic prior to commencement of active treatment and also, again, at the end of the study. This was to test if the patient's pain perception had changed during the study period. A total of 17 patients completed the study over 12 to 18 months. There was no significant change in the perception of cannulation pain and there was also no difference in pain perception between the two sites (artery and vein). However, percutaneous anaesthetic pain scores were significantly lower than the placebo pain scores.

The active preparation was applied some 6509 times during this trial and 66% of these applications showed no local skin reactions. The most frequently observed reaction was local paleness followed by local redness. Itching, burning and oedema were seldom seen. There was no correlation between local reaction and the number of applications, and no tolerance to the analgesic effect developed. Rather unusually, a statistical difference between EMLA® and placebo preparations was not obtained for applications made during the month of July. This was attributed to seasonal variation in skin thickness due to exposure to ultraviolet radiation during the summer.

Percutaneous local anaesthesia for pain relief when punctures are made through subcutaneous drug reservoirs was investigated by Halperin *et al.* (1988). Patients recruited into this study had previous experience of punctures made through their subcutaneous drug reservoir into the subclavicular area for the administration of chemotherapy. The study was double-blind and crossover in design. The percutaneous anaesthetic (EMLA®) or the placebo were applied for 60 minutes prior to puncture with 22-gauge curved needles specifically designed for use with the *Port-A-Cath* system. Pain was scored using a 10 cm VAS. The mean pain scores were 1.2 ± 1.8 with EMLA® and 3.9 ± 2.2 without. This difference was statistically significant, indicating that a worthwhile degree of pain relief could be obtained for this procedure using percutaneous local anaesthesia.

6.7 HARVESTING OF SPLIT SKIN GRAFTS USING PERCUTANEOUS LOCAL ANAESTHESIA

There are many situations where general anaesthesia is administered solely for the purpose of cutting a skin graft, a common surgical procedure with numerous and varied indications. There are two types of skin graft, split thickness and full thickness. Split skin grafts contain epidermis and an amount of dermis ranging from thin to thick depending on the method of harvesting. Full thickness grafts contain the entire dermis as well as the epidermis. With full thickness grafts the donor site must subsequently be closed or repaired with a skin flap or a split skin graft. With split skin grafts the donor site may be left to heal by granulation and re-epithelialisation. The majority of grafts routinely harvested are of the split skin type, with a typical thickness varying between about 0.35 mm and 0.45 mm.

Frequently the patient requiring a split skin graft is elderly and frail. Therefore, general anaesthesia, even of short duration, may be hazardous. A split skin graft may be cut using a conventional injectable local anaesthetic solution but there are drawbacks and limitations associated with this technique. In particular, multiple infiltration of the donor site is itself a painful and uncomfortable technique. Clearly, the use of a topically applied local anaesthetic would be advantageous for harvesting split skin grafts. The advantages accrue not only to the patient, in terms of increased safety and comfort, but also to the clinician in respect of a simpler preoperative procedure. There are also obvious economic benefits in reducing the use of general anaesthesia.

An investigation into the use of percutaneous anaesthesia for split skin grafts was made by Ohlsen *et al.* (1985). A total of 146 patients, 64 women and 82 men, were recruited into the study. Their ages were from nineteen to ninety-three years, with the age distribution tending towards the older end of the range. Premedication, consisting mainly of diazepam, was used in 50.5% of women and 64.6% of the men. The donor site was cleaned, shaved and a thick layer of percutaneous anaesthetic (EMLA®) was applied to a pre-marked area. The cream was covered with an occlusive dressing and slight compression was obtained by means of an elastic bandage. The application area varied from 50 cm^2 to in excess of 1 m^2, but the majority of grafts harvested were between 100 and 300 cm^2. In each case the skin graft was taken using an electrodermatome and the thickness varied from 0.41 mm to 0.53 mm. The most frequent donor site was the thigh. However the foreleg, upper arm and forearm were also used. EMLA® was applied for between 90 minutes and 460 minutes, with the mean application time being 200 minutes.

The results from this quite extensive study showed that only 1.6% of women and 6.1% of men stated that the cream caused a slight transient local irritation after application. This irritation only endured for a few seconds. During cutting of the skin graft 65.1% of all patients experienced no pain, 19.2% experienced slight pain but did not object, 13.7% described the pain as moderate and 2% described it as severe, thus needing additional local anaesthetic infiltration. Therefore, it was possible to carry out the planned operation in 98.0% of all cases and in 84.3% of these patients percutaneous local anaesthesia provided satisfactory protection from pain. Pain relief could not be related to premedication.

There was a statistically significant correlation of anaesthetic efficacy with application time. Moderate or severe pain was experienced more frequently by patients who had EMLA® applied for more than three hours. There was no association between pain and the thickness of the graft, and no obvious difference in the bleeding or healing times of patients with general or local anaesthesia. No allergic reactions or signs of toxicity were observed. Thus, the percutaneous anaesthetic was effective in blocking nerve endings. This was sufficient to permit the removal of split skin grafts with a thickness of at least 50-75% of the total thickness of the dermis. Local anaesthetics could be traced to a depth of about 1 mm in the skin, hence the lack of correlation of penetration depth to pain as the maximum graft harvested was only 0.53 mm in depth. A minimum application time of 60 to 90 minutes was necessary and duration of anaesthesia was reported to last for several hours. Patients who received EMLA® requested less analgesic subsequent to the procedure than would normally be expected.

In the eutectic system lignocaine and prilocaine are primarily released from the oil-in-water droplets in the emulsion to replenish the aqueous diffusion layer. A depletion of those droplets closest to the diffusion layer might be expected after long term application of EMLA®. This will cause a decrease in drug penetration as the concentration gradient falls across the diffusion layer/skin interface. Hence, a decrease in the local anaesthetic effect may be expected with this system with longer application times. This appears to occur with applications times of three hours and longer. Ohlsen *et al.* (1985) clearly demonstrated this effect by filling a glass tube with EMLA® and placing it over a silicone membrane separating the tube from a sink. The sink removed local anaesthetics from the droplets, thus resembling a membrane surface. After three hours, a clear zone was visible nearest the membrane, demonstrating the diminished effect of the eutectic system over longer application times. This process of diffusion layer depletion may well occur even faster *in vivo*. Hence, it was suggested that in clinical practice the bandage should be gently massaged at 60 minute intervals to homogenise the percutaneous anaesthetic cream.

Lahteenmaki *et al.* (1988) investigated the amount of EMLA® required for the painless harvesting of split skin grafts, together with the optimum application time for efficacy. Unlike the open study of Ohlsen *et al.* (1985), this investigation was a double-blind, multi-centre trial in adults, designed mainly to test the effect of dose variation on the efficacy of percutaneous anaesthesia. Dose was defined as the amount of the preparation applied to the donor site.

Application sites of 200 cm^2 and smaller were considered. The percutaneous anaesthetic was applied for between 2 and 6 hours at a dose of 30 g per 200 cm^2 (40 patients) or 60 g per 200 cm^2 (38 patients). The cream was covered with plastic film and an elastic bandage was applied to give an even distribution of cream and also to protect the site. Premedication was given to 32 patients in the lower dose group and to 27 patients in the higher dose group. The skin was cut with a dermatome and the patient was asked to assess the pain on a four point scale.

The results obtained by Lahteenmaki *et al.* (1988) showed that there was no statistical difference between applying the lower or higher doses of percutaneous anaesthetic (Fig. 6.7). The proportion of patients reporting either no or slight pain was 90% in each group. The results were similar in all four trial centres and ranged from 85 to 100% pain-free procedures. This is not surprising since much of the applied dose would not be in contact with the skin and, in thicker layers, would therefore make no contribution to the percutaneous delivery of the active local anaesthetics. The important factors are the drug concentration gradient achieved across the skin/diffusion layer interface and the availability of emulsified local anaesthetic droplets required for replenishment of the diffusion layer.

The application times used by Lahteenmaki *et al.* (1988) were between 2 and 5 hours with both doses of percutaneous anaesthetic. This contrasts with the earlier recommendations for EMLA® of Ohlsen *et al.* (1985) of between 60 and 90 minutes. Certainly, the longer times used seem excessive in view of the depletion of local

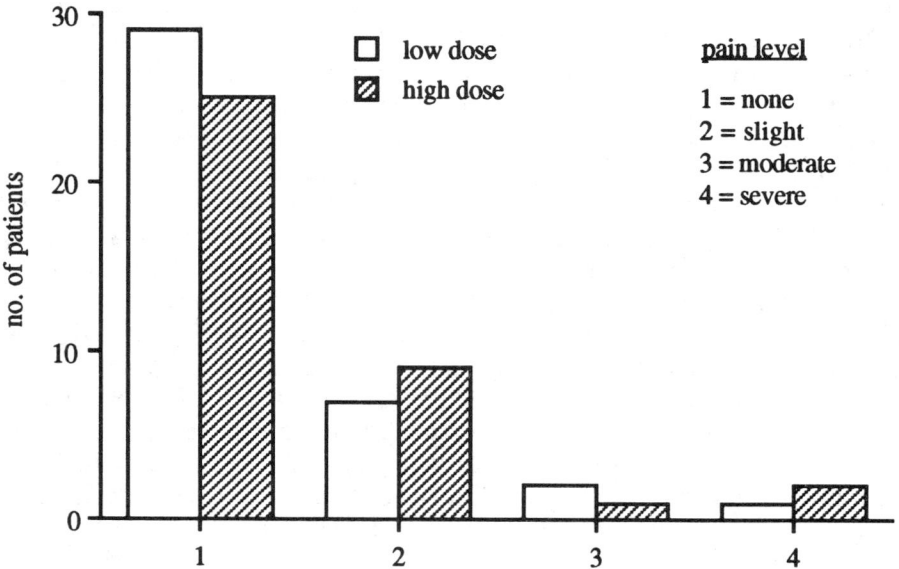

Fig. 6.7 — Patients' verbal rating of the pain experienced from the harvesting of a split-skin graft after treatment with EMLA® cream at two dose levels, high (60 g per 200 cm²) and low (30 g per 200 cm²). Reproduced from Lahteenmaki *et al.* (1988) with permission of the copyright holder, Williams and Wilkins, Baltimore

anaesthetics at the skin interface which can occur in this system. With respect to side effects, these were again minor, particularly considering the long application periods involved. A mild burning pain was felt in two patients in the lower dose group and in three patients who received the higher dose of EMLA®. Local pallor, redness and oedema were found in 35.9%, 43.6% and 9.0% of patients, respectively. These were probably due, in most cases, to the skin being occluded for a prolonged period under a substantial amount of a plastic dressing, cream and bandages. An interesting additional observation made during this study was that men are usually shaved prior to grafting. Shaving usually causes small wounds that may give a transient burning pain when a fluid with a high pH is applied. EMLA® has a reported pH of 9.7. As the local anaesthetic is absorbed, the burning pain usually disappears.

Goodacre *et al.* (1988) conducted a comparative study between percutaneous local anaesthesia with EMLA® and infiltration anaesthesia. The age range of the 80 patients considered was seventeen to eighty-seven years, with a mean age of forty-seven. A restriction was placed on the choice of application site, either the inner upper arm or the thigh being used, with a maximum area of 400 cm². The majority of cases were daycare patients (68.75%). Sedation with diazepam was required in only 4 patients.

Lignocaine and adrenaline were administered subcutaneously by infiltration, using a 25 g dental needle, 5 minutes prior to graft harvesting. For percutaneous anaesthesia the donor site was shaved, swabbed with alcohol and marked into a 100 cm² area. The local anaesthetic cream (30 g) was then applied to the site. This was probably an unnecessarily high dose in view of the results obtained by Lahteenmaki *et al.* (1988).

The donor site was then occluded with plastic food wrap. As the application time was 120 minutes, the cream was massaged hourly to ensure even distribution.

Split skin grafts were harvested conventionally using a Watson hand dermatome. Graft details are given in Table 6.9. Discomfort on preparation of the site was assessed using a 100 cm VAS, with 0 representing no pain and 100 being severe pain, and a VRS with four points from 0 (no pain) to 4 (severe pain). Statistical comparisons between the treatments were made using the Wilcoxon rank sum test with corrections for ties.

Table 6.9 — Details of split-skin grafts harvested using a percutaneous local anaesthetic cream (EMLA®)

graft details	no. of patients (infiltration)	no. of patients (percutaneous anaesthesia)
condition requiring graft:		
tattoo excision	13	15
basal/squamous ca.	10	7
burns	4	4
leg ulcers	5	3
traumatic loss	4	7
melanoma	2	1
others	2	3
donor sites:		
inner upper arm	23	24
thigh	17	16

Reproduced from Goodacre *et al.* (1988) with permission of the copyright owner, Churchill Livingstone

Although EMLA® caused no discomfort to any of the patients, infiltration anaesthesia resulted in varying degrees of pain ranging from 13 to 89 on a VAS. Pain on lignocaine infiltration was positively correlated to the volume of solution infiltrated. The mean application time for the percutaneous anaesthetic was 164 minutes. On harvesting the grafts the difference in VAS scores was not found to be statistically significant. Although patients appeared to record less pain on a VRS with EMLA® treatment, this difference again failed to reach statistical significance. However, the average application area for the percutaneous anaesthetic was 122.4 cm^2, compared with 69 cm^2 for infiltration. Thus, the comparison of pain felt during the graft cutting may reflect a treatment difference masked by differences in the size of graft cut.

Most of the patients in the study were attending for outpatient surgery and were therefore not premedicated, in contrast to most other studies of this type. Donor site bleeding was more profuse with the EMLA® group as this preparation contains no vasoactive compound (adrenaline), but this effect was no greater than with general anaesthesia. The general conclusion reached by Goodacre *et al.* (1988) is that a minimum of 15 g of EMLA® should be applied for 120 minutes per 100 cm^2 of donor site, in contrast to the 60-90 minute application period suggested by Ohlsen *et al.* (1985).

A potential problem with all percutaneous local anaesthetic treatments is the long waiting period for onset of anaesthesia to occur. Given the increased nature of the trauma involved, this period is further increased for the harvesting of split skin grafts compared to venepuncture and related applications. The amethocaine phase-change system is distinguished from EMLA® by, generally, having a shorter onset time and a longer duration of action. Its use for the harvesting of split skin grafts was therefore investigated by Small *et al.* (1988).

Over a one year period 80 patients were entered into the study involving the amethocaine percutaneous anaesthetic. The majority of these required the application of a split skin graft to a clean granulating wound. It was clearly a prerequisite that the wound did not require any surgical intervention and was in a suitable state to accept the graft. A lower age limit of twelve years was arbitrarily enforced but there was no upper age limit, the actual age range being from twelve to ninety-six years with a mean age of fifty-one. The main indications for grafting were in respect of burn wounds and blunt trauma. Excision of skin lesions, leg ulcers, tattoo excision and wound breakdown were also included in this series.

The donor site was marked out preoperatively, shaved and cleaned, and the amethocaine percutaneous anaesthetic applied as a 1 mm thick gel over the site. The area was covered with cling film and an elastic bandage. The minimum application time was 60 minutes, with the efficacy of the procedure being assessed by pinprick prior to cutting the graft at a mean delay time, measured from initial application, of 65 minutes. The procedure was abandoned if the attempted cutting of the graft elicited pain. Pain assessment during, and after, harvesting of the graft was made by the surgeon using a proforma sheet (Fig. 6.8).

In the pilot study reported by Small *et al.* (1988) the technique was completely successful in 80% of patients entered into the trial. Complete skin anaesthesia was established within 60 minutes from initial application, allowing pain-free cutting of the skin at all periods ranging from 60 to 300 minutes. In 10 patients there was still sensation to pinprick at 60 minutes from initial application and the method was therefore not attempted. In 6 patients there was complete cutaneous anaesthesia on testing but cutting of the graft was nevertheless resisted, once again emphasising the importance of psychological factors in this type of study. The authors considered that adequate preoperative explanation of the technique to patients was therefore essential as a confidence-building measure.

The largest graft harvested in this study measured 80 x 16 cm. Although the authors did not carry out specific assessments of donor site healing or graft take, routine clinical observations did not reveal any gross abnormalities in either area. There were no significant adverse reactions to the amethocaine percutaneous anaesthetic preparation. An occasional transient erythema was noted on removal of the preparation due to the

PROFORMA

NAME:
INDICATION FOR SKIN GRAFT:
DATE OF BIRTH:
NO:
DATE:
TIME CREAM APPLIED:

INTERVAL: APPLICATION - SENSORY TESTING

.....................Min

                                        total analgesia   ☐
                                        pain   ☐

INTERVAL: APPLICATION - CUTTING SKIN GRAFT

.....................Min

                                        total analgesia   ☐
                                        pain   ☐

                        skin thickness
                                        thin   ☐
                                        medium   ☐

                        procedure
                                        successful   ☐
                                        failed   ☐

COMMENT:

Fig. 6.8 — Proforma sheet for the assessment of skin analgesia to the harvesting of split-skin grafts. Reproduced from Small *et al.* (1988) with permission of the copyright owner, Churchill Livingstone Medical Journals

vasodilatory effect of the local anaesthetic.

Small *et al.* (1988) also reported, albeit on an anecdotal basis, the use of the amethocaine percutaneous anaesthetic for other topical surgical procedures, notably for laser treatment of skin lesions in order to render the laser beam painless. This makes treatment of large areas tolerable at a single session. Other applications that normally involve multiple local infiltration were also seen as areas where percutaneous anaesthesia would be beneficial. Finally, the authors concluded that, with the increasing tendency towards day-stay procedures, the use of percutaneous anaesthesia offers obvious benefits in increasing patient throughput.

The lack of any harmful effects of percutaneous local anaesthesia on subsequent wound healing is an important aspect of this technique in the harvesting of split skin grafts. The clinical observations to this effect are supported in a study by Nykanen *et al.* (1991) on the effects of EMLA® on wound healing in a rat animal model. In a comparison with local lignocaine infiltration, 36 wounds were assessed. No clinical or histological evidence of necrosis or infection was found in any wound. The authors concluded that the percutaneous anaesthetic had no effect on wound healing in the animal model studied and that its effects in this respect were comparable to lignocaine infiltration.

Percutaneous local anaesthesia, although effective in many cases for relatively superficial skin surgery, cannot completely replace local infiltration. This is particularly true where the surgical procedure is deep enough to involve the subcutis. In such cases local infiltration will be required. However, this procedure can be sufficiently painful enough in its own right to cause pain and anxiety, sometimes leading to vaso-vagal attacks. Therefore, Jones *et al.* (1990) investigated the use of percutaneous local anaesthesia in order to relieve or prevent the pain and discomfort associated with local infiltration.

Patients undergoing minor skin surgery were divided into two groups, according to the number of lesions requiring surgical treatment. The first group had a single lesion and were randomly allocated EMLA® or placebo. The second group, with two lesions, received the active agent for one lesion and placebo for the other. Unfortunately, the authors reported that in neither group was there a clinically useful reduction in discomfort, probably due to inadequate dermal anaesthesia. This rather surprising result appeared to be due to the application time of 60 minutes being too short to allow a sufficient penetration depth to be achieved. A longer application period for EMLA®, similar to that used in split skin grafting, would probably have produced a more clinically useful response. However, in this particular application the question of practicality arises when the application time becomes excessive. A more rapidly acting agent with increased anaesthetic potency is probably required for such applications.

6.8 PERCUTANEOUS LOCAL ANAESTHESIA FOR DEBRIDEMENT IN LEG ULCER TREATMENT

In Great Britain about 100,000 patients have active leg ulcers in a population of 400,000 leg ulcer patients. Two main types of leg ulcer tend to present at clinics. Venous leg ulcers have clinical signs of varicose veins. Pressure and arterial ulcers show no clinical signs of varicose veins with ankle pressure below 80 mm Hg. Factors which interfere with normal healing, such as necrotic tissue, need to be removed. If such tissue is left *in situ*, it promotes bacterial in-growth and retards epithelialisation. Surgical debridement of an ulcer has to be repeated many times. Due to pain, the cleansing may not always be as radical as is necessary.

A clean leg ulcer can sometimes be achieved by the use of enzyme preparations, repeated wet dressings or hydrocolloids. Holm *et al.* (1990) investigated the use of percutaneous local anaesthesia for ulcer cleaning. They used an open study with 50 patients and a double-blind, placebo control with 36 patients. In the open study the mean age was seventy years and with the double-blind group the mean was sixty-two years. All of the treatments were randomised except in respect of diabetic patients. A thick layer of test cream (EMLA®) was applied to the wound and covered with an occlusive dressing. A maximum of 5 g of cream was used in all but three patients who received 10 g. The application times were 10, 20 and 30 minutes in the open study and 30 minutes in the remainder of the study. Ulcer debridement was achieved with tweezers, scissors and curettes. The process was deemed completed when the ulcer was free from necrotic tissue, fibrin deposits and pus.

The patient assessed pain at debridement on a four point VRS (none to severe pain) and on a 100 mm VAS from 0 (no pain) to 100 (intolerable pain). Any differences in the groups were assessed using the Mann-Whitney U-test, the Wilcoxon matched pairs signed rank test or Fisher's exact test. Correlations between duration of symptoms and pain were tested by linear regression. In the open study, with percutaneous anaesthetic only, debridement was judged satisfactory in 98% of patients. With the double-blind study the median scores on the VAS were 18.5 mm (minimum 3, maximum 87) for EMLA® and 84 mm (minimum 12, maximum 95) for the placebo group. Among patients with venous ulcers, the median pair score was 17 mm with the active preparation and 89 mm for placebo. In arterial ulcers the values were 21.5 mm with EMLA® and 33.5 mm for the placebo. When diabetics were excluded, the median VAS scores for the percutaneous anaesthetic and placebo were 18.5 mm and 91 mm, respectively. Patients who reported pain to be as severe with the percutaneous anaesthetic as with placebo were given a second application, after which the reported pain was less.

Percutaneous local anaesthesia offered the majority of patients in this trial good pain relief and was thus important for the achievement of satisfactory debridement. The duration of the leg ulcer did not have any influence upon the degree of pain, nor did the initial pain reaction to debridement influence the analgesic response. However, diabetic patients tend not to feel as much pain as those without the condition.

The lignocaine and prilocaine plasma levels after application of lignocaine/prilocaine eutectic mixture (2% and 5%) to leg ulcers were determined by Malmros *et al.* (1990). This study also compared the effect of both concentrations of the preparation for the surgical cleansing of leg ulcers. The plasma concentrations were assessed in 8 patients aged sixty to eighty-five years who had leg ulcers measuring between 31 and 80 cm^2. Of these, 7 ulcers were sited on the lower leg and a single ulcer was located on the malleolus. Analgesic efficacy was assessed in 10 patients with ulcers measuring from 2 to 18 cm^2. Of these ulcers 6 were venous and 4 were immunological in origin. The lower leg contained 7 ulcers; the rest were located on the malleolus. Concomitant medication with analgesics or anti-inflammatory agents was continued in 5 patients in the plasma study and 5 in the efficacy study. This latter was of a double-blind design. For the plasma concentration study 8 - 10 g of the eutectic preparation (2%) was applied for 60 minutes. Blood samples were collected at 60, 90, 120, 150, 180 and 240 minutes after the application and the plasma analysed for local anaesthetics.

In the double-blind, crossover, four-period study both concentrations of percutaneous anaesthetic were applied. Each patient received both concentrations once during the first and second treatment and once during the third and fourth treatment. The application time was 30 minutes without occlusion, substantially different conditions to those required for achieving effective anaesthesia of intact healthy skin. In both studies pain was assessed on a VAS from 0 mm (no pain) to 100 mm (severe pain). The differences in VAS scores between the two anaesthetic concentrations were analysed by the Wilcoxon matched-pairs test.

The results of the plasma concentration assays of lignocaine and prilocaine are shown in Fig. 6.9. Lignocaine absorption appeared to be proportional to the ulcer size, whereas prilocaine absorption was not. The median prilocaine levels were only 17 - 30% that of the lignocaine levels. When a eutectic system containing 100 mg each of lignocaine and prilocaine was applied to leg ulcers measuring up to 80 cm^2 for 60 minutes, the resulting plasma concentrations were found to be 20 - 35 times lower than those associated with toxicity. The frequency of post cleansing pain may, however, be higher with the lower anaesthetic concentration, indicating a possible difference in the duration of analgesia. Also, in the double-blind study the third and fourth cleansing procedures were less painful than the first and second attempts. Possibly, this decrease is due to the psychological response to repeated debridement. The chronic nature of leg ulcers necessitates between one and three visits per week for several months for ambulatory patients. The only practical drawback with EMLA®, the authors concluded, was that a nurse may have to wait 30 minutes for it to take effect on a home visit.

An unusual method of treating leg ulcers with excessive granulation was suggested by McGrath and Scholfield (1990). This consisted of a percutaneous anaesthetic cream and 95% silver nitrate pencils. A thick layer (2 - 4 mm) of EMLA® was applied to the

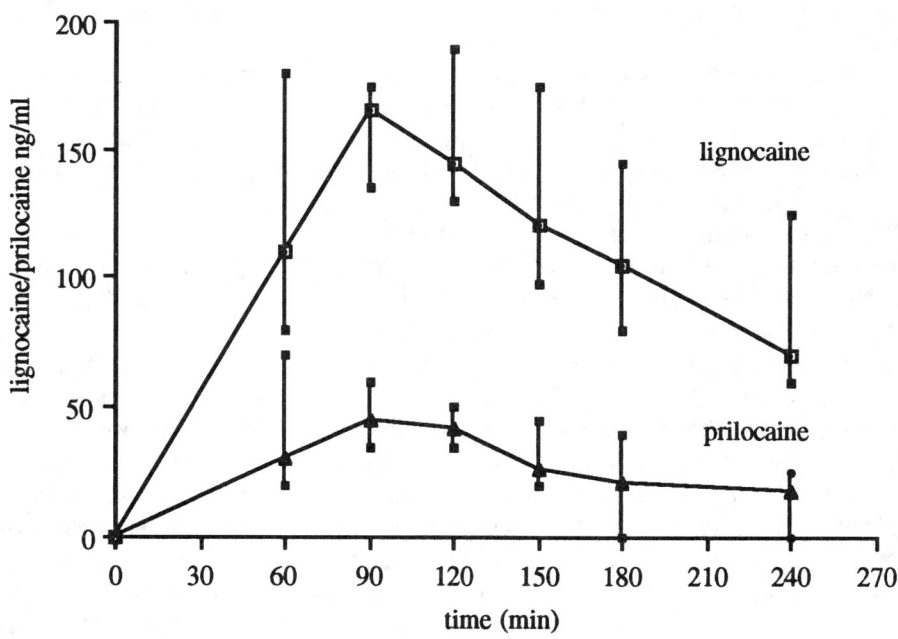

Fig. 6.9 — Plasma concentrations of lignocaine and prilocaine following the application of 8 - 10 g of lignocaine/prilocaine (2%) percutaneous anaesthetic cream for 60 minutes to leg ulcers measuring 31 - 80 cm^2. Reproduced from Malmros *et al.* (1990) with permission of the copyright holder

granulation tissue. After about one hour the area was treated with a wetted 95% silver nitrate pencil. The area was then covered with a non-adhesive dressing. This is not normal practice in leg ulcer treatment. After 24 hours the dressing was removed and a crust 1 - 3 mm thick was then easily peeled off in one piece. The whole procedure was then repeated 24 hours later. Re-epithelialisation can then take place much more satisfactorily over a flat ulcer bed. This method has been employed in dystrophic epidermolysis bullosa, junctional epidermolysis bullosa (non-Herlitz form) and pyoderma gangrenosum. Clinical trials have apparently shown this method to be superior to treatment with the more usual topical steroid and antibiotic combination.

6.9   TREATMENT OF MOLLUSCUM CONTAGIOSUM

The treatment of molluscum contagiosum is normally with a comedo extractor or a curette. Removal by either method is usually painful. It has been difficult to achieve satisfactory local analgesia in children with extensive lesions and general anaesthesia is,

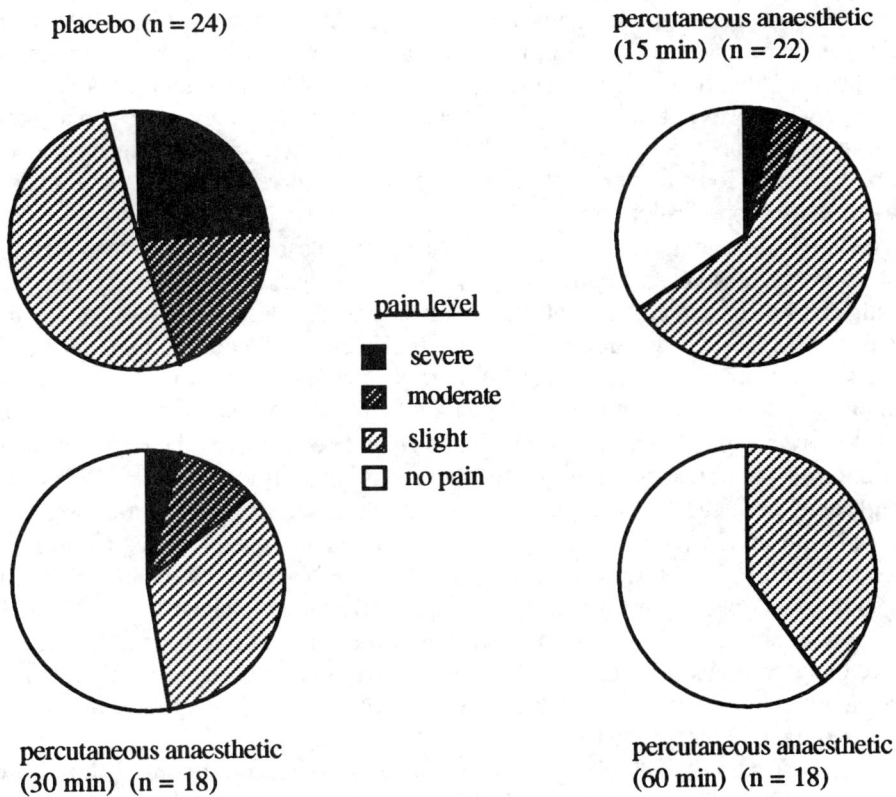

Fig. 6.10 — The effect of percutaneous local anaesthetic (EMLA[®]) application time on pain relief in curettage of molluscum contagiosum in children. Data from deWaard-van der Spek *et al.* (1990)

therefore, often required. Percutaneous local anaesthesia has been investigated for use in this area by de Waard-van der Spek *et al.* (1990) using a double-blind, placebo-controlled design. Children (83) aged from four to twelve years and with 5 or more molluscum contagiosum lesions were recruited. The children received an initial application of a percutaneous anaesthetic (EMLA®) or placebo preparation for 15, 30 or 60 minutes. A thick layer of cream was applied to the lesions at a dose of approximately 1 g per 10 cm^2 under occlusion. The maximum amount of any preparation used on each child was 10 g. The lesions were removed with a comedo extractor or curette and iodine was then applied. Both patient and physician assessed pain on a VRS as none, mild, moderate or severe. The patient also used a VAS of 100 mm. Statistical differences between active and placebo treatments, in respect of VAS scores and verbal pain assessments, were determined using the Mann-Whitney rank-sum test. The differences among the various application times within both groups were analysed with the Kruskal-Wallis and Terpstra-Jonckheere tests.

No significant differences in pain were observed among the various application times used in either the active or placebo groups. The latter were thus condensed into a single group for the purposes of analysis. The percutaneous anaesthetic treatment, using all three application times, significantly prevented pain compared with the placebo (Fig. 6.10). This was true for all methods of pain assessment. With the patients' VRS scores the frequency of totally pain-free procedures was 36% using a 15 minute percutaneous anaesthetic application. Thius increased to 61% with a 60 minute application, a difference which was not statistically significant. Of the children given the percutaneous anaesthetic treatment, 91% felt no or slight pain compared with 54% in the placebo group. Transient local redness was the only reaction observed, though this was absent with the shortest application time.

The surgical removal of mollusca requires a larger dose of EMLA® than for other applications such as venepuncture. This raises obvious questions of toxicity, an aspect investigated by Haugstvedt *et al.* (1990) in a two-part study. The first part consisted of 10 children (aged two to three years) with the second part comprising a further 10 subjects aged from six to eight years. A history of atopic dermatitis was present in 6 children, 3 in each study. In the first study a total of 10 g of percutaneous anaesthetic (EMLA®) was applied to normal skin at ten different body sites as the child was being anaesthetised for unrelated surgery. In the second study a total of 10 - 16 g of the percutaneous anaesthetic was applied to affected mollusca areas. The mollusca were removed with an Ewald pincette. The number of lesions treated in this manner was between 11 and 35. Pain was assessed using a 100 mm VAS and a 4-point verbal scale (no, slight, moderate or severe pain). The application times ranged from 120 to 130 minutes with occlusion. An intravenous cannula was inserted into a limb that had not received any previous percutaneous anaesthetic treatment in order to obtain a venous blood sample. The samples were taken between 2 and 5 hours post application and also prior to commencement of the treatment.

In the first study, the individual maximum plasma concentrations of lignocaine ranged from 92 to 315 ng ml^{-1}. For prilocaine the corresponding levels were from 45 to 215 ng ml^{-1}. In the second study, lignocaine concentrations ranged from 70 to 229 ng ml^{-1} and prilocaine levels were from 24 to 110 ng ml^{-1}. In both studies the maximum concentrations were found in the 120 or 180 minute (application time) samples.

Treatment with the percutaneous anaesthetic cream provided sufficient analgesia for the removal of mollusca. At a few sites with infected mollusca the cream was less effective. The dose of EMLA® administered per kilogram of body weight ranged from a total of 0.5 to 0.8 g in younger children up to 0.3 g kg^{-1} to 0.5 g kg^{-1} in the older age group. This corresponded to 8.6 - 20 mg kg^{-1} of lignocaine and prilocaine. The maximum plasma concentrations of lignocaine (315 ng ml^{-1}) and prilocaine (215 ng ml^{-1}) were 10 times less than those associated with toxic symptoms. An application time of 120 minutes for EMLA® was recommended when the Ewald pincette extraction technique is used. The advantages of EMLA® are that no general anaesthesia or other additional forms of pain relief were required. However, the authors did consider that, once again, the prolonged application time required may be disadvantageous under certain circumstances.

A further similar study was carried out by Rosdahl *et al.* (1988) on children aged between three and fourteen years with body weights ranging from 5 to 46 kg. A history of atopic dermatitis was present in 20 of the children. EMLA® was applied under occlusion at a dose of 10 g to the site some 60 minutes before the operation. It was assumed that 1 g covered an area of 2.5 x 2.5 cm. The molluscs were removed with a closed chalozion curette. Pain was assessed by both child and physician on a four point scale ranging from none to severe, the child also assessing the pain on a 100 mm VAS. In 93% of cases children self-assessed the pain as none or slight. The physician-assessed figure was 96%. The median VAS score for children was 3 mm. No general side effects were noted except for redness, pallor and oedema. There was no significant difference in the incidence of redness, pallor or oedema in patients with or without atopic dermatitis. The local reactions obtained in this study are summarised in Table 6.10.

Table 6.10 — Number of local reactions out of 397 individual assessments which occurred when EMLA® was applied for the curettage of molluscum contagiosum

| reaction | severity | | | | total | percentage |
	slight	moderate	severe	not assessed		
redness	46	47	16	3	112	28
pallor	63	97	2	1	163	41
oedema	9	36	0	1	46	12

The study, however, did not consider any other times for EMLA® application other than 60 minutes. With curette removal a shorter application time was suggested by de Waard-van der Spek *et al.* (1990). The use of percutaneous anaesthesia is an effective method of pain relief in the curettage of molluscum contagiosum in children. When using a curette removal method the application time should be between 15 and 60 minutes and with an Ewald pincette a longer application time appeared to be required.

6.10   CAUTERY OF GENITAL WARTS

The reported number of patients with genital warts (condylomata acuminata) is increasing. In 1987 the disease was three times as common as genital herpes (Hallen *et al.*, 1987). Classified as a sexually transmitted disease, it is caused by the human papillomavirus (HPV) which is probably associated with vulval and cervical cancer. Treatment is, therefore, important to avoid malignant transformation and to decrease the risk of further transmission. First line treatment is normally with cytotoxic agents such as podophyllotoxin. The remaining warts are usually removed surgically by cautery, diathermy, laser or excision. Intra-anal and intra-urethral condylomata, along with warts located in the vagina or cervix, are preferably removed without cytotoxics.

Cautery is painful and analgesia is normally provided by local infiltration anaesthesia. However, the genital area is extremely sensitive and injections can be unacceptably painful. General anaesthesia may, therefore, be required for cautery. Hallen *et al.* (1987) investigated the possibility of using percutaneous local anaesthesia for such operations. The study consisted of 57 men, aged from seventeen to fifty-nine years, and 51 women, aged from sixteen to forty-one years. Of the male group, 51 patients had warts in the preputial cavity, 7 in the urinary meatus, 20 on the penile shaft and 2 on the scrotum. In the female group warts were also present in more than one location. In 44 women warts were located on the mucous membranes of the vulva and in 34 there were warts on the skin, most often on the perineum or the perianal area. About 1 ml of EMLA® cream was applied to each lesion up to a maximum of 10 ml per patient. The

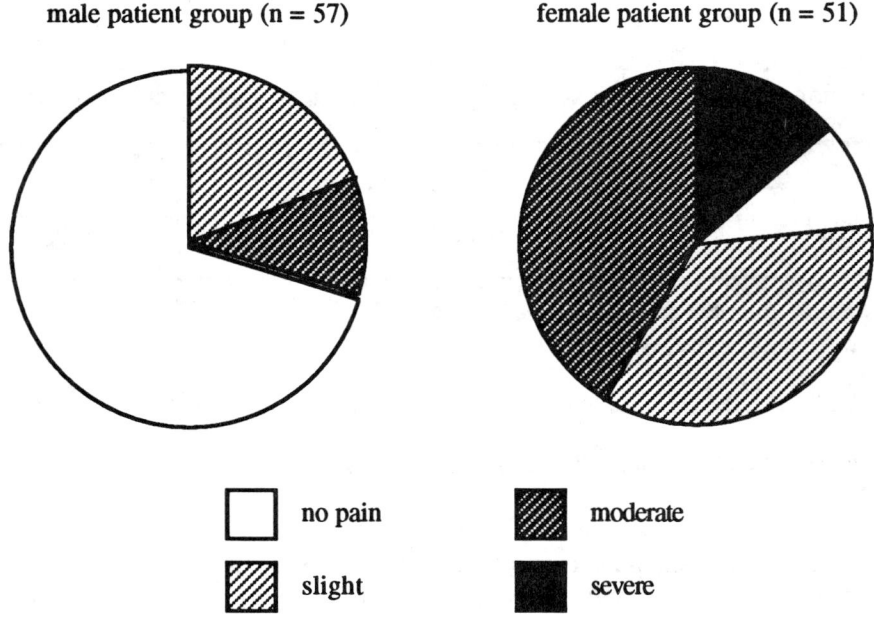

Fig. 6.11 — Physicians' pain evaluation of condyloma treatment following percutaneous local anaesthesia. Reproduced from Hallen *et al.* (1987) with permission of the copyright holder, The British Medical Association

application time was intended to be 30 minutes on mucus membranes and 60 minutes on normal skin. Plastic film was applied when natural occlusion was not available.

Thermocautery was used in 56 men, with both thermocautery and excision used in a single patient. Remnants of warts were scraped off with a curette in some of the operations. In women thermocautery was used in 48 patients, with 24 of the operations being completed by curettage. A carbon dioxide laser was used in a single female patient. The physician recorded pain on a four point scale and the pain perceived by patients was recorded on a five point scale.

In physician-analysed pain 90% of men felt no or only slight pain during treatment and none felt severe pain (Fig. 6.11). The corresponding figure in women, however, was only 45%. Patient-perceived pain correlated with the physician's observations. Additional analgesia was required in 60% of women. However, additional local anaesthetic infiltration was perceived as less painful after pretreatment with the percutaneous anaesthetic.

There was no obvious difference between male and female patients as to the efficacy of the percutaneous anaesthetic procedure. The median application times were 50 minutes (female group) and 35 minutes (male group). The study concluded that percutaneous local anaesthesia provided effective pain relief for the cautery of genital warts in men but was effective in only 40% of female patients.

A comparative study between percutaneous local anaesthesia with EMLA® and local infiltration in laser surgery of genital warts in men was compiled by Lassus *et al.* (1990). The study consisted of 100 men scheduled for the removal of mucosal genital warts. Infiltration anaesthesia was achieved using injections of between 2 and 6 ml of lignocaine hydrochloride solution. Occlusion with plastic film was required when natural occlusion was absent. After a 10 minute waiting period in both treatments, surgery was commenced using a CO_2 laser. Patients assessed pain on a 100 mm VAS and a four point VRS. Differences in pain scores were analysed by the Mann-Whitney two-tailed test.

During surgery, pain was found to be significantly less in the infiltration group compared to the percutaneous anaesthetic group. This was the case for both the verbal pain scores and the VAS. However, the combined VAS for pain during injection/application and during surgery was significantly less in the percutaneous anaesthetic group. Thus, the authors concluded that EMLA® is the anaesthetic of choice for treating mucosal genital warts with laser surgery. The 10 minute application time recommended was, however, different from that of Hallen *et al.* (1987) but similar to that recommended by Rylander *et al.* (1990), who, in a further study, demonstrated the efficacy of the method for pain relief in the laser treatment of condylomata acuminata on the genital mucosa.

A specific study on the onset time of anaesthesia with EMLA® for pain-free cautery of condylomata acuminata on the vulval mucosa was made by Ljunghall and Lillieborg (1989). Patients (52) aged from eighteen to twenty-eight years and with at least two condylomata were recruited into the study. The time of onset of anaesthesia after a 5 minute application of the percutaneous anaesthetic cream to the mucosa was established by pinching the area with a forceps at successive one minute intervals following removal of the cream. All 10 patients in a pilot study conducted in this manner were anaesthetised within 5 - 7 minutes. Subsequently, cautery was performed on 9 patients from this pilot group, with no, or only slight, pain being perceived in each case. In the main part of the study the percutaneous anaesthetic was applied to the mucosa for 10, 15 or 20 minutes. In 92% of these cases anaesthesia was satisfactory for cautery of the condylomata after a 10 minute application of the preparation. With longer application times beyond 15 minutes anaesthetic efficacy was found to gradually decrease.

The advantages of percutaneous local anaesthesia for pain-free vulval biopsies has now been demonstrated in studies by Ljunghall *et al.* (1990) and Byrne *et al.* (1988). In a vulval biopsy Ljunghall *et al.* (1990) stated that percutaneous anaesthetic treatment of 5 - 7 minutes duration achieved 100% analgesia for a forceps pinch. When EMLA® was applied for 5 - 10 minutes, the analgesia was satisfactory for thermocautery in 91% of women. The most effective application time was 4 - 5 minutes and analgesia diminished after 15 minutes.

A similar vulval biopsy study was performed by Byrne *et al.* (1989). The study consisted of 15 diagnostic punch biopsies and one excision biopsy which were performed on 10 patients. About 1 - 2 ml of EMLA® were applied under occlusion if this was not naturally available at the site. Pain was assessed on a five point scale. The mean time required for analgesia of the mucosal surface was 16 minutes. The biopsy was successfully performed in 88% of cases. In general, EMLA® seemed to be effective in relieving pain due to surgical intervention at the vulval mucosa when applied pre-operatively to the site for between 4 and 15 minutes.

In all studies involving the genital area it would appear that much shorter application times for EMLA® are required than would be the case with applications to intact skin, either on the arm or the dorsum of the hand. Duration of anaesthesia also appears to be shorter in these areas. This reflects the fact that the skin in the genital area is very thin or, in the majority of cases, applications have been made to mucosal epithelium rather than skin. In such cases the main barrier to drug penetration is absent and rapid absorption can be expected. The lack of any reservoir effect in the absence of the stratum corneum, together with a more rapid clearance of the anaesthetics from the site, probably accounts for the shorter duration of anaesthesia achieved in these applications.

6.11   POST-HERPETIC NEURALGIA

Herpes zoster occurs after the reactivation of the virus *Varicella zoster* in the dorsal root ganglion. The population incidence of this problem in the UK in 1989 was 3.4 per 1000, with more than 60% of those affected over fifty years old. Recovery is generally complete within a month. However, a small percentage of patients suffer for more than a year with post-herpetic neuralgia (PHN). The resulting pain can be disabling and often defies treatment. Stow *et al.* (1989) investigated percutaneous local anaesthesia in the treatment of PHN with 12 patients aged between fifty and eighty-five years. A baseline blood sample was taken after injection with lignocaine (1%) using a 16-gauge needle. EMLA®, 5 or 10 g, was applied to the hyperaesthetic area and covered with a clear plastic dressing, which was left in position for 24 hours. Pain was assessed using a 10 cm VAS. Blood lignocaine levels were assayed using mass fragmentography. Differences in pain were analysed by the Wilcoxon two-sample sign rank test for paired observations and plasma lignocaine levels by a two-way analysis of variance.

Mean pain intensity scores for all patients 6 hours after percutaneous anaesthetic treatment were significantly less than pretreatment values. This was also the case at the end of 24 hours. At the conclusion of the study 75% of patients continued to use percutaneous local anaesthesia for the condition. Lignocaine blood levels never reached toxic concentrations. A slight drawback, however, was that some discomfort did occur on removal of the occlusive dressing. The conclusion that EMLA® was beneficial for short-term treatment of PHN was confirmed in similar work by Collins (1991).

Latent human *Herpes simplex* (HHS) virus infections in the facial and genital areas of the skin are widespread in the population. Cassuto (1989) considered percutaneous local anaesthesia in the treatment of HHS in a randomised, double-blind, placebo-controlled crossover study with 12 patients. The mean yearly frequency of eruptions in the genital herpes group was 5.7 ± 1.3 and in the oral herpes group it was 3.3 ± 1.7. EMLA®, 0.5 - 1 g, was applied under occlusion for 90 minutes. The cream was applied starting from the first sensation of the next impending outbreak. Applications were repeated four times daily until lesions disappeared.

The mean duration of subjective symptoms in the oral group was 5.1 ± 0.4 days with the placebo and 2.1 ± 0.3 days with the percutaneous local anaesthetic. Eruptions lasted 7.3 ± 0.6 days after placebo and 2.6 ± 0.7 days with EMLA®. In genital herpes the duration of subjective symptoms was 4.9 ± 0.4 days with placebo and 1.8 ± 0.3 days with EMLA®. Eruptions lasted 6.8 ± 0.6 days with placebo and 1.6 ± 0.6 days with EMLA®. When the percutaneous anaesthetic was used at the onset of prodromal symptoms, eruptions were prevented in 29% of oral herpes cases and 50% of genital herpes cases. The only side effects reported in this study were hyperalgesia after the first application in two patients.

The author suggests that the inhibitory effects of a topical local anaesthetic on herpes simplex may involve mechanisms such as interruption of local axonic reflexes in the skin involved in the inflammatory response associated with virus activation. Alternatively, there may be interference with virus-membrane interactions important for virus penetration. By inhibiting capillary permeability, local anaesthetics may also interfere with virus spread through the lymph capillaries. Cassuto (1989) concluded that further consideration should be given to the use of percutaneous local anaesthesia in the treatment of *Herpes zoster* cases. More recently, Wheeler (1991) has recommended percutaneous anaesthesia for painful cases of shingles that had just passed the vesicular stage.

6.12   PAINFUL CONDITIONS OF THE EAR

Until recently there was no ideal method of painlessly achieving anaesthesia of the eardrum. The application of adequate local anaesthesia to the tympanic membrane, which is a relatively inaccessible structure, is a significant problem for otolaryngologists. Local anaesthesia is frequently required in outpatients for myringotomy and grommet insertion. Myringotomy has been performed since the mid-18th century for the treatment of acute otitis media but the procedure has now fallen into disuse. It is now largely used for the treatment of secondary otitis media, either with general anaesthesia, local anaesthesia or, in some cases, without any form of anaesthesia. Some patients would suggest that more discomfort was felt when the local anaesthetic was injected into the meatus than in the performance of the actual procedure itself.

Roberts and Carlin (1989) investigated the use of percutaneous local anaesthesia with EMLA® for anaesthetising the ear drum prior to myringotomy and grommet insertion. They considered any adult suffering from unilateral secretory otitis media requiring myringotomy and grommet insertion. The study was double-blind and consisted of twenty patients. Active and placebo creams were instilled into the external ear canal using a soft, silastic intravenous cannula and a 5 ml syringe. This procedure was performed under a microscope to ensure both immediate contact of the cream with the entire ear drum and that the ear canal was filled. The depth of cream provided self-occlusion. The pain of insertion of the cream was assessed on a VAS. After 30 minutes the cream was removed. Myringotomy was performed with a Beaver blade in the anterior quadrant. A Sheppard grommet was than inserted. The pain of both procedures was measured using a VAS. In addition to this study, a further twenty patients received anaesthesia with injected prilocaine and felypressin. The injection was performed using a dental syringe, injecting slowly at positions 12 o'clock and 6 o'clock in the meatus until blanching of the annulus was observed. Myringotomy and grommet insertion were carried out 5 minutes later.

The results obtained in this study showed that the insertion of the percutaneous anaesthetic was a relatively painless procedure. There was no significant difference between the pain of injecting local anaesthetics into the meatal skin and the pain of inserting a grommet without anaesthesia. Both the percutaneous anaesthetic and injected prilocaine were equally effective in anaesthetising the ear, and each was significantly better than the placebo.

Although injection of an anaesthetic is effective in achieving anaesthesia of the ear drum it is a painful procedure, similar to that of myringotomy and grommet insertion without anaesthesia. Although there was no significant difference between the anaesthesia achieved using EMLA® and that using an injection, there was much less pain with the percutaneous anaesthetic treatment in comparison to the injection. For the percutaneous anaesthetic to be effective an application time of at least 30 minutes was required but in this case such an application was less time consuming and also less difficult than injection of a local anaesthetic solution.

Bingham and Hawthorne (1988) and Bingham *et al.* (1991) also considered the use of percutaneous local anaesthesia for minor otological surgery such as myringotomy, grommet insertion and the repair of small perforations. The cream was syringed onto the tympanic membrane and external auditory canal with the use of an operating microscope. In contrast to the procedure of Roberts and Carlin (1989) the cream was left *in situ* for at least 60 minutes. The investigation consisted of 4 adults, in whom grommets had previously been inserted with other forms of anaesthesia, who had myringotomy and ventilation tubes inserted using EMLA®. Ring block was performed in a single patient at a previous grommet insertion. Topical cocaine was administered to a further 3 patients. In 3 adults myringotomies were performed for the first time and 2 of these patients had ventilation tubes inserted. All patients tolerated the procedure well. No patient volunteered that they felt pain or said that they felt pain in response to direct questioning. The advantages of percutaneous anaesthesia included a reduced risk of infection, as it is a non-invasive technique, and a high patient acceptability due to the sustained levels of adequate analgesia.

Iontophoresis is another well-documented method used to relieve pain at the tympanic membrane. In a comparative study Sirimanna *et al.* (1990) investigated the anaesthesia produced by EMLA® and iontophoresis. Adults (35) between twenty-six and eighty-eight years took part in this study. The reasons for grommet insertion were the presence of secretory otitis media, eustachian tube dysfunction and to help alleviate the symptoms of Menière's syndrome. Patients were asked to assess pain experienced at myringotomy on a 0 - 4 scale from no pain to severe pain. A 2 ml syringe, filled with EMLA®, was applied via a quill directly to the tympanic membrane using an operating microscope. The rest of the external canal was then filled, taking care to avoid the presence of air bubbles. The cream was allowed to remain *in situ* for 60 minutes before it was removed by suction.

In the iontophoresis group the external canal was filled with a mixture of equal quantities of 4% lignocaine and 1:1000 adrenaline solution that had previously been warmed to body temperature. A negative electrode was applied to the forearm and the positive electrode was placed into the anaesthetic solution in the external canal. A current of 0.5 nA maximum at 18 volts was then applied for 10 minutes. The current was allowed to rise gradually to a maximum over the first 30 seconds and then to gradually fall to a minimum value in the last 30 seconds. Following this procedure the fluid was removed from the external canal by suction.

All myringotomies were performed in the antero-inferior position of the tympanic membrane and fluid, if present, was aspirated. Percutaneous anaesthesia was administered to 15 patients and iontophoresis to 20. The pain scores were divided into two groups, 0 - 2 and 3 - 4. Pain levels of 0 - 2 were regarded as being clinically insignificant since they caused no interference with the procedure. Pain levels above this were associated with increased patient distress requiring temporary cessation of the operation. No statistically significant differences in pain stress were established between percutaneous and iontophoretic local anaesthesia.

Both percutaneous anaesthesia and iontophoretic injection have the advantage of allowing myringotomy and grommet insertion to be performed as an out-patient procedure, thus reducing the number of hospital admissions and freeing previously used operating time for other purposes. The major disadvantage with local anaesthetic methods is that they do not allow formal inspection of the post nasal space, which is obligatory in all cases of serious otitis media that fail to respond to an adequate course of conservative therapy. Thus, the surgeon must gain an adequate view of the post-nasal space through use of the post-nasal mirror or the fibre-optic nasoendoscope. Any suspicion of pathology in the post-nasal space would make a local anaesthetic procedure unsuitable since it would not allow adequate assessment and biopsy of the lesion.

Both iontophoresis and EMLA® were equally effective at inducing anaesthesia but the percutaneous anaesthetic seemed to provide a better anaesthetic effect on the skin of the external canal than iontophoresis. This suggested that percutaneous anaesthesia may be a more suitable preparation for more extensive external canal procedures such as the raising of the tympano-meatal flap.

Percutaneous local anaesthesia has been reported as useful in otitis externa by Premachandra *et al.* (1990). Acute inflammation of the external auditory meatus (EAM) is extremely painful. Inflammatory oedema of the external auditory meatal skin causes severe pain due to the stretching of the skin, which has a very rich nerve supply, lying directly on the perichondrium and periosteum of the EAM. Systemic analgesics for this small localised infection are often unrewarding and large doses may be needed. It is also necessary to clean the EAM for effective use of topical antibiotics.

EMLA® was used to treat 5 patients with painful otitis externa and an intact tympanic membrane. Of these patients, 3 had a furuncle and 2 had painful otitis externa. A syringe filled with EMLA® was attached to the EAM and closed with a cotton wool plug to prevent evaporation. After 60 minutes the patient was asked to mark the improvement in the level of pain on a five point scale from 1 (pain had worsened) to 5 (no pain). After this period, the patient's ear was cleared by microscopic suction. Those patients who had a furuncle were given antibiotics and a further instillation of EMLA®. Those with painful otitis externa were treated with topical antibiotics after meticulous cleaning of the EAM.

Percutaneous anaesthetic treatment was found to significantly reduce the pain experienced in acute otitis externa. All the patients noted on their pain scale that the ear felt much better. Pain during jaw movement was also a little better in 3 patients and much better in 2. Without EMLA® the tenderness of the EAM is often intolerable, thus preventing effective cleaning. However, the value of percutaneous local anaesthesia in otitis externa is limited to those who have a painful ear without perforation since local anaesthetics can be absorbed in high concentrations by the middle ear with a consequent risk of ototoxicity.

Two main routes exist by which agents injurious to the inner ear can gain access to the membranous labyrinth. These are via the blood stream and from the middle ear cavity by direct penetration through the round and oval windows. The ototoxic potential of EMLA® was investigated by Anniko et al. (1988). The study consisted of 25 pigmented guinea pigs. EMLA®, its cream base and saline were administered under general anaesthesia into the left tympanic cavity (bulla tympanica) through the tympanic membrane, guided by an operating microscope. A single application of EMLA® was given to 6 animals and 2 animals received the drug-free base. Repeated applications (four applications at two week intervals) of EMLA® were administered to 6 animals, its cream base to 2 animals and the placebo to 4 animals. In 5 animals EMLA® was instilled into the left external auditory canal with an intact tympanic membrane. The animals were anaesthetised with ether and decapitated. The temporal bone was removed and analysed with scanning electron microscopy and light microscopy.

The study concluded that EMLA® is potentially ototoxic, inducing inner ear damage, which was morphologically localised in the basal hook region and approximately 2 mm above this area. The area of the organ of Corti closest to the round window showed the most severe damage. The organ degenerated completely and only a thin layer of epithelium covered the basilar membrane. No difference was found in the extent of ototoxic effects between a single administration of EMLA® and repeated applications.

In inner ear fluid dynamics both radial and longitudinal flows of endolymph occur. The authors point out that this may help limit the ototoxic effect of EMLA® as it becomes diluted with increasing distance from the round window. The portal of entry to the inner ear for EMLA® is the round window and, to a certain extent, the annular ligament of the stapes footplate. EMLA® caused reversible effects on hearing thresholds and latencies at all levels in the basal coil. Also, the outer rows of the third coil suffered extensive damage and only minor changes occurred in the middle ear. EMLA® appeared to be toxic to the inner ear but did not induce formation of new bone in the middle ear.

A similar study was conducted by Schmidt et al. (1988) and considered the effects of EMLA® on the tympanic membrane using both the rat and the guinea pig as animal models. The alterations were confined mainly to the connective tissue layer, which was considerably thicker. The main use of EMLA® in the ear is in myringotomies, which are performed mainly in inflammatory conditions of the middle ear. EMLA® is applied on an intact membrane over a middle ear with a considerably thickened mucosa. The risk of penetration of local anaesthetics to the inner ear should be minimal, these authors concluded. EMLA® seemed to induce minimal changes in the tympanic membrane structure in either animal model. The relevance of both these studies to the use of the lignocaine-prilocaine eutectic system in normal concentrations in the human ear does, however, remain to be established. Nevertheless, given that the ototoxicity of local anaesthetic agents is well established in animal models (Schmidt and Hellstrom, 1986; Schmidt et al., 1984, 1986) caution is certainly advisable in this particular application in respect of all percutaneous local anaesthetics.

6.13   LASER-INDUCED PAIN

Cutaneous thermoreceptors can be tested by detecting the warmth and cold thresholds, or determination of the interval between warmth and cold thresholds to thermode stimulation. Warmth is transmitted by unmyelinated C fibres whereas the sensation of cold is transmitted by thin myelinated Aδ-fibres. The introduction of lasers for thermal stimulation has made it possible to activate the thin afferents selectively and determine sensory and pricking pain thresholds without mechanically touching the skin. Arendt-Nielsen and Bjerring (1988, 1989) conducted two studies into the use of laser-induced pain for the evaluation of percutaneous local anaesthesia with EMLA®. Both studies were similar in design and apparatus. In the 1989 human volunteer study a visible argon laser light and a thermode produced heat/cold to analyse the penetration characteristics and the anaesthetic properties of EMLA®.

EMLA® (5 g) was applied to a 10 cm^2 area of skin under occlusion. The study was of a double-blind design using a placebo cream. After removal, thermode stimulation was performed on human volunteers with a Marstock stimulator where the Peltier device (area 8 cm^2) was either heated or cooled depending on the direction of the electrical current. A thermocouple measured the surface temperature of the skin. The pressure of the thermode on the skin was standardised by adding a fixed weight to the thermode. The rate of temperature change was individually calibrated to 1°C per second and a small thumb switch was activated as soon as a sensation of warmth or cold was perceived. This immediately reversed the current to the thermode. Temperature limits of 20 or 40°C were established in order to increase the sensitivity of the system to a maximum in the temperature span of interest and to avoid a general cooling of the tissue, burning lesions or eliciting of pain.

The laser stimulus for determination of the sensory and pain thresholds was of 200 ms duration and a maximum power of 2.4 W. The stimulus was applied to the dorsal area of the lower mid-forearm. The sensory and pain thresholds were calculated as the mean of five ascending, and five descending, series of stimulations. The sensory threshold was defined as warmth and the pain threshold as a painful pin prick.

The warmth and cold thresholds were measured every 15 minutes for a period of 105 minutes. The placebo or percutaneous anaesthetic under occlusion was removed from the target area immediately before each occasion on which the thresholds were determined.

The cream was applied to the area again after approximately 3 minutes. The experiment included 10 patients of mean age thirty-three years with a range of twenty-five to forty years.

The results of this study showed that the warmth threshold was significantly increased after 45 minutes of EMLA® application by 12% and the cold threshold was significantly increased by 3% after 60 minutes. The placebo did not affect the thresholds. The difference in warmth threshold between placebo and active cream was 3.4 ± 1.5°C after 105 minutes and 6.2 ± 1.8°C for the cold threshold. The sensory and pain thresholds were increased significantly after 45 minutes with EMLA® application compared to placebo. Also, the sensory and pain thresholds to the placebo remained constant during the experiment with coefficients of variation below 11.9% and 8.5%, respectively. The sensory and pain thresholds increased linearly with increasing application time of the active preparation and correlation coefficients were 0.98 and 0.94. After 60 minutes of EMLA® application the pain threshold exceeded the skin destruction level of 2.4 W in 30% of volunteers. After 80 minutes the pain threshold reached skin destruction level in all patients but a sensory threshold was still detected in 80% of these cases. The study concluded that laser and thermode stimulation supported the concept that topical application of EMLA® blocks free nerve endings rather than nerve fibres and induces a sequence of sensory loss which differs in some respects from that typically observed after perineural application of local anaesthetics. This is of importance in selecting the optimal procedures for anaesthetising the skin prior to laser or cryosurgery.

Arendt-Nielsen and Bjerring (1988) also compared EMLA® with local infiltration of lignocaine in prevention of laser-induced pain. The cutaneous nociceptors were selectively stimulated with high-energy argon laser pulses and the pain sensation, pain thresholds and pain-related cortical evoked responses were measured. The study determined the duration of the analgesic effect of EMLA® when applied for 30 minutes. This was evaluated by pain-related cortical responses. A 30 minute application time was considered because pain block could be selectively produced. The cortical projection of non-painful sensation was compared to the threshold findings. The study consisted of 6 patients aged from twenty-three to thirty-three years.

Results from this study showed that the cortical responses decreased gradually for the first 60 - 90 minutes after EMLA® was removed. After 60 - 90 minutes the analgesia began to be less effective and the fixed stimulus intensity was perceived as being more and more painful. This increase in pain intensity was related to a corresponding increase in cortical amplitude. Recordings of cortical responses are often preferable to threshold determinations because the shape of the cortical response contains information on perceptual changes to the stimulus whereas the threshold measurements mainly reflect changes in sensitivity to the stimulus. High-energy argon laser stimulation is recommended as a thermal stimulator in the study of local analgesia because the laser light penetrates through the epidermis and reaches the deeper dermal layers where part of the receptors might be located. It therefore appears to be a suitable model for the measurement of pain arising from surgical skin incisions.

There are a number of specific clinical applications involving laser treatment. The use of a pulsed dye laser for treatment of port-wine stains is one such example Ashinoff and Geronemus (1990) considered 8 patients, aged between four and thirty-two years, for the pulsed dye laser treatment of port-wine stains with EMLA® pretreatment. Blanching or pallor of the skin, often seen subsequent to EMLA® treatment, is thought to be due to vasoconstriction. This posed the question as to whether or not prior treatment with this percutaneous anaesthetic system would decrease the efficacy of pulsed dye laser treatment (PDL) since this laser's energy is selectively absorbed by haemoglobin.

The lesions treated in this study comprised five on the face and neck, two on the trunk and one on the leg. A flashlamp-pumped dye laser with a pulse duration of 450 µs and a circular spot size of 5 mm were used. Two test sites were performed in the same area of the port-wine stain on the same anatomical area of the body, 2 x 2 cm^2 in size, using the same power density. The percutaneous anaesthetic was applied under occlusion for 60 minutes and then left unoccluded for a further 15 minutes prior to laser treatment. Photographs were taken of all patients before and 6-8 weeks after each treatment.

Immediately post-treatment there were no differences noted between percutaneous anaesthetic treated sites and non-pretreated sites except that the treated sites were surrounded by a zone of paleness after 60 minutes occlusion. Both sites were characteristically blue-grey immediately after treatment but turned purpuric in a few hours and remained so for 7-10 days. As the purpura disappeared, the area lightened progressively. After treatment, the test sites were covered with a hydrogel surgical dressing.

No distinction could be made between the pretreated and non-pretreated sites on follow-up visits in any of the patients in the study. This was also found on viewing the photographs taken. Both areas had the same degree of lightening. All patients, however, noted less pain when the percutaneous anaesthetic treated site was exposed to the laser. No depressions, epidermal alterations, sclerosis, hypertrophic scars, hypo- or hyperpigmentation was noted at either test site. The authors concluded that prior treatment with a percutaneous anaesthetic was a safe and effective method for pain relief in the pulsed dye laser treatment of port-wine stains.

Carbon dioxide laser treatment for the treatment of various classes of cervical intraepithelial neoplasia (CIN) is now a recognised out-patient clinical procedure. Various attempts have been made to control the associated pain by infiltration of local anaesthetics. This itself is painful, making the patient apprehensive. It may also prolong the overall treatment because of bleeding from the infiltration. Sarkar (1990) suggested the use of percutaneous local anaesthesia with laser treatment of the cervix. Their open study consisted of ten patients scheduled for laser treatment for a premalignant condition of the cervix. EMLA® was applied to the cervix and left for 10 minutes with the help of a cotton wool ball. The study group was compared with a control group of ten patients who received no treatment prior to laser vaporisation. A carbon dioxide laser with a power density setting of 25 W/cm^2 and a spot size 1.8 mm was used. The pain experienced was assessed by the patient on a VAS (0 - 110 mm) and a VRS (0 - 5).

The percutaneous anaesthetic treated group felt less pain both during, and after, treatment compared to the control group. However, the difference between the groups was not statistically significant. Nevertheless, the results did suggest that the use of the percutaneous anaesthetic did reduce the severity of pain associated with this particular application of laser treatment.

The use of percutaneous local anaesthesia as a diagnostic procedure for Ehlers Danlos Type III (EDS) syndrome has been reported by Arendt-Nielsen *et al.* (1991). The disease involves hyperextensibility of the joints, hyperelasticity and fragility of the skin. It is often difficult to distinguish from the more common simple hypermobility. The study design used laser stimulation and controlled needle insertions to quantitatively investigate if EDS patients responded differently to percutaneous anaesthesia than hypermobile patients, the aim being to determine if these parameters could be used as a new differential diagnostic test between the two disease states.

EMLA® was applied to seven EDS patients, ten hypermobile patients and fifteen controls. Anaesthetic efficiency was evaluated by sensory and pain thresholds to brief argon laser stimuli, with the depth of skin anaesthesia being measured by controlled needle insertions. Control and hypermobile patients did not differ in their response to percutaneous anaesthesia. However, the thresholds to cutaneous laser stimulation and the depth of analgesia increased significantly less in EDS patients compared to the other two groups. In clinical practice the authors concluded that a needle insertion test could be easily applied to determine if patients were responders or non-responders to percutaneous local anaesthesia, thus forming the basis of a differential diagnostic test for EDS.

6.14   MANIPULATION OF NASAL FRACTURES

Reduction of a simple fracture of the nasal bone under local anaesthesia avoids hospitalisation and the risks of general anaesthesia. Local anaesthesia for the reduction of fractured nasal bone is usually achieved by blocking of the infra-orbital, intra-trochlear and external nasal nerves, along with cocainisation of the nasal mucosa. This procedure has many disadvantages. It is invasive, painful and the patient will receive six injections. Local infiltration will also cause a swelling over the nasal bridge, thus impairing the accurate assessment of the final result. In addition, the procedure may cause injury to the nerves. El-Kholy (1989) suggested the use of percutaneous local anaesthesia with EMLA® as an alternative method.

The study consisted of 12 patients with ages ranging from sixteen to thirty years who had their fractured nasal bones reduced under topical local anaesthesia using EMLA® plus cocainisation of the nasal mucosa. The reduction was done between the fifth and eleventh day post injury and the patient had only simple fractures of the nasal bones without fractures of the facial bones. The area surrounding the bridge of the nose was cleaned with an alcohol swab. The percutaneous anaesthetic was applied in a thick layer (60 mg) and covered for one hour. The nasal mucosa was cocainised using 4 ml of a 5% cocaine solution. Of the twelve patients in the study, seven needed only slight pressure with the thumb to put the nasal bridge into the midline. Deviation of the nasal bridge associated with depression of one of the nasal bones occurred in five patients. The depressed nasal bone was elevated using Hill's elevator and the nasal bridge was pushed to the midline at the same time.

All of the patients tolerated the procedure well and all denied suffering pain. None would have preferred general anaesthesia as an alternative. There were no complications and good cosmetic results were obtained as all of the patients were happy about the finished manipulation, with the exception of one patient where the manipulation failed due to a previous old fracture. Thus, the study concluded that the use of a percutaneous local anaesthetic plus cocainisation of the nasal mucosa was painless, economical and recommended for adult patients requiring this painful manipulative procedure.

6.15   TOPICAL ANAESTHESIA OF THE GINGIVAL MUCOSA

Haasio *et al.* (1990) compared the effectiveness of EMLA® and a 10% lignocaine spray on the gingival mucosa. Specifically designed electrodes connected to the constant current stimulator of an electromotive generator were used to test pain thresholds. The study was randomised and no premedication was used. During the sensory and pain threshold studies the subjects were lying in a comfortable supine position with a cubital vein cannulation for blood sampling. The pH of the saliva was estimated with pH-indicator strips before local anaesthetic application. The two stimulating electrodes were made of stainless steel and were held in contact with the gingival mucosa by the volunteer. Stimulating pulses were of 0.2 ms duration in the current range of 0 - 100 mA at a frequency of 1Hz. Both sensory and pain thresholds were measured. The volunteers were also asked to report when the stimulus was first perceived as painful in order to improve the distinction between tolerable and intolerable pain. After drug applications, threshold tests were performed at 5 minute intervals until complete recovery, or a level within 20% of the starting level and which remained constant for 15 minutes, was achieved.

The percutaneous local anaesthetic (4 g) was divided into 3 - 4 portions and applied to the upper gingiva with an electric toothbrush for 4 minutes. The mouth was then emptied. For volunteers receiving lignocaine spray, a single application of 50 mg was applied at each of four sites on the upper gingiva. Venous blood samples were drawn at 5, 10, 20 and 30 minutes after application and plasma lignocaine and prilocaine concentrations were determined.

There was no difference between the topical analgesic efficiency of the two drug applications. Aδ and C fibre blockade was of short duration, usually less than 30 minutes. In the dosages used the absorption of lignocaine/prilocaine from the eutectic system was more rapid than lignocaine absorption after spray application. Although the eutectic system contained half of the lignocaine content of the spray, the patients had approximately similar plasma levels of lignocaine after both applications. This observation is a good illustration of the efficiency of the specifically formulated percutaneous system at delivering the local anaesthetic agents compared with a standard aqueous salt formulation. It does mean, however, that extra care must always be taken when such products are applied topically to areas where the stratum corneum barrier to absorption is absent, as, of course, is the case with applications made to mucosal epithelium. Nevertheless, in this case there were no signs of any mucosal damage of the gingiva caused by the presence of relatively high local anaesthetic concentrations.

The study concluded that small and relatively short surgical procedures could be performed using either of these two topical anaesthetic methods. As both EMLA® and 10% lignocaine spray were equally effective in these applications, the choice was really one of subjective preference. However, all volunteers in this particular study preferred the use of the percutaneous anaesthetic.

6.16   ALLEVIATION OF PAIN DUE TO RETROBULBAR INJECTION

Day case cataract surgery is now commonly performed in the USA and Canada (Sunderraj *et al.* 1991). It is now becoming more popular in the UK with increasing use of local anaesthesia, either retrobulbar or peribulbar. Both of these injections involve the insertion of a needle through the skin of the periocular region and can be very painful. Pain increases anxiety in the elderly, causing the experience to be unpleasant and the procedure potentially more difficult for the surgeon. Sunderraj *et al.* (1991) investigated the use of a percutaneous local anaesthetic, EMLA®, in such procedures.

The study consisted of 115 patients between the ages of fifty-seven and ninety-five years who were scheduled for day case cataract surgery. The study was double-masked and placebo-controlled. The percutaneous anaesthetic was administered to 63 patients and placebo to 52. Oral premedication was not used for any patient. About 2 ml of EMLA® was applied under occlusion to the skin in the region of the outer half of the inferior orbital margin at least one hour preoperatively.

Retrobulbar injections were performed with a 23 standard wire gauge, 30 mm long disposable needle. The needle was introduced at the junction of the lateral one-third and the medial two-thirds of the inferior orbital rim. Up to 5 ml of 0.5% bupivacaine hydrochloride with 1500 units hyaluronidase was slowly injected after aspiration to eliminate possible intravascular injection. The surgeon assessed the patient's reaction at skin penetration on a 0-2 point scale. The patient also assessed pain on a 0-10 point scale and the results from both assessments were analysed statistically.

Treatment with the percutaneous local anaesthetic cream resulted in significantly less pain on retrobulbar injection compared with placebo. The individual pain scores after the application of the placebo cream were scattered over the whole scale whereas the majority of scores after EMLA® pretreatment were near the "no pain" end of the scale. No significant local side effects were noted and there were no cases of marked erythema, scaling, oedema or allergic reactions with either treatment. Some EMLA® inadvertently leaked on to the eyes of three patients between application and arrival at the operating theatre. All three eyes showed congestive conjunctiva with loss of the corneal epithelium in one eye. The latter could have been due either to the preoperative ocular biometry or to EMLA®. The percutaneous anaesthetic treatment did produce transient stinging but in all patients uncomplicated cataract-intraocular lens surgery was possible. The authors now use this method of pain relief for all patients requiring local anaesthetic treatment prior to intraocular surgery.

6.17   TOURNIQUET PAIN

The use of a pneumatic tourniquet to facilitate limb surgery is often complicated by the development of tourniquet pain. Various methods have failed to alleviate this pain. Lowrie *et al.* (1989) suggested the use of percutaneous local anaesthesia for attenuating tourniquet pain. Their double-blind, randomised, placebo-controlled, crossover study consisted of 10 male patients aged from twenty-four to thirty-six years. The study sessions for each subject were one week apart. EMLA® (50 - 60 g) or placebo were applied circumferentially under occlusion to the non-dominant upper arm before the study. An in-dwelling cannula was placed in a vein of the dorsum of both hands. A tourniquet cuff (8 cm) was then applied over a double layer of plaster wool and occlusive dressing, to be positioned directly over the area of skin covered by cream. Systemic arterial pressure was measured non-invasively at 5 minute intervals on the opposite arm.

Tourniquet pain was assessed by means of a 100 mm VAS recorded at 5 minute intervals. Following a 10 minute period of stabilisation the arm was exsanguinated by elevation and the tourniquet inflated to the systolic pressure plus 100 mm Hg. Prilocaine (0.25%), at a dose of 0.5 ml/kg, was injected into the isolated forearm. The study was terminated when the patient reported pain as intolerable.

The duration of the tourniquet inflation tolerated in the percutaneous anaesthetic group was 46 ± 3.5 minutes compared with 37 ± 2.7 minutes with placebo ($P < 0.05$). EMLA® was tolerated longer than placebo by 80% of patients (Fig. 6.12). VAS scores were comparable in both groups before inflation of the tourniquet and, although they also increased in both groups over the study period, they were significantly lower with EMLA®. For example, after 40 minutes the mean placebo VAS was 73.33 ± 4.9 compared to the percutaneous anaesthetic group mean VAS of 42.43 ± 6.9 mm. Blanching or reddening of the skin occurred in some subjects in the active treatment group. These changes were noticeable only after the cream had been removed at the end of the first study period. The significant increase in mean tourniquet time tolerated with percutaneous anaesthetic treatment and the apparent decrease in the severity of the pain felt under the cuff may, however, be of limited clinical relevance. Nevertheless, the authors point out that there is clearly a small but significant cutaneous component to pain experienced with the use of a pneumatic tourniquet.

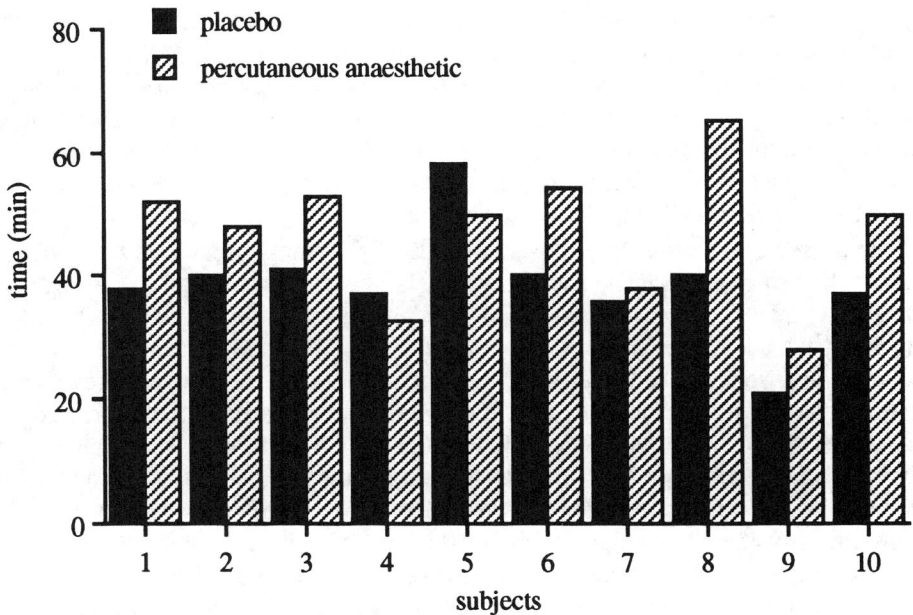

Fig. 6.12 — Duration of tourniquet inflation tolerated by each subject with either percutaneous anaesthetic or placebo pretreatment. Reproduced from Lowrie *et al.* (1989) with permission of the copyright holder

6.18   EXPERIMENTALLY INDUCED PRURITUS

Pruritus is common in dermatological disease, but there are few ways of alleviating this symptom other than by removing the disorder causing it. The sensation of itch appears to be mediated by the same neural pathways as those responsible for pain. Hence, Shuttleworth *et al.* (1988) investigated the use of percutaneous anaesthesia in such cases. Their study consisted of 20 patients aged between nineteen and fifty years. The histamine-induced itch threshold was determined for each subject. Test solutions of histamine, as histamine acid phosphate diluted in sterile water, were prepared in increasing concentration from 0.013 µmol to 3.26 µmol. An area of 1.5 x 15 cm was delineated on the volar aspect of the forearm and 1200 µl of the most dilute test solution was applied to a 1 cm^2 area within this region. The skin was scarified using a hypodermic needle, disrupting the stratum corneum and allowing the test material to pass into the viable cell layers. After two minutes the subject was asked to report any itching or stinging. The concentration of histamine applied was increased until stinging or itching occurred.

To determine the effect of percutaneous anaesthetic pretreatment with EMLA®, or of placebo, on the itch threshold, two further 1.5 x 15 cm areas were delineated. One site received EMLA® applied and the other had a placebo cream applied. Each application site was occluded. The effect of the percutaneous anaesthetic on itching induced by artificial pruritogens was investigated on a separate 1.5 x 15 cm delineated area. The subjects received cowhage and papain. Sufficient of these artificial pruritogens were applied to produce itching. The area was then treated with percutaneous anaesthetic or placebo as with the itch threshold study. The test was open in regard to the operator. Patients assessed the degree of itching on a 100 nm VAS and a 4 point VRS.

Following percutaneous anaesthetic treatment all subjects were less sensitive to histamine, with 70% requiring a solution two or three concentration increments stronger than on the untreated site to provoke a reaction. Placebo treatment showed no loss of sensitivity. Only six subjects required a solution of more than one concentration increment stronger than the original concentration.

The decrease in sensitivity to histamine was significantly greater on the EMLA® treated site than on the placebo site. In consideration of the sensitivity to cowhage and papain, all patients in the percutaneous anaesthetic group experienced less itching or stinging than the untreated group. The cowhage and papain groups were tested separately and all comparisons showed significantly greater irritation on the untreated area than on the treated area. Mild redness and oedema occurred in two patients in the percutaneous anaesthetic group. The authors concluded that the differences in sensitivity to the pruritogens was probably due to inter-subject variation. Percutaneous local anaesthetic treatment was effective in reducing pruritis induced by histamine, cowhage and papain. It was also very effective in eliminating or reducing the itching in such cases.

This study raises the possibility of the use of percutaneous anaesthetic treatment in those conditions where persistent itching can be traumatic, often resulting in painful lesions to the skin due to persistent scratching. Atopic eczema is one such condition. However, as the skin is often broken in such cases, the risk of significant systemic absorption of local anaesthetics is greatly increased. This may limit the possibility of applying percutaneous anaesthesia to this area, though it would at least seem to warrant some specific further investigations.

6.19   EXTRA-CORPOREAL SHOCK WAVE LITHOTRIPSY

Extra-corporeal shock wave lithotripsy (ESWL) can be painful. In the treatment of uncomplicated urinary tract calculi with a Siemens lithostar device, Bierkens *et al.* (1991) found that 51.4% of patients needed intravenous analgesia. This group carried out a double-blind, placebo-controlled, randomised trial to determine the efficacy of percutaneous local anaesthetic treatment in ESWL for urinary calculi. EMLA® or placebo cream (30 g) was applied for 50 minutes before treatment on the skin (100 cm²) at the site of shock-head coupling under an occlusive dressing. The number of shocks per treatment varied from 1,000 to 4,000. The shocks began at 13.9 kV and increased to 17.5 kV. After 500 shocks pain was recorded on a VAS and fentanyl citrate (0.05 mg intravenously) was given to the patient on demand.

EMLA® was administered to 40 patients and a further 43 patients received placebo cream. In the percutaneous anaesthetic group 30% of patients needed intravenous fentanyl citrate compared with 53% in the placebo. There was a significant decrease in the pain due to ESWL experienced by those patients receiving the active treatment compared to placebo. The study recommended, however, that percutaneous anaesthetic treatment should not be applied routinely in all patients undergoing ESWL but rather reserved for those patients in whom intravenous anaesthesia cannot be used.

6.20   ADVERSE REACTIONS DUE TO PERCUTANEOUS LOCAL ANAESTHESIA

Given the vasoactive nature of local anaesthetics (Section 3.6.4), the most frequently seen reactions with percutaneous delivery are either local pallor or erythema, depending on the local anaesthetics involved. Typical of this are the observations on local skin reactions of Woolfson *et al.* (1990) based on their extensive clinical experience with a percutaneous anaesthetic gel derived from the amethocaine phase-change system. Children up to the age of sixteen who had received this preparation on a named patient basis were carefully monitored for possible adverse reactions. All applications were made to healthy, intact skin. As would be expected, there were no systemic effects. Local skin reactions were classified into three possible classes. Class A was a severe hypersensitivity reaction, precluding further use of the preparation. Class B was an urticarial reaction, generally presenting with localised oedema and itch. This type of reaction disappeared spontaneously within about two hours. Patients who exhibited this reaction were not subsequently sensitised to amethocaine and could receive further applications of the preparation. These patients did not necessarily have a Class B reaction on subsequent exposures to the drug. Class C was a slight, transient erythema of the treated site, disappearing rapidly following removal of the preparation. Interestingly, despite the history of amethocaine as a potential sensitising agent, no class A reactions were recorded, and only 0.6% of patients had a Class B reaction. A detailed breakdown of the reactions recorded in various age groups is shown in Table 6.11. Given that amethocaine is a potential sensitiser, it is clearly important to consider the effect of repeated applications of the drug to the same individual. Table 6.12 reveals no evidence of sensitisation in 123 patients, drawn from the overall trial group, who received more than one application of the preparation.

Table 6.11 — Incidence of adverse local skin reactions to a percutaneous amethocaine preparation

age (years)	no. of applications	severity of reaction					
		class A no.	class A %	class B no.	class B %	class C no.	class C %
0-2	68	0	0	0	0	3	4.4
3-5	405	0	0	4	1.0	15	3.7
6-10	499	0	0	2	0.4	32	6.4
> 10	269	0	0	2	0.7	28	10.4
total or mean %	1241	0	0	8	0.6	78	6.3

Reproduced from Woolfson *et al.* (1990). with permission of the copyright holder

Table 6.12 — Influence of repeated applications on the incidence of adverse reactions with a percutaneous amethocaine preparation

no. of repeat applications	no. of subjects	severity of reaction					
		class A no.	class A %	class B no.	class B %	class C no.	class C %
1	123	0	0	0	0	7	5.7
2	123	0	0	1	0.8	12	9.8
3	59	0	0	2	3.4	7	11.9
4	37	0	0	0	0	4	10.8
5	21	0	0	1	4.8	4	19.0
6	11	0	0	0	0	0	0
> 6	2	0	0	0	0	1	50.0

Reproduced from Woolfson *et al.* (1990). with permission of the copyright holder

It is, perhaps, significant that a drug, long classified as a potent sensitiser, failed to produce any evidence in this study of local dermatitis due to a hypersensitivity reaction. The importance of the treated site, in this case healthy skin rather than damaged or sensitive areas, is clear. Nevertheless, any percutaneous anaesthetic preparations should, of course, be withdrawn from an individual if there are clear signs of skin symptoms pointing to an overt hypersensitivity reaction.

In contrast to the amethocaine system, the lignocaine-prilocaine eutectic mixture tends to produce a localised, transient blanching of the skin at the application site. Studies aimed at finding the best method of administration for EMLA® have shown that application under occlusion for one hour yielded the greatest rate of blanching immediately after the application period. This rate decreased for longer times, with no blanching after a four hour application. This was probably due to exhaustion of local anaesthetics from the skin boundary layer, with the initial reaction simply having passed over this prolonged period. In 25 - 55% of cases the rate of blanching did vary significantly with the dose applied (Evers *et al.*, 1985).

Blanching of the skin due to treatment with the lignocaine-prilocaine system appears to be a transient reaction, disappearing about two hours after the end of the application. This blanching effect may have been caused by a number of factors, including the anaesthetic mixture, the vehicle and occlusion of the site. Indeed, blanching has been observed when the vehicle alone is occluded. Villada *et al.* (1990), in a double-blind, randomised trial with 50 volunteers, investigated the cause of blanching. All patients recruited into this trial were Caucasian in respect of skin type and were not receiving any concomitant medication. Each patient had EMLA® (0.5 ml) applied on two 5 cm^2 areas of the forearm under an occlusive dressing for 60 minutes. The active preparation was applied to one site and the vehicle alone to the other. Reading of any subsequent skin reactions was done using visual evaluation by the same operator after one, two and three hours. Quantifying blanching was difficult because of the induction of erythema by the tape used to limit the area around the zone.

After application of EMLA®, blanching was observed in 66% of cases compared with 6% of cases treated with the vehicle alone. This difference had a high degree of statistical significance. In almost every case the blanching was present at the end of the application period following removal of the occlusive dressing (58% out of 66%). In four cases blanching developed one hour later. In all cases the blanching was transient and disappeared before three hours had elapsed from the end of the application period. In 26% of cases the initial blanching was followed by an erythema. Erythema was observed in 34% of patients compared to 2% with vehicle alone, the difference again being statistically significant. The erythematous response, which gradually faded, was slight, symptomless and observed at the greatest rate two hours after the conclusion of the application period. The study clearly demonstrated that the local circulatory effects, blanching and erythema, were caused by the active ingredients, lignocaine and prilocaine. However, the mechanism of this circulatory action is unknown. One likely hypothesis seems to be that lignocaine has a vasoconstrictor effect at low concentration and a vasodilator effect at higher concentrations, a so-called biphasic effect. Thus, erythema following initial blanching is observed even after the cream has been removed. This factor has been attributed to storage of lignocaine in the stratum corneum. A second theory is that the local anaesthetic would first reach the sympathetic nervous system leading to vasoconstriction and only then the parasympathetic system leading to a vasodilation. This concept seems rather less credible, though, given the slow rate of absorption of the drugs and the very low systemic blood levels that are eventually achieved.

A rather similar study was conducted by Bjerring *et al.* (1989), again comparing EMLA® with a placebo cream. The authors concluded that it was EMLA® which was responsible for the pallor and erythema. The pallor occurred maximally following a ninety minute application period, with erythema seen at two hours onwards. This earlier study did not break down EMLA® into its components in order to establish which substituent caused the local circulatory effects.

Juhlin and Rollman (1984) investigated abnormal vascular reactions in atopic dermatitis following application of EMLA®. Ten patients, aged from eighteen to twenty-five years, who had atopic dermatitis since childhood were considered. They all had lichenified plaques with dry, rough skin on the trunk and arms. Three patients, with chronic, generalised eczema of unknown cause, aged from fifty-one to seventy years, were also studied. The control group consisted of ten healthy patients aged twenty to forty years. In the healthy subjects EMLA® was applied under occlusion for 30 - 60 minutes. This produced a slight blanching and analgesia, which lasted 1 - 2 hours. When applied for 2 - 4 hours, the blanching was more pronounced and was replaced in 0.5 - 2 hours by a slight to moderate erythema, which persisted for 1 - 3 hours.

When the percutaneous anaesthetic was applied for one minute on dry, itching skin and lichenified patches of atopic dermatitis, blanching was seen in four patients 1 - 5 minutes after removal of the dressing. The pale areas did not attain analgesia and the blanching disappeared after 15 minutes. Application for 5 - 10 minutes was followed within 5 - 15 minutes by blanching and analgesia in all patients with atopic dermatitis and chronic eczema. After prolonged exposures (30 - 60 minutes) to EMLA®, the white area turned pale red or red and 60 minutes after removal of cream the test area was markedly red centrally. Sometimes there was a 2 - 3 mm white border. In one patient purpura appeared 60 minutes after application. This faded slowly within a week. The white dermographism, observed in all atopics, was inhibited or immediately turned red in areas treated with EMLA® for between 15 and 60 minutes. The anaesthesia and reddening persisted for about two hours.

In atopic dermatitis patients there was a quicker onset of blanching and anaesthesia. Hence, a more rapid percutaneous absorption of the drugs occurred than is seen with applications to normal skin. The blood levels of lignocaine and prilocaine were not investigated but it was suggested that these might be quite high as a result of enhanced percutaneous absorption. Hence, a shortened application time for EMLA® is recommended in patients with atopic dermatitis. Once again, the extra care needed when using percutaneous anaesthetic preparations on damaged skin is emphasised in this study and it is always well to remember that these formulations are specifically designed to promote drug penetration through healthy, intact skin.

Systemic absorption from percutaneous local anaesthetic preparations is not normally a significant clinical problem. This is emphasised in a study on lignocaine and prilocaine absorption by Juhlin *et al.* (1989). They investigated the absorption of the anaesthetics from normal facial skin, arm skin and diseased skin. Thirteen patients aged from twenty to sixty years with normal skin served as the control group. Eight patients, aged from twenty to sixty-three years, with chronic, plaque-type, psoriatic lesions on the hands or lower arms were also investigated. The study further considered three women aged from eighteen to twenty-four years, two of whom had atopic dermatitis and one who had contact dermatitis of the lower arms.

EMLA® (10 g) was applied, under occlusion, on 100 cm^2 of the face or forearm for two hours in a study of crossover design. Blood was drawn from an antecubital vein in the arm into heparinised vacuum tubes at varying times of application from 0.5 - 12 hours. With respect to diseased skin, some 4 - 6 g of the percutaneous anaesthetic were applied to 25 cm^2 under occlusion for one hour. The sites of application were the dorsal and volar aspects of the lower arm. The degree of blanching or reddening was noted (0 to +++) between 30 and 120 minutes. The analgesic effect was assessed using a sequence of ten pin pricks and a blood sample was also taken in these cases. The lignocaine and prilocaine concentrations in plasma were subsequently determined.

Mean maximum plasma levels, following a 100 cm^2 application on the face, were found to be 150 ng ml^{-1} of lignocaine and 58 ng ml^{-1} of prilocaine. On the forearm, following a five hour application, the corresponding mean value for lignocaine was 18 ng ml^{-1} whereas for prilocaine levels were too low for measurement even by mass fragmentography. When the percutaneous anaesthetic was applied on a 25 cm^2 area in three healthy volunteers for one hour, neither lignocaine nor prilocaine were detected in the general circulation within three hours using an assay with a sensitivity limit of 10 ng ml^{-1}. After applications to patients with psoriasis and dermatitis, detectable levels of lignocaine (16 - 450 ng ml^{-1}) were found after one hour in all patients and for prilocaine in 73% of cases. When EMLA$^®$ was applied on the facial skin, the maximum lignocaine levels in the plasma occurred within two hours and the maximum levels were reached in the arm after five hours. Hence, lignocaine and prilocaine are more rapidly absorbed from the face. After EMLA$^®$ had been applied on diseased skin the plasma concentrations of both drugs increased more rapidly and reached higher levels than those found for normal skin. The plasma levels were, however, still 100 times lower than those associated with toxicity. Nevertheless, these observations give further emphasis to the care that must be taken if applying preparations such as EMLA$^®$ to large areas of diseased skin.

Although percutaneous local anaesthesia of intact, healthy skin does not normally result in systemic complications, there is a specific danger associated with the topical use of prilocaine, notably in the very young. However, Jakobson and Nilsson (1985) reported a case of moderate methaemoglobinaemia associated with the use of the lignocaine-prilocaine eutectic. A twelve-week-old boy (weight 5.3 kg) was scheduled for elective reimplantation of the right ureter. He was being treated preoperatively with a trimethoprim-suxamethoxazole mixture, having had pyelitis at the age of three weeks. Otherwise, the child was healthy. EMLA$^®$ (5 g) was applied on the back of the hands and in the cubital regions. However, the operation was delayed and the percutaneous anaesthetic was left *in situ* for five hours. The anaesthetist noticed the patient's skin was pale and his lips had a brownish, cyanotic colour. Vital signs were normal and the condition was ascribed to a combination of starvation and hypothermia. Cystoscopy was performed but the laparotomy was postponed because of the cyanosis, which did not improve following ventilation with pure oxygen.

Suspicion of methaemoglobinaemia warranted blood sampling and methylene blue at a dose of 1 mg kg^{-1} was infused intravenously at a slow rate. After 30 minutes the cyanosis had virtually disappeared. The methaemoglobin level was then 28%. Throughout the operation there were no signs of hypoxaemia. The slight metabolic acidosis was considered to be related to the long starvation.

Methaemoglobin, which is formed by the oxidation of haemoglobin, has a minimal oxygen carrying capacity (Fig. 6.13). High levels can cause tissue hypoxia. It is normally formed in the erythrocytes but is maintained at a minimal level by constant reduction back to haemoglobin. This reaction is catalysed by the enzyme NADH-dehydrogenase, with cytochrome b-5 as the electron carrier. The reaction can also be catalysed by NADP-diaphorase, if methylene blue is administered as an electron carrier.

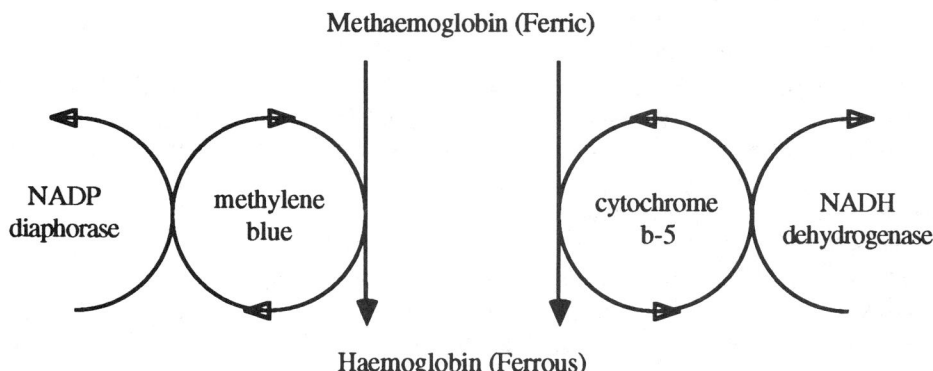

Methaemoglobin (Ferric)

Haemoglobin (Ferrous)

Fig. 6.13 — The relationship between haemoglobin and methaemoglobin with associated enzymes and electron carriers. Reproduced from Jakobsen and Nilsson (1985) with permission of the copyright holder, Acta Anaesthesiologica Scandinavica

Congenital forms of methaemoglobinaemia can occur, as in haemoglobin-M disease and in hereditary deficiency of NADH-dehydrogenase. Small infants, however, have a lower activity of NADH-dehydrogenase and are therefore more susceptible to oxidative stress. Consequently, they can develop methaemoglobinaemia more readily. A variety of agents are known to cause methaemoglobin formation including sulphonamides, prilocaine, benzocaine, aniline dyes, nitrites and nitrates. Prilocaine is implicated as a potential causative agent (Section 3.11.3) since it is metabolised to ortho-toluidine, a methaemoglobin-inducing agent. In the case reported by Jakobson and Nilsson (1985) the child received sulphonamides and prilocaine. The former had been administered for more than two months without signs of methaemaglobinaemia. The authors therefore concluded that there was probably an additive effect between the antibacterial agent and prilocaine. No attempt to determine the prilocaine plasma level was made in this study.

More detailed information on the risks associated with the topical administration of prilocaine in the very young was obtained in a later investigation by Engberg *et al.* (1987). Their study consisted of 22 infants divided into two groups, three to six months and six to twelve months, who were scheduled for surgery, mainly hernia repair and cystoscopy. Pethidine was administered to most infants above 6 months. EMLA® (2 ml) was applied on four skin areas, mainly the dorsum of the foot and the cubital fossa, with a total surface area of 16 cm² under occlusion. The application times varied between two and four hours. A time of two hours was chosen to begin with. Since the methaemoglobin levels were found to be below toxic levels in these cases, the application time was subsequently increased to four hours. Plasma levels of methaemoglobin were determined spectrophotometrically.

The main application times used in the study fell between 230 and 265 minutes. Some kind of local reaction was observed in 32% of infants. The most common reaction was hyperaemia. The venous plasma concentrations of lignocaine and prilocaine were in all cases below 200 ng ml^{-1}. The maximum lignocaine level in children under 6 months was 127 ng ml^{-1} and for prilocaine the value was 131 ng ml^{-1}, both occurring after four hour applications of EMLA®. In the lower age group the maximum lignocaine level was 155 ng ml^{-1} compared to a prilocaine concentration of 79 ng ml^{-1}, both again occurring after a four hour application period. The baseline level of methaemoglobin varied between 0.16% and 1.53%, with the median for children under 6 months being 0.8% and 1% for those in the higher age group. There was a larger spread of methaemoglobin concentration in children over 6 months. The median value of 1.7% at eight hours was higher than the baseline median. This increase was statistically significant. No correlation was found between the plasma concentration of prilocaine and the methaemoglobin level.

Due to the risk of methaemoglobinaemia the use of EMLA® is now restricted in infants younger than twelve months and is not recommended in those below the age of six months. In the study by Engberg et al. (1987) the concentrations of methaemoglobin were found to be within the normal range in all infants. The study concluded that EMLA® could safely be used in infants over three months if they were not receiving concomitant medication of a methaemoglobin-inducing agent. A further specification was that the amount applied should be less than 2 g and the total skin area covered not greater than 16 cm^2 for a period not longer than four hours. Although the use of the lignocaine-prilocaine system in very young children must, therefore, be viewed with some caution and the clinician needs to be aware of the risk of methaemoglobinaemia, the condition, if it occurs, can rapidly and safely be reversed without damage by the intravenous infusion of methylene blue.

Powell et al. (1991) investigated the application of a percutaneous anaesthetic to wound sites in order to determine if such preparations, although designed for use on intact skin, could also safely be used for anaesthesia of wounds. In vitro studies were designed to determine the influence of EMLA® on bacterial growth, either by monitoring growth in bacterial suspensions incubated with EMLA® or by measuring the magnitude of a zone of bacterial growth inhibition on an agar streak plate subsequently surface-treated with the percutaneous anaesthetic.

To test the toxicity of the percutaneous anaesthetic in wounds female Hartley guinea pigs were used. Two parallel incisions were made in the paravertebral skin and extended through the panniculus carnosus. The wounds were contaminated with 0.05 ml of designated concentrations of bacteria. After 15 minutes EMLA® (0.25 ml) was added via a 1 ml syringe. A saline control was also similarly set up. Inflammatory responses were assessed four days later. To assess wound-breaking strength EMLA® (0.25 ml) was applied to one wound and saline was added to the contralateral wound. The wound-breaking strength was recorded seven days after wounding. Parallel incisions were made, on each side of the healing wound, 6 mm from the edge. One lip of the wound edge was kept stationary and the other was attached to a continuous drive motor with a screw gear advance. This was connected in turn to a recorder to measure the force required to disrupt the wound.

Percutaneous anaesthetic treatment resulted in a significant reduction in bacterial growth in vitro. When EMLA® was extruded onto an agar plate containing a confluent growth of bacteria, a zone of inhibition measuring 2.9 ± 0.5 mm was observed. No such zone was observed with saline. In wounds treated with percutaneous anaesthetic or saline the inflammatory response parameters were proportional to the size of the inoculum.

EMLA® was shown in this study to have antibacterial properties *in vitro*, in keeping with the properties of many local anaesthetic agents (Section 5.7). However, this was of little clinical value in contaminated wounds since the preparation was found to damage host tissue defences. In percutaneous anaesthetic-treated wounds the inflammatory responses to subinfective doses of bacterial inocula were significantly greater than those encountered in wounds subjected to saline irrigation. However, wound repair in wounds not subjected to bacterial contamination was not interfered with. The breaking strength of EMLA®-treated wounds seven days after surgery was significantly greater than control wounds and this enhanced breaking strength was associated with an exaggerated inflammatory response. The authors concluded that the infection-potentiating properties of EMLA® militated against its use in wounds. They emphasised that the main application of such preparations was for anaesthesia of intact skin.

Apart from specific cases of adverse reactions to percutaneous anaesthetics, or their use in situations for which these preparations were never intentionally designed, there have been some additional minor complications seen in a few patients, mainly in respect of the preparation being ingested orally. Norman and Jones (1990) reported three cases where the occlusive plastic dressing covering an area treated with EMLA® became detached and affected other areas of the body. The first such case involved a severely brain-damaged, twenty-four year old man who presented for knee surgery. He was aphonic and communication was impossible. The patient was premedicated with diazepam and the percutaneous anaesthetic was applied to the dorsum of both hands. On arrival in the anaesthetic room EMLA® was found to be present on only one hand. During general anaesthesia the larynx was inspected. It was seen to be partially occluded by a greyish mass which lay beyond the cords. This mass proved to be the occlusive dressing of EMLA®, which the patient had ingested orally.

In the second of these cases a child of two years was premedicated two hours before an operation. EMLA® was applied to the dorsum of each hand under occlusion. On arrival in the anaesthetic room one of the dressings had been punctured and the cream was dissipated. It was suspected that the child had chewed the dressing and swallowed the cream. Thus, a laryngoscopy was performed. It appeared that the upper airway had become effectively anaesthetised. This is a reflection of the comparatively large bulk of material which must be applied in even routine applications of EMLA® cream.

Finally, a small child arriving in the anaesthetic room two hours after premedication, having had bilateral application of EMLA® cream to the hand, continued to rub his left eye vigorously with the back of his left hand. The dressing was found to have been loosened. The eyelids and adjacent area were smeared with the cream. The area was subsequently bathed and the cornea inspected for abrasion which may have occurred when it was anaesthetised. No injury was found.

The study concluded that, to prevent the removal of the occlusive dressing by the patient, a secondary protective dressing of conforming (crepe) cotton bandage should be applied over the plastic film. This is probably not necessary for the majority of patients. In any case, a more convenient dosage form for the application of percutaneous anaesthetics probably represents a safer solution to this type of occasional problem.

6.21   CONCLUSIONS

There is no doubt that percutaneous local anaesthesia is a safe and effective means of preventing the pain associated with various invasive procedures of the skin. These preparations are designed for use on intact, healthy skin and they should probably be restricted to such applications unless there are sufficient benefits to be gained from their application to broken skin or mucosal surfaces. In such cases greater care and awareness of possible adverse reactions, including the increased risk of significant systemic absorption, is required. Most clinical applications to date have related to the use of the lignocaine-prilocaine eutectic system, and there is no doubt that the availability of this first percutaneous anaesthetic preparation represents a major step forward in the field. The main areas of improvement which we can look forward to will be in respect of a shorter and more clinically convenient application time, greater duration of effect and a more convenient presentation, particularly important when large areas must be treated. Although there will always be some time delay to onset of full skin anaesthesia, ultimately it should be possible for patients to routinely self-apply preparations of this type before leaving home for the clinic. This will, of course, require a window of activity of sufficient length to allow for any delays. The advantages of pain-free procedures, such as venepuncture or the taking of split skin grafts, should, by now, be obvious both for children and adults alike, and also for clinical and nursing staff presented with a more compliant and less traumatised patient.

REFERENCES

Anniko, M. and Schmidt, S.H. (1988) The ototoxic potential of EMLA. *Acta Otolaryngol. (Stockh.)* **105** 255-265.

Arendt-Nielsen, L. and Bjerring, P. (1988) Laser-induced pain for evaluation of local analgesia: A comparison of topical application (EMLA) and local injection (lidocaine). *Anesth. Analg.* **67** 115-23.

Arendt-Nielson, L. and Bjerring, P. (1989) The effect of topically applied anaesthetics (EMLA cream) on thresholds to thermode and argon laser stimulation. *Acta Anaesthesiol. Scand.* **33** 469-473.

Arendt-Nielson, L., Kaalund, S., Hogsaa, B., Bjerring, P. and Grevy, C. (1991) The response to local anaesthetics (EMLA cream) as a clinical test to diagnose between hypermobility and Ehlers Danlos Type III syndrome. *Scand. J. Rheumatol.* **20** 190-195.

Ashinoff, R. and Geronemus, R.G. (1990) Effect of the topical anaesthetic EMLA on the efficacy of pulsed dye laser treatment of port-wine stains. *J. Dermatol. Surg. Oncol.* **16** 1008-1081.

Bianchetti, M.B., Speck, S. and Oetliker, O.H. (1990) Topical skin anaesthesia before inserting haemodialysis cannula. *Pediatrics* **85** 624.

Bierkens, A.F., Maes, R.M., Hendrikx, A.J.M., Erdos, A.F., de Vries, J.D.M. and Debruyne F.M.J. (1991) The use of local anesthesia in second generation extracorporeal shock wave lithotripsy: eutectic mixture of local anesthetics. *J. Urol.* **146** 287-289.

Bingham, B. and Hawthorne, M. (1988) The use of anaesthetic EMLA cream in minor otological surgery. *J. Laryngol. Otol.* **102** 517.

Bingham, B., Hawke, M. and Halik, J. (1991) The safety and efficacy of EMLA cream topical anesthesia for myringotomy and ventilation tube insertion. *J. Otolaryngol.* **20** 193-195.

Bjerring, P., Andersen, P.H. and Arendt-Nielsen, L. (1989) Vascular response of human skin after analgesia with EMLA cream. *Br. J. Anaesth.* **63** 655-660.

Byrne, M.A., Taylor-Robinson, D., Pryce, D. and Harris, J.R.W. (1989) Topical anaesthesia with lidocaine-prilocaine cream for vulval biopsy. *Brit. J. Obstet. Gynaecol.* **96** 497-199.

Cassuto, J. (1989) Topical local anaesthetics and herpes simplex. *Lancet* i 100-101.

Collins, P.D. (1991) EMLA cream and herpetic neuralgia. *Med. J. Australia* **155** 206-7.

Cooper, C.N., Gerrish, S.P., Hardwick, M. and Kay, R. (1987) EMLA cream reduces the pain of venepuncture in children. *Eur. J. Anaesthesiol.* **4** 441-448.

de Waard-van der Spek, F.B., Oranje, A.P., Lillieborg, S., Hop, W.C.J. and Stolz, E. (1990) Treatment of molluscum contagiosum using a lidocaine/prilocaine cream (EMLA) for analgesia. *J. Amer. Acad. Dermatol.* **23** 685-688.

Ehrenstrom-Reiz, G.M.E. and Reiz, S.L.A. (1982) EMLA - a eutectic mixture of local anaesthetics for topical anaesthesia. *Acta Anaesth. Scand.* **26** 596-598.

El-Kholy, A. (1989) Manipulation of the fractured nose using topical local anaesthesia. *J. Laryngol. Otol.* **103** 580-581.

Elland, J.N. and Anderson, J.E. (1977) The experience of pain in children. In: Jacox, A.K. (ed.) *Pain: A Source Book for Nurses and Other Health Professionals.* Little, Brown and Co., Boston, pp. 453-473.

Engberg, G., Danielson, K., Henneberg, S. and Nilsson, A. (1987) Plasma concentrations of prilocaine and lidocaine and methaemoglobin formation in infants after epicutaneous application of a 5% lidocaine-prilocaine cream (EMLA). *Acta Anaesthesiol. Scand.* **31** 624-628.

Evers, H., Von Dardel, O. and Juhlin, M. (1985) Dermal effects of compositions based on the eutectic mixture of lignocaine and prilocaine (EMLA). Studies in volunteers. *Br. J. Anaesth.* **57** 997-1005.

Goodacre, T.E.E., Sanders, R., Watts, D.H. and Stoker, M. (1988) Split skin grafting using topical local anaesthesia (EMLA): a comparison with infiltrated anaesthesia. *Brit J. Plastic Surgery,* **41** 533-538.

Gunawardene, R.D. (1990) Local application of EMLA and glyceryl trinitrate ointment before venepuncture. *Anaesthesia* **45** 52-54.

Haasio, J., Jokinen, T., Numminen, M. and Rosenberg, P.H. (1990) Topical anaesthesia of gingival mucosa by 5% eutectic mixture of lignocaine and prilocaine or by 10% lignocaine spray. *Brit. J. Oral Maxillofacial Surg.* **28** 99-101.

Hallen, B., Carlsson, P. and Uppfeldt, A. (1985) Clinical study of a lignocaine-prilocaine cream to relieve the pain of venepuncture. *Br. J. Anaesth.* **57** 326-328.

Hallen, A., Ljunghall, K. and Wallin, J. (1987) Topical anaesthesia with local anaesthetic (lidocaine and prilocaine, EMLA) cream for cautery of genital warts. *Genitourinary Med.* **63** 316-319.

Halperin, D.L., Koren, G., Attias, D., Pellegrini, E., Greenberg, M.L. and Wyss, M. (1989) Topical skin anesthesia for venous, subcutaneous drug reservoir and lumbar punctures in children. *Pediatrics* **84** 281-284.

Haugstvedt, S., Friman, A.M. and Danielson, K. (1990) Plasma concentrations of lidocaine and prilocaine and analgesic effect after dermal application of EMLA cream 5% for surgical removal of mollusca in children. *Z. Kinderchir.* **45** 148-150.

Holm, J., Andren, B., and Grafford, K. (1990) Pain control in surgical debridement of leg ulcers by the use of a topical lidocaine-prilocaine cream, EMLA. *Acta Derm. Venereol.* **70** 132-136.

Hopkins, C.S., Buckley, C.J. and Bush, G.H. (1988) Pain-free injections in infants. *Anaesthesia,* **43** 198-201.

Jakobson, B. and Nilsson, A. (1985) Methemoglobinemia associated with a prilocaine-lidocaine cream and trimetoprim sulphamethoxazole. A case report. *Acta Anaesthesiol. Scand.* **29** 453-455.

Jones, S.K., Handfield-Jones, S. and Kennedy, C.T.C. (1990) Does EMLA reduce the discomfort associated with local-anesthetic infiltration? *Clin. Experiment. Dermatol.* **15** 177-179.

Juhlin, L. and Rollman, O. (1984) Vascular effects of a local anaesthetic mixture in atopic dermatitis. *Acta Derm. Venereol. (Stockh.)* **64** 439-440.

Juhlin, L., Hagglund, G. and Evers, H. (1989) Absorption of lidocaine and prilocaine after application of a eutectic mixture of local anaesthetics (EMLA) on normal and diseased skin. *Acta Derm. Venereol. (Stockh.)* **69** 18-22.

Kapelushnik, J., Koren, G., Solh, H., Greenberg, M. and DeVeber, L. (1990) Evaluating the efficiency of EMLA in alleviating pain associated with lumbar puncture; comparison of open and double-blinded protocols in children. *Pain* **42** 31-34.

Lahteenmaki, T., Lillieberg, S., Ohlsen, L., Olenius M. and Strombeck, J.O. (1988) Topical analgesia for the cutting of split-skin grafts: a multicenter comparison of two doses of a lidocaine/prilocaine cream. *Plastic Reconstruct. Surg.* **82**. 458-463.

Lassus, A., Kartamaa, M. and Happonen, H.P. (1990) A comparative study of topical analgesia with a lidocaine/prilocaine cream (EMLA) and infiltration anesthesia for laser surgery of genital warts in men. *Sex. Trans. Dis.* **17** 130-132.

Ljunghall, K. and Lillieborg, S. (1989) Local anaesthesia with a lidocaine/prilocaine cream (EMLA) for cautery of condylomata acuminata on the vulval mucosa. The effect of timing of application of the cream. *Acta Derm. Venereol.* **69** 362-365.

Ljunghall, K., Rylander, E., Sjoberg, I. and Lillieborg, S. (1990) Topical anaesthesia with lidocaine-prilocaine cream for vulval biopsy. *Brit. J. Obstet. Gynaecol.* **97** 864-865.

Lowrie, A., Jones, M.J. and Eastley, R.J. (1989) Effect of a eutectic mixture of local anaesthetic agents (EMLA) on tourniquet pain in volunteers. *Brit. J. Anaesth.* **63** 751-753.

Malmros, E., Nilsen, T. and Lillieborg, S. (1990) Plasma concentrations and analgesic effect of EMLA (lidocaine/prilocaine) cream for the cleansing of leg ulcers. *Acta Derm. Venereol.* **70** 227-230.

Manner, T., Kanto, J., Iisalo, E., Lindberg, R., Viinamaki, O. and Scheinin, N. (1987) Reduction of pain at venous cannulation in children with a eutectic mixture of lidocaine and prilocaine (EMLA cream): comparison with placebo cream and no local premedication. *Acta Anaesthesiol. Scand.* **31** 735-739.

McCafferty, D.F., Woolfson, A.D. and Boston, V. (1989) *In-vivo* assessment of percutaneous local anaesthetic preparations. *Brit. J. Anaesth.* **62** 17-21.

McGrath, J. and Scholfield, O. (1990) Treatment of excessive granulation tissue with

EMLA cream and 95% silver-nitrate pencils. *Clin. Exper. Dermatol.* **15** 468.

Nilsson, A., Danielson, K., Engberg, G. and Henneberg, S. (1990) EMLA for pain relief during arterial cannulation. *Uppsala J. Med. Sci.* **95** 87-94.

Norman, J. and Jones, P.L. (1990) Complications of the use of EMLA. *Br. J. Anaesth.* **64** 403.

Nott, M.R. and Peacock, J.L. (1990) Relief of injection pain in adults. EMLA cream for 5 minutes before venepuncture. *Anaesthesia* **45** 772-774.

Nykanen, D., Kissoon, N., Rieder, M. and Armstrong, R. (1991) Comparison of a topical mixture of lidocaine and prilocaine (EMLA) versus 1% lidocaine infiltration on wound healing. *Ped. Emerg. Care* **7** 15-17.

Ohlsen, L., Englesson, S. and Evers, H. (1985) An anaesthetic lidocaine/prilocaine cream (EMLA) for epicutaneous application tested for cutting split skin grafts. *Scand. J. Plast. Reconstr. Surg.* **19** 201-209.

Page, B. and Morgan-Hughes, J.O. (1990) Behaviour of small children before induction. The effect of parental presence with EMLA and premedication with triclofos or a placebo. *Anaesthesia* **45** 821-825.

Premachandra, D.J. (1990) Use of EMLA cream as an analgesic in the management of painful otitis externa. *J. Laryngol. Otol.* **104** 887-888.

Price, H.V. (1988) Lignocaine-prilocaine cream for lumbar puncture in children. *Lancet* i 1174.

Powell, D.M., Rodeheaver, G.T., Foresman, P.A., Hankins, C.L., Bellian, K.T., Zimmer, C.A., Becker, D.G. and Edlich, R.F. (1991) Damage to tissue defences by EMLA cream. *J. Emerg. Med.* **9** 205-209.

Roberts, C. and Carlin W.V. (1989) A comparison of topical EMLA cream and prilocaine injection for anaesthesia of the tympanic membrane in adults. *Acta Otolaryngol. (Stockh.)* **108** 431-433.

Rosdahl, I., Edmar, B., Gisslen, H., Nordin P. and Lillieborg, S. (1988) Curettage of molluscum contagiosum in children: Analgesia by topical application of a lidocaine/prilocaine cream (EMLA). *Acta Derm. Venereol.* **68** 1439-153.

Rylander, L., Sjoberg, I., Lillieborg, S. and Stockman, O. (1990) Local anesthesia of the genital mucosa with a lidocaine/prilocaine cream (EMLA) for laser treatment of condylomata acuminata: A placebo-controlled study. *Obstet. Gynecol.* **75** 302-306.

Sarkar, P.K. (1990) Topical anaesthesia with lignocaine-prilocaine cream (EMLA) for carbon dioxide treatment to the cervix - a pilot study. *Brit. J. Clin. Pract.* **44** 353-353.

Schmidt, S.H., Hellstrom, S. and Carlsoo, B. (1984) Short-term effects of local anaesthetic agents on the structure of the rat tympanic membrane. *Arch. Otorhinolaryngol.* **240** 159-166.

Schmidt, S.H. and Hellstrom, S. (1986) Late effects of local anesthetics on tympanic membrane structure. A study in the rat. *Am. J. Otolarygol.* **7** 346-352.

Schmidt, S.H., Hellstrom, S. and Carlsoo, B. (1986) Fine structure of the rat tympanic membrane after treatment with local anesthetics. *Acta Otolaryngol.* **101** 88-95.

Schmidt, S.H., Hellstrom, S. and Anniko, M. (1988) Structural effects of the topical lidocaine-prilocaine anesthetic EMLA on the tympanic membrane. *Arch. Otorhinolaryngol.* **254** 136-141.

Shuttleworth, D., Hill, S., Marks, R. and Connelly, D.M. (1988) Relief of experimentally induced pruritus with a novel eutectic mixture of local anaesthetic agents. *Brit. J. Dermatol.* **119** 535-540.

Sirimanna, K.S., Madden, G.J. and Miles, S. (1990) Anaesthesia of the tympanic membrane: Comparison of EMLA cream and iontophoresis. *J. Laryngol. Otol.* **104** 195-196.

Small, J., Wallace, R.G., Millar, R., Woolfson, A.D. and McCafferty, D.F. (1988) Pain-free cutting of split-skin grafts by application of a percutaneous anaesthetic cream. *Brit. J. Plastic Surgery* **41** 539-543.

Smith, M., Gray, B.M., Ingram, S. and Jewkes, D.A. (1990) Double-blind comparison of topical lignocaine-prilocaine cream (EMLA) and lignocaine infiltration for arterial cannulation in adults. *Br. J. Anaesth.* **65** 240-242.

Soliman, I.E., Broadman, L.M., Hannallah, R.S. and McGill, W.A. (1988) Comparison of the analgesic effects of EMLA (Eutectic Mixture of Local Anaesthetics) to intradermal lidocaine infiltration prior to venous cannulation in unpremedicated children. *Anaesthesiology* **68** 804-806.

Spitz, L. and Thomas, D.F.M. (1992) Paediatric surgery. In: Kyle, J., Smith, J.A.R. and Johnston, D.H. (eds) *Pye's Surgical Handicraft.* Butterworth-Heinemann Ltd., Oxford, pp. 389-414.

Stow, P.J., Glynn, C.J. and Minor, B. (1989) EMLA cream in the treatment of post-herpetic neuralgia. Efficacy and pharmacokinetic profile. *Pain* **39** 301-305.

Sunderraj, P., Kirby, J., Joyce, P.W. and Watson, A. (1991) A double-masked evaluation of lignocaine-prilocaine cream (EMLA) used to alleviate the pain of retrobulbar injection. *Brit. J. Ophthalmol.* **75** 130-132.

Villada, G., Zetlaoui, J. and Revuz, J. (1990) Local blanching after epicutaneous application of EMLA cream. *Dermatologica* **181** 38-40.

Wahlstedt, C., Kollberg, H., Moller, C. and Uppfeldt, A. (1984) Lignocaine-prilocaine cream reduces venepuncture pain. *Lancet* ii 106.

Wehle, B., Bjornstrom, M., Cedgard, M., Danielsson, K., Ekernas, A., Gutierrez, A., Petterson, U. and Lindholm, T. (1989) Repeated application of EMLA cream 5% for the alleviation of cannulation pain in haemodialysis. *Scand. J. Urol. Nephrol.* **23** 299-302.

Wheeler, J.G. (1991) EMLA cream and herpetic neuralgia. *Med. J. Australia* **154** 781.

Wig, J. and Johl, K.S. (1990) Our experience with EMLA cream for painless venous cannulation in children. *Ind. J. Physiol. Pharmac.* **34** 130-132.

Woolfson, A.D., McCafferty, D.F. and Boston, V. (1990) Clinical experiences with a novel percutaneous amethocaine preparation: prevention of pain due to venepuncture in children. *Br. J. Clin. Pharmac.* **30** 273-279.

Young, A.C., Shorthall, A., Haynes, W. and Young, G. (1987) Lignocaine-prilocaine cream for lumbar puncture. *Lancet* ii 1533.

Index